20 001 639 63

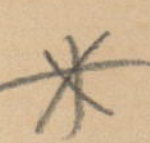

AF606240

The Instruments of Psychiatric Research

The Instruments of Psychiatric Research

Edited by

Chris Thompson
Professor of Psychiatry
Southampton University
Royal South Hants Hospital
Southampton
UK

A Wiley Medical Publication

JOHN WILEY & SONS
Chichester · New York · Brisbane · Toronto · Singapore

Library of Congress Cataloging in Publication Data:

The instruments of psychiatric research / edited by Chris Thompson
p. cm.—(A Wiley medical publication)
Includes bibliographies and index
ISBN 0-471-91794-X.
1. Psychiatric rating scales. 2. Psychiatry—Research—Methodology. 1. Thompson, Chris. II. Series.
[DNLM: 1. Mental Disorders—diagnosis. 2. Psychiatric Status Rating Scales. WM 141 I59]
RC473.P78I57 1989
616.89'075—dc19
DNLM/DLC
for Library of Congress

British Library Cataloguing in Publication Data:

Thompson, Chris
The instruments of psychiatric research.
1. Medicine. Psychiatry. Methodology
I. Title
616.89'001'8

ISBN 0 471 91794 X

Phototypeset by Input Typesetting Ltd, London
Printed at Biddles Ltd, Guildford, Surrey

Contents

List of contributors

Adrian Angold BSc MBBS MRCPsych, Associate Professor of Child Psychiatry, Duke University Medical Centre, Department of Psychiatry, Box 3454, Durham, N. Carolina 27710, U.S.A.

Thomas R. E. Barnes MBBS MRCPsych, Senior Lecturer in Psychiatry, Charing Cross and Westminster Medical School, London, UK

Brendan Bradley PhD, Lecturer in Experimental Psychology, University of Cambridge, Cambridge, UK

Keith Bridges BSc MBChB MSc MRCPsych, CertHE, Consultant Psychiatrist and Honorary Associate Lecturer, Manchester Royal Infirmary and University of Manchester, Manchester, UK

Traolach S. Brugha MB BCh MD MRCPsych, Senior Lecturer in Psychiatry, Leicester Royal Infirmary, Leicester, UK

John R. M. Copeland MA MD FRCP FRCPsych, Professor and Head of University Department of Psychiatry, Director, Institute of Human Aging, University of Liverpool, Liverpool, UK

Brian Ferguson MBBCh MRCGP MRCPsych, Consultant Psychiatrist, Mapperley Hospital, Nottingham, UK

David Goldberg MA DM MSc FRCP FRCPsych, Professor of Psychiatry, University Hospital of South Manchester and University of Manchester, Manchester, UK

Deborah S. Hasin PhD, Assistant Professor of Clinical Public Health, College of Physicians and Surgeons and School of Public Health, Columbia University, New York, USA

Keith Hawton DM MRCPsych DPM, Consultant Psychiatrist and Clinical Lecturer, University Department of Psychiatry and Warneford Hospital, Oxford, UK

Steven R. Hirsch BA MD MPhil FRCP FRCPsych, Professor of Psychiatry, Charing Cross and Westminster Medical School, London, UK

Rahul Manchanda MBBS MD MRCPsych, Assistant Professor of Psychiatry, University of Western Ontario, St Thomas Psychiatric Hospital, St Thomas, Ontario, Canada

Andrew E. Skodol MD, Associate Clinical Professor of Psychiatry, College of Physicians and Surgeons, Columbia University, New York, USA

Tim Stockwell PhD, Deputy Director, National Centre for Research into the Prevention of Drug Abuse, South Perth 6151, Australia

John Strang MBBS MRCPsych, Director, Drug Dependence Clinical Research and Treatment Unit, Maudsley Hospital, London, UK

George I. Szmukler MD DPM MRCPsych FRANZCP, Consultant Psychiatrist, Royal Melbourne Hospital, Parkville, Victoria and University of Melbourne, Melbourne, Australia

Chris Thompson MBBS BSc MPhil MD MRCPsych, Professor of Psychiatry, Southampton University, Royal South Hants Hospital, Southampton, UK

Peter Tyrer BA, MD, MRCP FRCPsych, Senior Lecturer in Psychiatry, St Mary's Hospital, London, UK

K. C. M. Wilson MB MPhil MRCPsych, Consultant in Psychiatry of Old Age, Royal Liverpool Hospital and Clinical Lecturer in Psychiatry, University of Liverpool, Liverpool, UK

The Instruments of Psychiatric Research
Edited by C. Thompson

CHAPTER 1

Introduction

CHRIS THOMPSON
Southampton University
Royal South Hants Hospital,
Southampton, UK

The idea for this book came about when my own research began to branch out from narrowly biological studies on depression, utilizing a few standard instruments, to include studies on general hospital psychiatry, neurosis, general practice psychiatry and other fields in which I hadn't a clue at first how to measure what I wanted to measure. I was lucky at the time to be working at the Institute of Psychiatry, where I could walk along the corridor and find someone who knew what I needed, or thought they did. However, it soon became clear that, although psychologists can find an index of tests in print, psychiatrists usually have to chase an obscure literature to find the tests they need, an even more obscure one to find the correct way to use and score them, and an almost submerged literature on their psychometric properties. There are a few highlights which researchers tend to know, such as Hamilton's papers of the 1960s. However, it may be that the lack of knowledge about the principles of measurement and the instruments already developed has inhibited research by putting off some young researchers and inducing others to reinvent the wheel.

One aim of this book is therefore to provide an inventory of the available instruments, at least the most prominent ones. The subject has been divided into sections representing not only the major psychiatric conditions but also disciplines within general psychiatry such as social psychiatry, old age psychiatry and child psychiatry. Of course developments in the technology of measurement are continuing all the time and new conditions are being recognized which require instruments to make operational definitions and measurements of severity. Limits have therefore had to be set and there may well be instruments which the reader seeks and does not find. It is not in that sense an exhaustive dictionary of the available tests. However, it does have the advantage over a dictionary that there is space to discuss the tests in the light of studies which have used them and, in some cases, studies which have used more than one instrument to measure the same thing, thus allowing a comparison of two or more instruments.

In most cases it has not been possible to print the instrument itself because of copyright restrictions, although examples of the items are often given. Details of the administration are given and, where available, reliability and validity under appropriate conditions.

The book begins with a theoretical introduction which contains nearly all of the technical terms which are used in the later part of the book, as well as a brief description of the main problems in measuring psychiatric symptoms. Each subsequent chapter deals with a specific area of psychiatric research in which there is a literature on measurement. There are some areas which have been left out because they are not specifically psychiatric but have a more general psychological importance. An example of this is the technique of measuring personal constructs. In most chapters there is an introduction to familiarize the reader with the background to that field and where necessary an extended section on methodological issues which are not covered in the introduction. Finally the most prominent instruments in that field are described, with their psychometric properties where known. An extensive list of references then allows a relatively painless entry into the important literature.

THEORY OF RATING SCALES

All science depends on the ability to measure natural phenomena. If psychiatric knowledge is to develop, then accurate definition and measurement are essential. Since the 1960s there has been an accelerating drive within psychiatry to objectify and operationalize diagnoses, treatments and judgements about severity, particularly in the research context but also in clinical practice, for example in the *Diagnostic and Statistical Manual* (American Psychiatric Association, 1980). Thus, much psychiatric research in the last two decades has been concerned with the first task of a science, that of learning how to define and measure the phenomena with which it deals. In psychiatry this is particularly difficult.

Physical medicine, in contrast, is better off. For example, blood pressure can be measured relative to certain well-defined and easily observable criteria, such as the amount of pressure necessary to occlude the brachial artery at the upper arm. The meaning of the figures derived in this way can be specified physiologically as systolic and diastolic blood pressure, and can be related to cardiac output and peripheral resistance. The severity of pathological processes which raise blood pressure can be described numerically, and the necessity for treatment can be decided on that basis.

The psychiatrist has no such advantages. Firstly there are few tests of any diagnostic utility which can distinguish between different types of mental disorder. In general the psychiatrist relies upon the consensus among his colleagues that a particular constellation of symptoms or phenomena tend to occur together and can be recognized as a syndrome. The validity of this syndrome and of the boundaries between it and other syndromes can be tested to some extent by examination of related features such as the demographic characteristics of sufferers, the prognosis or the response to treatment. In this process the syndrome may become refined and changed. Some of the symptoms may be found to be unreliably identified, such as the fundamental symptoms of schizophrenia (Bleuler, 1911). Others may be found to be unrelated or only weakly related to core symptoms of the disorder.

Not only does the psychiatrist have no ultimately validated diagnostic boundaries, but also the severity of the conditions cannot be related to the severity of a pathological change in the function of a physiological system, as would be the case in hypertension. An exception is dementia, in which the severity of intellectual deterioration correlates with the cholinergic abnormalities (Perry *et al.*, 1978). In this situation it is hardly surprising that there are no ratings of severity of psychiatric conditions which are firmly based on natural interval scales (one in which the differences between each consecutive point on the scale are equal). For example, in the measurement of blood pressure the difference between 80 and 81 mmHg is of the same magnitude as the difference between 120 and 121 mmHg. In contrast, there is no way of knowing if the difference between 0 and 5 on the Hamilton Rating Scale for depression is the same as the difference between 20 and 25.

One implication of these considerations is that psychiatric ratings can only be expected to have limited transferability between one situation and another, for example between different groups of patients, between different raters, between different cultures and in the same groups at different times.

So how have psychiatrists attempted to overcome such enormous disabilities? The short answer is by a mixture of pragmatism and diligence of definition. The lengthy answer is what constitutes the remainder of this volume. The pragmatic researcher accepts the inadequacies of knowledge in his subject and measures as accurately as possible under the circumstances—the proof of the pudding is then in the eating. If the measures were inappropriate or inaccurate then results will be insignificant or unreplicable. Diligence in defining terms (operationalizing them) is the most important element of this pragmatic approach, for a common understanding is crucial to the communicability and the general applicability of results. The extent to which this essentially pragmatic approach has succeeded is shown by the advances in knowledge in the last three decades, but the limits are readily shown by the large number of questions as yet unanswered and unanswerable.

So the development of rating scales in psychiatry begins and ends as a standardization of clinical practice and understanding. There are few external criteria against which diagnoses can be judged and only the crudest of criteria against which severity scores can be validated. Not only is the target of our rating scales invisible but it is also constantly shifting. One only has to look at the change in the concept of schizophrenia in clinical research over the last two decades to realize this. This change has been mirrored by a multiplication of diagnostic criteria (and to some extent rating scales) to cope with the different conceptions of the disease. However much one applies sophisticated statistics to the results of rating scales, nothing can be learned in this way about the underlying nature of psychiatric conditions because the process is inherently tautological.

It is for this reason that we must disagree with Hamilton when he writes: 'A rating scale is, in a sense, an end product of the development of psychiatry. When the phenomena to be studied have been completely defined in nature and range then it is possible to construct a scale to evaluate them' (Hamilton, 1972).

On the contrary, we must agree with Wing (1978), who treats the process of disease naming and measuring with greater caution: 'Diseases are names for theories rather than names for things.'

In this way it is possible to overcome the paradox of trying to measure something whose true identity one doesn't know. Rating scales operationalize diseases, i.e. they define what the researcher means by the term 'depression' and by defining the cues to be used to judge severity they make communicable statements about the severity of the condition. In other words it is not necessary to know the nature of things before acting upon them. Rather the nature of things becomes apparent after interactions have taken place between the scientist and the phenomena.

In the next part of the Introduction we will consider some ways of describing rating scales which are important in assessing how good or bad the scale is at the job for which it was designed. Examples will be drawn predominantly from the depression literature, since it is highly developed.

There are two main types of scale which are used in psychiatry:

1. Likert scales: these are categorical scales, i.e. they consist of a number of categories (symptoms), each of which is rated in terms of severity, often, as recommended by Likert, on a five-point scale (0–4) (Likert, 1932).
2. Analogue or graphic scales: in these scales a straight line is combined

with verbal cues, and the rater places a mark on the line to indicate where they lie on the dimension of severity. These are of several types, for example:

(a) Unipolar:
Not at all sad ______________________ Extremely sad

(b) Bipolar:
As happy as I have ever been ______________________ As sad as I have ever been

(c) Discretized analogue scale:

0	1	2	3	4	5	6	7	8	9	10
no depression		mild depression			moderate depression			severe depression		

(see Bech *et al.*, 1986).

DESCRIPTIVE DIMENSIONS OF RATING SCALES

Item Bias

Item bias or orientation (Carroll *et al.*, 1973) refers to the scale's content and which part of the syndrome is best represented in it. In Table 1 a number of scales are shown, with the percentage of the theoretical maximum score which is made up by each category of symptom.

Table 1

Category	HDRS	Bech	MADRS	BDI	Zung	Wake	Carroll
Mood	8	18	30	9.5	15	25	8
Vegetative	28	18	30	29	35	33	35
Motor	12	18	0	0	5	8	15
Social	8	9	0	5	0	8	0
Cognitive	28	27	30	52	35	0	27
Anxiety	16	9	10	0	5	17	15
Irritability	0	0	0	5	5	8	0

Percentage contributed to the theoretical maximum score by each of seven categories of symptom for each of seven rating scales.

Mood includes sadness, loss of enjoyment, distinct quality to mood, weeping and diurnal variation.

Vegetative includes sleep disturbance, appetite change, weight change, loss of libido, constipation and fatigue.

Motor includes retardation, agitation and restlessness.

Social includes withdrawal, isolation and inability to function at work or other tasks.

Cognitive includes thoughts of hopelessness and helplessness, suicide, illness and guilt, as well as loss of insight and indecision.

Anxiety includes psychic and somatic and phobic anxiety.

Irritability includes both inwardly and outwardly directed hostility.

Abbreviations: HDRS = Hamilton Rating Scale; Bech = Bech–Rafaelson Melancholia Rating Scale; MADRS = Montgomery Asberg Depression Rating Scale; BDI = Beck Depression Inventory; Wake = Wakefield Depression Inventory.

The item bias of the scales is determined by several factors. In the case of the HDRS, Hamilton (1967) was concerned to represent a broad range of symptoms, and it can be seen that this was more or less achieved. Beck *et al.* (1961) developed the BDI while at the same time exploring his cognitive theory and therapy, and it is therefore no surprise that the BDI is heavily loaded with cognitive symptoms (over 50% of the theoretical maximum score). Montgomery and Asberg (1979), in creating a scale to be particularly sensitive to change in severity during a treatment trial, were concerned to ensure that it did not turn out to be just composed of items which recorded side effects such as sedation. From Table 1 it can be seen that 60% of the maximum score is made up of mood items or vegetative symptoms, i.e. core symptoms of the depressive state, showing that they have avoided the pitfall. Item content is therefore determined by the mode of development of the scale as well as the recognized symptoms of the condition to which it is applied.

The usefulness of individual items can be tested on three criteria:

1. Calibration: does the item occur frequently enough in the population for which the scale is used to warrant inclusion. An arbitrary cut-off of 10% has been used in the past (Bech *et al.*, 1975).
2. Ascending monotonicity: the item score should significantly correlate with the total score (see 'Internal consistency or homogeneity' below).
3. Dispersion about the regression line given by the above correlation should not be too high, indicating reasonable reliability of the item score.

For self rating scales more than observer ratings the scale constructor must beware of obscure or technical wording which will make an item incomprehensible to the general public. For example 'subsequent to' should be 'since'. It is also better use of English. The understandability of the item can be worked out using the Flesch Reading Ease Scale, which is derived as follows:

Average number of syllables in 100 words = W
Average length of a sentence in words = S

$$W = \frac{\text{Syllables}}{\text{Words}}$$

$$S = \frac{\text{Words}}{\text{Sentences}}$$

$$\text{Reading ease} = 206.4 - 0.85W - 1.02S$$

Score	% of population understanding
0–30	4.5
31–50	24
51–60	40
61–70	75
71–80	80
81–90	86
91–100	90

Scoring of Items

Each item of a scale is scored according to defined criteria. Hamilton (1972) discusses several ways of establishing the criteria. The simplest is to score each item present or absent. This is the method used in check-lists of symptoms where the total score is the same as the number of symptoms present. However, this method does not take into account the relative severity of each symptom or the fact that it may occasionally be difficult to decide if a symptom is present or not.

Hamilton (1968) recommends a three-stage rating of absent, doubtful and present. 'Present' can then be subdivided into mild, moderate and severe. Numerical values of 0 (absent), 1 (doubtful), 2 (mild), 3 (moderate) and 4 (severe) can then be assigned. To assign numerical values to a scale of this kind, however, is to make a number of unwarranted assumptions; it is to convert a nominal scale to an interval scale. In what sense is 'doubtful' half as severe as 'mild'? This is the most obvious example of error being introduced by the spurious use of an interval scale. In this scale there is no way of telling whether 2 (mild) really is half as severe as 4 (severe). It has to be accepted that a 'ratio' or 'natural interval' scale in psychiatry is not presently possible (and may never be possible). However, as described above, there is a practical need to measure the severity of psychiatric conditions, so rating scales must be developed which have the minimum of distortion.

Apart from this basic issue of converting a nominal into an interval scale there are a number of other issues in the rating of individual items which must be considered. First is the criteria on which the ratings are made. Hamilton (1967) leaves this up to the discretion of the raters, all of whom should be expert psychiatrists. However, he does provide guidance for rating most items.

On what criteria should the severity of a symptom be judged? Is it severe if it is present all of the time or if it is unbearable when present but only present infrequently? Some scales have used the duration of the symptom almost exclusively (e.g. Zung, 1965); for example: never (0), some of the time (1), often (2), always (3). Others have used the severity of the symptom when present (e.g. Beck *et al.*, 1961). The Hamilton scale allows discretion to be used but it is specified that only expert raters should use the scale. Some symptoms do not lend themselves to duration ratings, for example panic attacks, while others do, for example free-floating anxiety symptoms, so each item should be worded to make sense of that individual symptom.

How closely should the criteria necessary to reach each grade of severity be specified? This depends largely on the expertise of the raters. With expert raters, all trained in the same way, it can be left more flexible so that the raters can use the whole range of their experience in making the judgement. Miller *et al.* (1985), in constructing a version of the HDRS for non-expert raters, had to specify rather more carefully, and in self-rating scales such as the Carroll scale (Carroll *et al.*, 1973), in which the patient would otherwise use only their own experience, it might be thought that even closer definition would be required. In practice, with self rating scales, the patient is allowed to make their own judgement of severity, using phrases like ‘a little’, ‘a great deal’, because self rating scales have to speak the patient’s language as a priority, and most patients have only their own lay experience on which to base their judgements.

How many grades should there be for each item? The maximum number depends on the ingenuity of the constructor in devising definitions of the different points. However, the optimum number depends on the experience of the raters. More experienced raters can use more grades without too much loss of reliability. The optimum rating is usually around 5 or 6, above which reliability tends to fall. Other factors have to be taken into account. An odd number of ratings has a central point which will be over-used owing to the so-called ‘central tendency error’ (see below). This is the reason why some scales (the General Health Questionnaire is a particularly good example; Goldberg, 1972) have been designed with four point ratings. Scales which are designed to be sensitive to change often use more rating points. If seven points are included only five of them will be used regularly because of the reluctance of raters to use the end ratings, but there will still be a greater number of points in use than in a five-point scale, when only three will be used with any great frequency.

The Meaning of the Total Score

What is the justification for adding together all of the scores of individual items in order to derive an overall score of severity? Critics have drawn attention to the illogicality of adding scores on such disparate items as loss of weight, anxiety and suicidal thoughts, saying that it is like adding the weight of chalk and cheese. Is this really a problem? There are at least three counter-arguments.

1. In some circumstances it may indeed be meaningful to add chalk and

cheese, for example if they are both in the same truck. If it can be shown that all of the items being summed are in some sense in the same category then it makes sense to add them even if it is not exactly statistically or mathematically correct. In this case it makes sense if it can be shown that all of the items relate in the same way and in the same direction to the concept we want to measure (Snaith, 1981). There are several ways of doing this, and they are covered under the headings 'Specific objectivity' and 'Internal consistency or homogeneity' below.
2. The pudding argument: after more than 25 years of rating scale use in psychiatry it can be stated unambiguously that rating scales work; they distinguish between populations and demonstrate changes over time. Therefore 'the proof of the pudding is in the eating'.
3. The validity of the results depends to some extent on the statistics used to analyse them. As rating scale scores are really rank scores, i.e. 'severe' is worse than 'mild' but not necessarily twice as bad, then it follows that non-parametric statistics should be used to analyse all results. However, many researchers, especially if they have gathered a large amount of data, will use parametric statistics. This is only strictly allowable if the populations being tested can be shown to have a normal distribution with respect to the rating scale scores (Hamilton 1968, Bech *et al.*, 1981). Also the mean of the population under test should be close to the theoretical mean of the rating scale which is half maximum score. In addition, the population scores should spread over the whole range of scores and adopt a non-skewed distribution (Guilford, 1954). In reality these strict criteria are never met (see Bech, 1981).

Information Access

This simply means the information which the scale can provide and is dependent upon choice of items and method of administration. A self-rating scale cannot meaningfully ask about insight and can only circumstantially enquire about *signs* such as agitation or retardation (Carroll *et al.*, 1973).

Utility

In this context utility refers to the ease of administration (Carroll *et al.*, 1973). However, it should be noted that utility has another meaning (Rowlands, 1985). In this other sense it refers to the actuarial utility of a measure—how useful are the conclusions which can be drawn from a single observation, for example a score of 7 on the General Health Questionnaire?

Validity

There are two obvious types of validity which cannot be tested:

1. Content validity: the scale contains the number and content of questions appropriate to the attribute to be measured.
2. Face validity: the scale appears to measure what it is supposed to measure.

There are three types of validity which can be tested and will be discussed. They have all been used in standardization of rating scales:

1. Criterion validity: the agreement between the scale score and some external criterion. For example, in neuropsychological tests this can be the demonstration of a lesion in the brain. In psychiatric rating scales no such external criterion is available so a rather more tautological approach is taken. One criterion which has been used depends upon the assumption that patients in high-dependency care are more severely ill than those in lower-dependency care. Thus the prediction would be that a valid scale should show the scores of in-patients to be higher than day patients, which are higher than out-patients, which are in turn higher than general practice patients, which are themselves higher than the general community. Although there are flaws in the argument it generally holds and scales which fail on this simple task must be suspected of invalidity (e.g. Carroll *et al.*, 1973).

   The usual method is to test a scale against expert clinicians global judgements of severity as recorded on a numerical scale varying from 3 to 11 gradations. The reliability with which clinicians make such global judgements must be tested in each study, to ensure that the validating criterion is at least reliable.

Construct validity embraces both of the following:

2. Concurrent validity: in this method the scale is tested against already established instruments. Most new depression instruments, for example, are tested against the HDRS because it is the most commonly used of the scales. Several studies are available to show a generally high concurrent validity for the commonly used rating scales (Davies *et al.*, 1975; Kearns *et al.*, 1982).
3. Predictive validity: few psychiatric rating scales are separately validated in this way. One or two scales have been designed to predict the outcome of a particular treatment, for example ECT (Carney *et al.*, 1965) or antidepressants (Burrows *et al.*, 1976).

Reliability

Reliability is the extent to which the score on a scale reflects the hypothetical 'true' score and how much interference there is from extraneous influences. Once again there are a number of ways of establishing the reliability of a scale:

1. Inter-rater reliability. This is only applicable to observer-rated scales. It is the degree to which two raters give a subject the same score. The value of the reliability statistic can be maximized by having the two raters rating the same interview, thus controlling the variance which is due to the amount of information available. Lower reliabilities are usually obtained when the two raters conduct separate interviews.
2. Test–retest reliability. The test is given on two separate occasions to the same subjects, and the similarity in scores is the degree to which the test is reliable over time. While this is a useful measure in personality testing in which the traits are meant to remain stable over time, it is less useful in a scale for a changing attribute like depression or anxiety. Many scales are designed specifically to follow changes in state. If the test and retest are given very close together then memory factors come into play, the patients attempting to answer consistently. If they are given far enough apart to overcome this then real changes in the clinical state might account for changes in the ratings.

   Two attempts have been made to get around these problems. Snaith *et al.* (1971) gave the first self rating scale of depression immediately before an ECT and repeated the administration soon after it in the expectation that one ECT would cause a retrograde amnesia for the first administration while not significantly altering the clinical state. Acceptable reliability was found for this particular scale, arguing to some extent in favour of the usefulness of the technique. On the other hand two extraneous variables were introduced—the therapeutic and amnesiogenic effects of ECT—the combined effects of which were unknown.

   In another attempt to get around the problem Sheffield and Kellner (1970) used a version of the Symptom Rating Test which enquired about the previous week. He gave this to the same patients on subsequent days and employed irrelevant tests in between in an attempt to mask the memory for the first set of answers. Once again it is uncertain how effective this manoeuvre was. Although the scale appeared to have high reliability was this because the masking tests failed?
3. Split half reliability: in tests which have a large number of items all of which measure the same variable it is possible to split the test into two equivalent sections and examine the correlation of the scores on the

two halves. This is seldom possible with rating scales, which aim to be as brief as possible to spare patients effort. There are therefore seldom two equivalent items to be separated.

Errors

What are the errors in rating which can operate to reduce reliability? (see Rowlands, 1985). Individual raters may have a *bias* (generosity or leniency error) to rate high or low, and this is the reason for standardization sessions before the start of a study, when inter-rater reliabilities are calculated and those raters who are outliers in the distribution of scores are asked to modify their rating criteria.

A response set is the tendency to rate more to the left than the right of a scale or vice versa. It is particularly a problem when one end is always the 'desirable' end. It can be overcome by arranging desirable responses first to left then right of the items.

A special type of bias is known as the *central tendency error*, i.e. the reluctance to use the ends or extremes of a scale in preference to the central points. The *halo effect* is the tendency to make a global judgement early in the process of rating and then apply that to all of the subsequent items. Thus if the rater decides the patient is severely ill they will be biased towards high ratings on all items. The *logical error* is the tendency to assume that all items which seem on the face of it to be related will score similarly. It might be assumed that if a patient scores highly on 'guilty delusions' they will also score highly on 'worthlessness'. The *proximity error* is the tendency to rate adjacent items similarly.

In more general terms disagreement on ratings may be due to:

1. Information variance: the raters have different information available to them about the patient owing to differences in interview style or skill. This can be overcome to some extent by providing an interview schedule to go with the rating scale. In a study by Beck *et al.* (1962) only 5% of diagnostic disagreements were due to actual inconsistency on the part of the patient.
2. Observation variance: the raters observe the same thing but observe it differently. For example, when two raters rate the same interview, one is observing, interviewing and rating at the same time while the other is only observing and rating. Therefore they see the interview from a different perspective. Inconsistency of the interviewer from one patient to the next accounts for approximately 32% of diagnostic disagreement.
3. Terminology variance: the raters observe the same phenomena in the same way but come to apparently different conclusions because they use words differently. A glossary of terms can overcome this variety of

error to some extent, especially if training is provided, for example the Present State Examination (Wing *et al.*, 1974). 63% of diagnostic disagreements are due to nosological inadequacy, i.e. inadequate definition, when standard scales are not used (Beck *et al.*, 1962).

4. Ignorance of clinical phenomena: this is a particularly difficult source of variance in self-rating scales and when inexperienced raters are used.

When self rating scales are considered several other sources of error become important (Cronbach, 1946). Patients have an overall *agreement set*. If you ask 'do you . . .?' they will tend to answer yes more than no. There is also a *social desirability set* (Langevin and Stancer, 1979); so if a patient considers one response to be more socially acceptable than another, that is the one he will tend to choose. These extra sources of variance tend to make self-rating scales somewhat less reliable (Boyle, 1985).

Sensitivity to Change

In scales which are designed to measure severity, sensitivity to change is an important variety of validity. Does the scale record change as the condition changes clinically? To test this, global ratings of severity are obtained from independent raters, and the correlations between the change in global ratings and the change in scale scores are calculated. Using several outcome measures can demonstrate differences in sensitivity between them (Montgomery and Asberg, 1979; Kellner, 1972; Lipman *et al.*, 1965). Some writers use this term to describe sensitivity to differences between groups as in criterion validity. In addition sensitivity is used in epidemiological research referring to the proportion of true cases correctly identified by a test (see Ch. 6).

Specificity

Most scales of severity are designed for use with already diagnosed populations, so that as long as the items cover the correct symptoms of the condition that is sufficient (Hamilton, 1967). However, in some circumstances it is important to know that the scale does not also yield high scores for patients suffering from other disorders. In practice specificity (high scores only in the target condition) is difficult to achieve in psychiatry and the use of a diagnostic interview before application of a severity scale is important. Like sensitivity this word has another meaning in epidemiological research, being the proportion of true normal subjects correctly identified as such by a test (see Ch. 6).

Specific Objectivity

To what extent is the scale score a sufficient measure of, say, depression in all groups of patients and in all circumstances? To take an analogy the amount of expansion in the mercury of the thermometer is a sufficient measure of body temperature in clinical medicine all over the world in any patient. To meet criteria for specific objectivity and be a sufficient measure of a psychiatric condition, a scale must be:

1. Homogeneous, i.e. internally consistent (see below).
2. Transferable: a given score has the same meaning in groups of patients of all ages and both sexes. Some scales give correction values for some groups (e.g. Zung, 1967), and this clearly shows they have low transferability.

Rasch (1960) has provided complicated statistical models to test these attributes but to date the only scales to which they have been applied are the Hamilton and the Bech scales (Bech *et al.*, 1981).

Internal Consistency or Homogeneity

The extent to which all of the items agree determines the acceptability of the operation of summing item scores to obtain a single severity score:

1. Item–total correlation. The usual way of assessing internal consistency is to correlate the scores of each item with the total score of the scale. Those items which do not correlate significantly should probably be dropped.
2. Another way of checking the usefulness of the total score is to factor analyse the scale results in a diagnosed population. If all items load positively on the first factor extracted then it can be said that the most important factor contributing to the variance is one of severity.

The paradox of internal consistency is that highly intercorrelated items are redundant, i.e. they give no more information than a single item. However, absolute homogeneity is never achieved. Even when items are highly intercorrelated there is still a point in including several items in the scale. With only one item the score is equivalent to a global rating and, like the global rating, gives little clue about the principles or cues which have been used to assign ratings to patients. When the item content of a scale is low the information content of the results of its use will be correspondingly low. That is why most scales have at least six items, the minimum required to make any sense of severity ratings of a complicated psychiatric condition. The ideal is a moderate degree of homogeneity since a high degree indicates redundancy of items and a low degree indicates a lack of a common dimension.

So far the points we have discussed have applied mainly to scales which are used to score severity. However, the process of standardization also applies to diagnostic instruments. Many of the above considerations also apply to these instruments. However, there are other important definitions for diagnostic instruments which are not used in rating scales.

Restrictiveness

In 100 cases of depression diagnosed on clinical grounds how many will be classed as cases of depression by the instrument? The term restrictiveness is used because it is simpler and carries the meaning we need here. Some instruments, such as the Newcastle scale for endogenous depression (Carney *et al.*, 1965) and the Present State Examination (Wing *et al.*, 1974), are more restrictive than others and give the diagnosis only to 'gold-plated cases'. Others are too loose, i.e. not at all restrictive, and therefore have little utility. In epidemiological research this would be referred to as the instrument's specificity and sensitivity for detecting cases. However, in the more complex field of standardization of *clinical* diagnosis restrictiveness has extra meaning because of the variety of definitions of the syndrome to be detected. Each may have some degree of validity but some may exclude more individuals than others.

Exclusion Clause

This is similar to the specificity item in severity rating scales. To make a diagnosis of depression you must exclude the diagnosis of schizophrenia but not necessarily that of anxiety state. The exclusion clauses vary in their adequacy, for example, from a plain statement to exclude schizophrenia to a list of the symptoms. Exclusion clauses appear to be essential for specificity in a diagnostic instrument. In the development of the WHO schedule for standardized assessment of depressive disorders the specificity of diagnosis fell from 90% to 20% when the four exclusion categories were removed (Gastpar, 1979).

REFERENCES

American Psychiatric Association (1980). *Diagnostic and Statistical Manual of Mental Disorders*, 3rd edn, American Psychiatric Association, Washington.

Bech, P., Gram, L. F., Dein, E., Jacobsen, O., Vitger, J. and Bolwig, T. G. (1975). Quantitative rating of depressive states. *Acta Psychiatr. Scand.* **51**, 161–170.

Bech, P., Allerup, P., Gram, L. F., Reisby, N., Rosenberg, R., Jacobsen, O. and Nagy, A. (1981). The Hamilton Depression Scale: evaluation of objectivity using logistic models. *Acta Psychiatr. Scand.* **63**, 290–299.

Bech, P., Kastrup, M. and Rafaelson, O. J. (1986). Mini Compendium of Rating Scales for states of anxiety, depression, mania, schizophrenia with corresponding DSM III syndromes. *Acta Psychiat. Scand.* **73**, Suppl. 326.

Beck, A. T., Ward, C. H., Mendelson, M., Mock, J. and Erbaugh, J. (1961). An inventory for measuring depression. *Arch. Gen. Psychiatry* **4**, 561–571.

Beck, A. T., Ward, C., Hendelson, M., Mock, J. and Erbaugh, J. (1962). Reliability of psychiatric diagnoses: a study of consistency of clinical judgements and ratings. *Am. J. Psychiatry* **119**, 351–356.

Bleuler, E. (1911). The fundamental symptoms of dementia praecox or the group of schizophrenias. *Trans. Zinkin J.*; International University Press, New York (1950).

Boyle, G. J. (1985). Self report measures of depression: some psychometric considerations. *Br. J. Clin. Psychol.* **24**, 45–59.

Burrows, G. D., Foenander, G., Davies, B. *et al.* (1976). Rating scales as predictors of response to tricyclic antidepressants. *Aust. NZ J. Psychiat.* **10**, 53–56.

Carney, M. W. P., Roth, M. and Garside, R. F. (1965). The diagnosis of depressive syndromes and the prediction of ECT response. *Br. J. Psychiatry* **111**, 659–674.

Carroll, B. J., Fielding, J. M. and Blashki, T. G. (1973). Depression rating scales: a critical review. *Arch. Gen. Psychiatry* **28**, 361–366.

Cronbach, L. J. (1946) Response set and test validity. *Ed. Psych. Measurement* **6**, 475–495.

Davies, B., Burrows, G. and Poynton, C. A. (1975). Comparative study of four depression rating scales. *Aust. NZ J. Psychiat.* **9**, 21–24.

Gastpar, M. (1979). Diagnose und therapie depressiver patienten in der praxis. In *Habilitation*, University of Basle.

Goldberg, D. P. (1972). The detection of psychiatric illness by questionnaire, *Maudsley Monograph 21*, Oxford University Press, London.

Guilford, J. P. (1954). *Psychometric Methods*, McGraw-Hill, New York.

Hamilton, M. (1967). Development of a rating scale for primary depressive illness. *Br. J. Soc. Clin. Pychiat.* **6**, 278–296.

Hamilton, M. (1968). Some notes on rating scales. *Statistician* **18**, 11–17.

Hamilton, M. (1972). Rating scales in depression. In *Depressive Illness* (P. Kielholz, ed.), Huber, Berlin.

Kearns, N. P., Cruickshank, C. A., McGuigan, K. J., Riley, S. A., Shaw, S. P. and Snaith, R. P. (1982). A comparison of depression rating scales. *Br. J. Psychiatry* **141**, 45–49.

Kellner, R. (1972). Part 2: Improvement criteria in drug trials with neurotic patients. *Psychiat. Med.* **2**, 73–80.

Langevin, R. and Stancer, H. (1979). Evidence that depression rating scales primarily measure a social undesirability response set. *Acta Psychiat. Scand.* **59**, 70–79.

Liekert, R. (1932). A technique for the measurement of attitudes. *Arch. Psychol.* **140**, 1–55.

Lipman, R. S., Cole, O. J., Park, L. D. and Rickels, K. (1965). Sensitivity of symptom and non symptom focused criteria of out patient drug efficacy. *Am. J. Psychiatry* **122**, 24–27.

Miller, I. W., Bishop, S., Norman, W. H. and Maddever, H. (1985). The modified

Hamilton Rating Scale for Depression: reliability and validity. *Psychiatr. Res.* **14**, 131–142.

Montgomery, S. A. and Asberg, M. (1979). A new depression rating scale designed to be sensitive to change. *Br. J. Psychiatry* **134**, 382–389.

Perry, E. K., Tomlinson, B. E., Blessed, G., Bergmann, K., Gibson, P. H. and Perry, R. H. (1978). Correlation of cholinergic abnormalities with senile plaques and mental test scores in senile dementia. *Br. Med. J.*, 1457–1459.

Rasch, G. (1960). *Probabilistic Model for Some Intelligence and Attainment Tests*, Danish Institute for Educational Research, Copenhagen.

Rowlands, L. (1985). Assessment. In *Psychological Applications in Psychiatry* (B. Bradley and C. Thompson, eds), Wiley, Chichester.

Sheffield, B. F. and Kellner, R. (1970). The temporal stability of self ratings of neurotic symptoms, *Br. J. Soc. Clin. Psychol.* **9**, 46–53.

Snaith, R. P. (1981). Rating scales. *Br. J. Psychiatry* **138**, 512–514.

Snaith, R. P., Ahmed, S. N., Mehta, S. and Hamilton, M. (1971). Assessment of the severity of primary depressive illness: the Wakefield self assessment depression inventory. *Psychol. Med.* **1**, 143–149.

Wing, J. K., Cooper, J. E. and Sartorius, N. (1974). *The Measurement and Classification of Psychiatric Symptoms*, Cambridge University Press, Cambridge.

Wing, J. K. (1978). *Reasoning about Madness*, Oxford University Press, London.

Zung, W. W. K. (1965). A self rating depression scale. *Arch. Gen. Psychiatry* **12**, 63–70.

Zung, W. W. K. (1967). Factors influencing the self rating depression scale. *Arch. Gen. Psychiatry* **16**, 543–547.

The Instruments of Psychiatric Research
Edited by C. Thompson

CHAPTER 2

Standardized diagnostic interviews for psychiatric research

DEBORAH S. HASIN[1,2,3] and ANDREW E. SKODOL[1,3]
[1]*College of Physicians and Surgeons,
Columbia University,
New York, USA*

[2]*School of Public Health (Epidemiology),
Columbia University,
New York, USA*

[3]*New York State Psychiatric Institute,
New York, USA*

INTRODUCTION

Over the last twenty-five years the assessment of psychopathology for research purposes has undergone considerable change and improvement. Psychiatric diagnoses are now made according to specified criteria, with the result that mental disorders can be assessed much more reliably than had previously been possible. In addition, due in part to international collaboration in research, conceptualizations in the USA and the UK of the symptoms that constitute the major psychiatric disorders have converged to a large extent, although differences remain. Dimensional ratings of aspects of psychopathology have also been developed, some of which are incorporated into interviews that also produce dichotomous diagnoses.

While researchers needing assessments of psychopathology once faced a bleak picture, i.e. a lack of useful procedures, their problems now are different. Many assessment procedures have been developed, each with different strengths, weaknesses and practical problems. Currently, the difficulty lies in choosing the best procedure for the research problem at hand, given the time and financial resources available to the investigator.

In this chapter, we have provided information intended to reduce the difficulties in beginning the decision-making process. We have focused on assessment procedures that cover a wide variety of areas of psychopathology, rather than questionnaires or interviews that focus on only one area. We have limited our coverage to procedures that are administered by interviewers and that yield, as at least part of their output, psychiatric diagnoses according to specified criteria. Thus, we are not discussing many psychopathology rating scales, such as the Delusions Symptoms States Inventory (DSSI) used to generate the Foulds and Bedford hierarchy (Foulds and Bedford, 1975; Foulds, 1976), the Comprehensive Psychopathological Rating Scale (CPRS) (Asberg *et al.*, 1978), or the Hopkin's Symptom Checklist-90 (SCL-90) (Derogatis *et al.*, 1974). Although such instruments yield descriptive data on a wide range of psychiatric symptoms and are sometimes administered by interviewers, they were designed as self-report questionnaires and do not yield psychiatric diagnoses according to any generally accepted classification of mental disorders. Some scales, such as the Current and Past Psychopathology Scales (CAPPS) (Endicott and Spitzer, 1972b), were forerunners of structured interviews and will be mentioned in their historical contexts.

For each of the procedures we do discuss, we provide a brief background; a description of the procedure itself and its diagnostic coverage; indications of the types of subjects for which the procedure is suitable, the interviewers required and the training needed by these interviewers; data on reliability and validity; and information on associated assessment procedures and future directions of development. The instruments we have covered are the Schedule for Affective Disorders and Schizophrenia, the Diagnostic Interview Schedule, the Structured Clinical Interview for DSM-III-R and the Present State Examination.

SCHEDULE FOR AFFECTIVE DISORDERS AND SCHIZOPHRENIA

The Schedule for Affective Disorders and Schizophrenia (SADS) (Endicott and Spitzer, 1978) is a semi-structured interview designed for use by interviewers with clinical experience. It was initially developed at Columbia University in New York City (USA) for use by the National Institute of Mental Health (NIMH) Clinical Studies Branch for the Collaborative Study on the Psychobiology of Depression (Katz *et al.*, 1979). The SADS was designed to evaluate the symptoms of disorders as defined by the Research Diagnostic Criteria (RDC) (Spitzer *et al.*, 1978), the intermediate set of diagnostic criteria between the earlier Feighner Criteria (Feighner *et al.*, 1972) and DSM-III (American Psychiatric Association, 1980). The developers of the SADS had had many years of experience developing interviews and rating scales to assess various dimensions of psychopathology. Some of the instruments which can be considered 'forerunners' of the SADS include the Mental

Status Schedule (MSS) (Spitzer *et al.*, 1967), the Current and Past Psychopathology Scales (CAPPS) (Endicott and Spitzer, 1972b), the Psychiatric Evaluation Form (PEF) (Endicott and Spitzer, 1972a) and the Psychiatric Status Schedule (PSS) (Spitzer *et al.*, 1970).

The full SADS interview is intended for use with psychiatric patients, or with other subjects currently experiencing some psychopathology. It consists of two main sections. Both sections cover a number of areas to be clinically explored with subjects in order to determine the most valid ratings.

The first section contains multi-point items (mostly six-point items) for rating the severity of subjects' *current* conditions. These items cover symptoms and other aspects of affective disorders, anxiety disorders and psychosis in considerable detail. A few items are provided for less detailed ratings of alcohol, drug and antisocial problems, and psychosocial functioning. The symptoms and associated features are rated in two ways in Part 1 of the SADS: when each was at its most severe level during the current episode, and the level of each in the week prior to the interview. Note that the severity levels of the items are defined with 'anchor points' and are not left to unspecified clinical judgement.

Fig. 1 provides examples of an item from Part 1 of the SADS: insomnia. By the time the interviewer arrives at this point, he or she will already have explored the subject's current condition, treatment status, affective state, and a number of other cognitive and somatic features of depression and anxiety. If sleep disturbance has been mentioned in the preceding discussion, the interviewer reminds the subject about it, and if not, asks the initial probe provided for the insomnia item. The interviewer then asks questions to ascertain the detail necessary to rate the severity of sleep disturbance when at its worst during the current episode. Some patients may have experienced a peak in severity of all their symptoms at the same time, and hence all severity items cover the same time period. Others may have experienced peak severity of some symptoms at one point in an episode, and peak severity of others at a different point, and hence the ratings do not necessarily all refer to exactly the same time, although they do all refer to the same episode. If the subject has no current episode, or if the current episode has lasted longer than a year, then the item is rated for when the symptom was at its worst in the year prior to the interview.

After rating the item at its worst (and noting the types of insomnia), the interviewer then asks about insomnia during the week prior to the interview, which is rated on the horizontal scale seen at the bottom of the figure. This provides a cross-sectional picture of symptom severity at a consistent time point for all subjects.

The items from the first part of the SADS can be used to make diagnoses of most of the disorders covered by the RDC (Spitzer *et al.*, 1978). They can also be combined to yield summary scale scores on symptom dimensions,

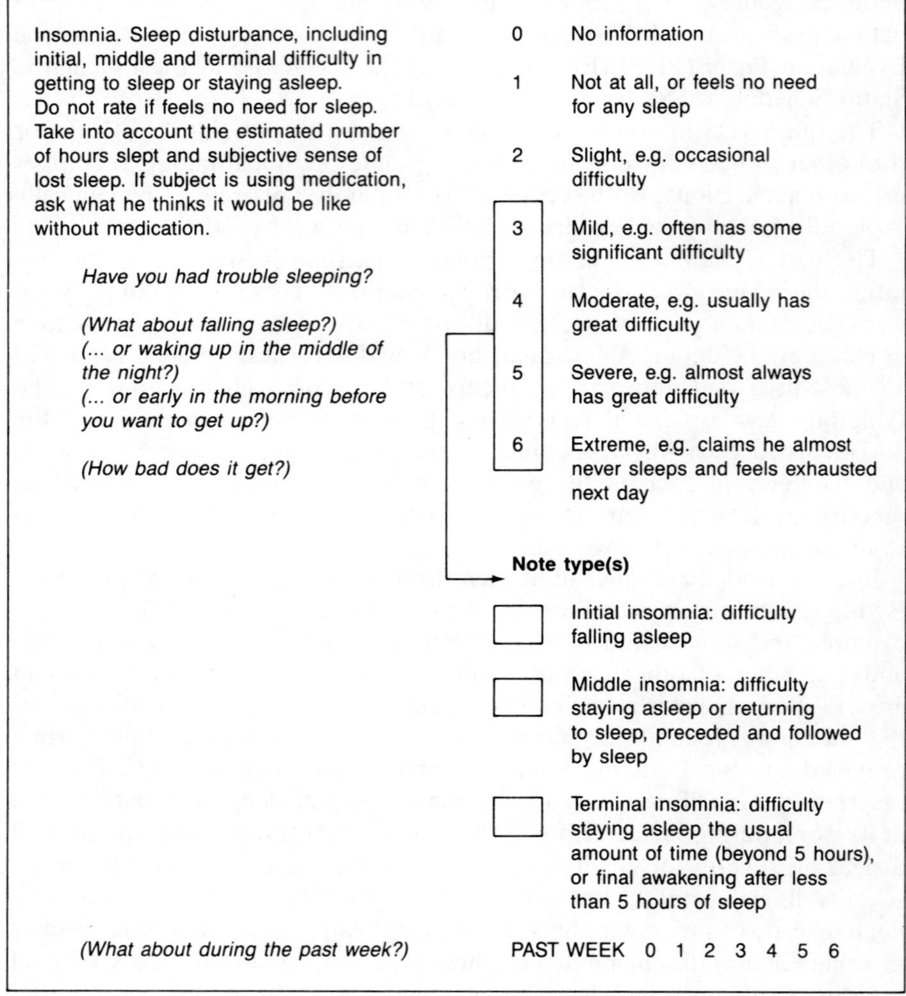

Insomnia. Sleep disturbance, including initial, middle and terminal difficulty in getting to sleep or staying asleep. Do not rate if feels no need for sleep. Take into account the estimated number of hours slept and subjective sense of lost sleep. If subject is using medication, ask what he thinks it would be like without medication.

Have you had trouble sleeping?

(What about falling asleep?)
(... or waking up in the middle of the night?)
(... or early in the morning before you want to get up?)

(How bad does it get?)

0 No information

1 Not at all, or feels no need for any sleep

2 Slight, e.g. occasional difficulty

3 Mild, e.g. often has some significant difficulty

4 Moderate, e.g. usually has great difficulty

5 Severe, e.g. almost always has great difficulty

6 Extreme, e.g. claims he almost never sleeps and feels exhausted next day

Note type(s)

☐ Initial insomnia: difficulty falling asleep

☐ Middle insomnia: difficulty staying asleep or returning to sleep, preceded and followed by sleep

☐ Terminal insomnia: difficulty staying asleep the usual amount of time (beyond 5 hours), or final awakening after less than 5 hours of sleep

(What about during the past week?) PAST WEEK 0 1 2 3 4 5 6

Fig. 1. Example of an item from the SADS: insomnia. The vertical ratings are for the symptom at its worst during the current episode, or the past year. The horizontal 'past week' ratings are for the symptom at its worst during the week prior to the interview

such as current depressive mood and ideation, current manic syndrome and current formal thought disorder.

The second part of the SADS covers subjects' lifetime history of RDC mental disorders prior to the year before the interview. The items are clustered into diagnostic-specific sections, and are largely rated as dichotomous (present or absent). The general rule in determining whether a symptom receives a positive rating in this section is that it must have occurred at a severe enough level to warrant a clinically significant rating on the corresponding multi-level item from the first part of the SADS. Most diagnostic sections begin with a few screening questions. If these elicit negative responses the interviewer skips to the next section.

When used together, the first and second parts of the SADS provide information for making both current and lifetime psychiatric diagnoses. Interviewers may take more than one session to administer the SADS, if necessary. They also consult charts or records and speak with staff, family members or significant others who can provide additional information or clarifications to aid in making the most valid ratings on the SADS. The interview takes a minimum of an hour to administer, and may require 2 or 3 hours when subjects have had complex or confusing psychiatric histories.

After all items in the SADS have been rated, the rater consults the RDC and makes the diagnoses according to these diagnostic criteria. A score-sheet is provided with the SADS to note the presence or absence of all current, past and lifetime diagnoses, as well as age at onset of the first episode, subtypes of the disorder (if applicable) and duration (in weeks) of current episodes. Table 1 shows the major diagnoses covered by SADS.

Our description of the full SADS facilitates the description of other forms of the interview. Perhaps the most commonly used of these is the SADS-L (lifetime version of the SADS) (Endicott and Spitzer, 1978). The SADS-L ascertains information necessary to make both current and lifetime diagnoses. However, the amount of information recorded on current psychopathology is much less detailed than in the full SADS. The format of the SADS-L is nearly identical to the second (past) section of the full SADS, supplemented to rate the presence and absence of current as well as past disorders. This instrument was intended for use with subjects who are not expected to evidence much current psychopathology. The SADS-L was originally designed to evaluate the lifetime psychiatric histories of the relatives of index subjects in the NIMH Collaborative Study of Depression.

The SADS-C (change version) (Endicott *et al.*, 1981) consists of items from the first section of the SADS. These items rate symptoms such as depressed mood, worry or blunted affect at their highest level of severity in the week prior to the interview. When used at multiple points in time, this version of the SADS allows the detailed recording of changes in status.

Two other versions of the SADS-L have been developed recently and warrant mentioning. The SADS-LA (anxiety) (Manuzza *et al.*, 1986) was designed for a family study of anxiety disorders, and provides for the recording of a great deal of information on subclinical and clinical manifestations of anxiety disorders. The SADS-LB (bipolar) was recently designed for a study on the molecular genetics of bipolar disorders. This version of the SADS-L elicits information on subclinical and clinical manifestations of bipolar disorders (J. Endicott, New York State Psychiatric Institute).

Table 1. Diagnoses and subtypes covered by the SADS and SADS-L interviews. All diagnoses made according to Research Diagnostic Criteria[a]

Non-affective disorders	Affective disorders
Schizophrenia	Manic disorder
Acute–chronic	Hypomanic disorder
Paranoid	Bipolar with mania (bipolar I)
Disorganized	Bipolar with hypomania (bipolar II)
Catatonic	
Mixed (undifferentiated)	Major depressive disorder
Residual	Primary
	Secondary
Unspecified functional psychosis	Recurrent unipolar
Schizotypal features	Psychotic
	Incapacitating
Briquet's disorder (somatization disorder)	Endogenous
	Agitated
Alcoholism	Retarded
	Situational
Drug use disorder	Simple
Sedatives/hypnotics/tranquillizers	
Narcotics	Minor depressive disorder
Cocaine	Intermittent depressive disorder
Amphetamines	(dysthymic disorder)
Hallucinogens	Cyclothymic personality
Cannabis	Labile personality
Solvents	
Poly-drug	Depressive syndrome superimposed on residual schizophrenia
Antisocial personality disorder	
	Schizoaffective disorder
Panic disorder	Manic
Obsessive-compulsive disorder	Repressed
Phobic disorder	
Generalized anxiety disorder	
Other psychiatric disorder	

[a] Categories also include currently not mentally ill and never mentally ill.

As mentioned above, the SADS and the SADS-type interviews were designed to elicit the information necessary to make psychiatric diagnoses according to RDC criteria. Since publication of the SADS, newer nomenclatures have been introduced such as DSM-III (American Psychiatric Association, 1980), and DSM-III-R (American Psychiatric Association, 1987). Some sections of the SADS and SADS-type interviews can be modified easily to make the newer diagnoses. However, other sections would require substantial modification to elicit the information for the newer nomenclatures (primarily alcohol, drug and antisocial personality diagnoses).

Note that no computer program is available to make RDC diagnoses from SADS data. The authors of the SADS, disappointed by earlier efforts to produce diagnostic programs (Spitzer *et al.*, 1974), take the position that subtle diagnostic distinctions cannot be made by computer. Other investigators have had concerns about the problem of rater error in making diagnoses by the complex RDC rules and have developed computer programs to generate RDC diagnoses. Researchers who develop computer algorithms for diagnoses should check computer diagnoses carefully against expert clinical diagnosis on the most complex of cases, in order to eliminate errors in their diagnostic algorithms.

Interviewer Qualifications

SADS interviewers should have had clinical experience prior to commencing SADS training, and some part of this experience should have been in making judgements about manifest psychopathology. Ideally, SADS interviewers will have had experience with the types of subjects they will be interviewing for a study. Psychiatrists and doctoral-level clinical psychologists usually have the background needed to use the SADS. Masters-level clinicians, including social workers and clinical psychologists, also make good SADS interviewers. Masters-level nurses and counsellors can also be trained to administer the SADS, although raters with these training backgrounds are less likely to have had experience with psychiatric diagnoses and may need additional training. Non-clinicians will have to be trained not only in diagnosis but also in the clinical skills necessary to elicit the required information. While non-clinicians can be trained to be good SADS interviewers, investigators should realize that the training necessary for non-clinicians will be considerably longer and more complicated than for raters with the appropriate clinical background. Finally, we note that for the SADS, as well as for the other diagnostic procedures discussed below, some people simply cannot be trained to administer the interview well. They may have had considerable clinical experience, but still cannot master the organization of the interview, or cannot take the information recorded in the SADS and put it together correctly according to RDC rules to assign diagnoses.

Interviewer Training

Interviewers begin SADS training (Gibbon *et al.*, 1981) by reading case vignettes and making RDC diagnoses based on these vignettes. The diagnoses are checked with an answer key. Any problems are discussed with an experienced SADS rater. Trainees then watch a set of videotaped interviews, and rate these interviews in SADS booklets. They make diagnoses based on the interview material, and compare all item and diagnostic ratings to answer keys. Once again, any areas of difficulty are discussed with an experienced rater.

After the preliminary portions of training are complete, trainees then administer the SADS under the observation of an experienced SADS interviewer. (These can be audiotaped, videotaped or observed 'live'.) Additional help is usually needed at this point to encourage raters to probe areas more fully, or to conform more closely to the interview format. Sometimes advice is needed, based on experience, about how to handle certain aspects of the interview. Once trainees have completed these practice interviews, they are ready for an inter-rater reliability study, which (it is hoped) will demonstrate that they are rating and diagnosing consistently.

Reliability of the SADS and SADS-type Interviews

Initial results from New York indicated that the test–retest reliability of summary scale scores from Part 1 of the SADS were excellent, with intraclass correlation coefficients (ICC) (Shrout and Fleiss, 1979) greater than 0.78, with the exception of anxiety (ICC=0.67) and formal thought disorder (ICC=0.49) (Endicott and Spitzer, 1978). Test–retest examination of RDC diagnoses from the SADS showed that most disorders and subtypes of affective disorders could be diagnosed at a good to excellent level of inter-rater reliability, with kappa levels of agreement (Cohen, 1960) greater than 0.65, with the exceptions of hypomania ($\kappa=0.57$) (Spitzer *et al.*, 1978). Agreement was also good to excellent for most subtypes of affective disorder (Spitzer *et al.*, 1978). Additional studies on the reliability of the SADS have used raters from several different cities. When raters diagnosed from videotapes, agreement was found to be good to excellent (Andreasen *et al.*, 1982). Another study, using a morning versus afternoon test–retest design with live interviews, showed good to excellent agreement on affective diagnoses and SADS summary scales (Keller *et al.*, 1981). A complex design was used to study inter-rater agreement on the SADS-L, comparing morning versus afternoon ratings and initial versus 6-month ratings made by raters from different cities. The reliabilities of SADS-L diagnoses were good to excellent for most disorders except bipolar II (Andreasen *et al.*, 1981).

More recent studies of the reliability of SADS-L lifetime diagnoses have shown less encouraging results when the interval between interviews was long or when community residents were the subjects, rather than psychiatric patients or their relatives. Bromet *et al.* (1986) found a kappa of only 0.41 for major depression with a re-interview at 18 months. Preliminary analysis by John Rice and colleagues in the NIMH Collaborative Depression Study of re-interviews 6 years later of 1682 relatives of psychiatric patients found the following kappas: 0.57 for major depression, 0.66 for mania, 0.33 for hypomania, 0.69 for alcoholism and 0.29 for generalized anxiety disorder.

Further analyses of these data are currently underway to identify factors predicting diagnostic inconsistency over time. However, initial analyses on a subsample of these subjects showed that disorders which were severe or treated showed better reliability over 6 years than mild or untreated cases (Rice *et al.*, 1987a).

Validity

While research on reliability can be complex, the usual reliability study produces coefficients with fairly standard interpretations, and the results are thus quantified. The study of validity is much more complex and less easily quantifiable. Validity cannot be achieved without reliability, but reliability does not guarantee validity.

SADS and SADS-L diagnoses have been shown to cluster generally within families (Andreasen *et al.*, 1987; Weissman *et al.*, 1984). Many subtypes of affective disorders have been shown to be differentially familial (Rice *et al.*, 1987b; Coryell *et al.*, 1984a; Endicott *et al.*, 1986b), although this was not the case for all subtypes examined (Andreasen *et al.*, 1986). The prognostic significance of subtypes such as schizoaffective disorder compared to psychotic and non-psychotic depression (Coryell *et al.*, 1984b) has been demonstrated. Additional research has shown differences in the clinical course of bipolar 1, bipolar 2 and unipolar depression (Coryell *et al.*, 1987) and the poor prognosis of cycling between affective poles within a bipolar episode (Keller *et al.*, 1986). Certain configurations of SADS-L diagnoses have been shown to predict good outcome of treatment for opiate addicts, while other diagnostic groupings do not (Woody *et al.*, 1985). SADS items and scale scores measuring depressive features have been shown as sensitive to change in drug–placebo studies. The SADS (supplemented with a few additional items) produced data on the diagnosis of schizophrenia showing that DSM-III criteria were more highly predictive of outcome than were several other sets of diagnostic criteria (Endicott *et al.*, 1986a).

Associated Procedures

To achieve the goals of the NIMH Collaborative Study of Depression, a number of other assessment procedures were developed. Perhaps the two with the greatest utility to other researchers are the Family History–RDC (FH–RDC) (Andreasen *et al.*, 1977) and the Longitudinal Interval Follow-up Evaluation (LIFE) (Keller *et al.*, 1987).

FH–RDC

The FH–RDC was designed to obtain information on the lifetime psychiatric histories (diagnoses, treatment, suicidal behaviour) of the relatives of an index subject, usually a patient with a given disorder. This procedure elicits detailed information on each first-degree relative individually, and in less detail on second-degree relatives. The diagnostic coverage of the FH–RDC is less extensive and specific than the SADS. Interviewers for the FH–RDC are usually SADS or SADS-L interviewers. The FH–RDC can be taught fairly quickly to interviewers who are familiar with the SADS or SADS-L. The major advantages of the FH–RDC procedure for assessing family history are:

1. It is considerably easier and less expensive to carry out than a study in which all relatives are interviewed directly.
2. It may be the only way to get information on relatives who have died, who refuse to participate in an interview, or are otherwise unavailable for a family study.

As might be expected, the main problem with the FH–RDC is low sensitivity (Andreasen *et al.*, 1986; Thompson *et al.*, 1982; Orvashel *et al.*, 1982). The FH–RDC methodology may be adequate for assessing gross differences in family history of certain disorders between subgroups of subjects (if no reason exists to suspect that differential sensitivity to the psychiatric histories of relatives exists between the subgroups). The FH–RDC serves as an important adjunct to direct interviews in a family/genetics study for relatives who cannot be interviewed. Use of the FH–RDC alone as a source of information on family psychiatric histories may be warranted for study of a particular research question that has not yet been explored; the results of the FH–RDC may indicate that further study with direct interviews would serve a worthwhile purpose. However, one should not rely on FH–RDC information alone for complex genetic analyses.

Longitudinal Interval Follow-up Evaluation (LIFE)

The LIFE was developed in response to the need for a procedure to make detailed assessments of the course of disorders over time. The LIFE provides a means for recording the status of RDC disorders at weekly intervals after intake into a study. Interviewers question subjects about major changes in the status of disorders previously diagnosed, as well as about the occurrence of any new conditions. If changes or new conditions have occurred, the interviewer then probes to locate these as accurately in time as possible, relating changes to holidays, seasons, etc., if necessary. These weekly ratings allow the statistical analysis of the number of weeks to remission or relapse by survival analytic techniques. These techniques, in turn, allow the use and presentation of considerably more information about the course of a mental disorder than the simple assessment of recovery (or some other event, such as relapse) by a given point in time. A joint-rating reliability study using videotaped interviews showed good to excellent inter-rater reliability on most aspects of the LIFE, including the timing of change points and the severity of illness.

Thus far, data from the LIFE have been used primarily for analyses of the course of affective disorders (most studies cited above on the prognostic validation of aspects of the SADS used data collected with the LIFE, and several others have been published). However, the LIFE has recently proved useful in examining the course of RDC alcoholism in patients with affective syndromes (Hasin *et al.*, 1989), and therefore has considerable potential for studying the course of other disorders.

Further Information

For information on the SADS and related procedures, contact Dr Jean Endicott, Columbia University College of Physicians and Surgeons, New York State Psychiatric Institute, 722 W 168th Street, Box 123, New York, New York 10032, USA; telephone (212) 960–2270.

DIAGNOSTIC INTERVIEW SCHEDULE

The Diagnostic Interview Schedule (DIS) was developed by researchers at Washington University in St Louis, Missouri (Robins *et al.*, 1981). This research centre was the setting for pioneering work in the development of specified diagnostic criteria for psychiatric disorders, as represented by the Feighner Criteria (Feighner *et al.*, 1972). The DIS, a fully structured diagnostic interview designed for administration by non-clinicians, was developed in response to an NIMH request for a relatively inexpensive procedure that could be used for assessing the current and lifetime psychiatric histories of many thousands of subjects in a large-scale epidemiological survey (Regier *et al.*, 1984). Since the introduction of the DIS, its developers have endorsed it for use in clinical, as well as epidemiological, research. The DIS *Newsletter*, which describes studies using the DIS and lists publications of such studies, indicates that some researchers have adapted this instrument for use in clinical studies. (The newsletter is available from the address given below for Dr Robins.) The only subjects for which the DIS is not recommended are those showing such severe symptoms of organic mental syndrome that an interviewer cannot proceed.

The DIS consists of numerous diagnostic sections. The coverage of the instrument is noted in Table 2. The DIS is an extension of an instrument previously developed by the same research group, the Renard Diagnostic Interview (Helzer *et al.*, 1981), which was designed to make assessments of diagnoses by the Feighner Criteria. However (as shown in Table 2), the DIS

Table 2. Diagnoses and subtypes covered by the DIS interview. All diagnoses made according to DSM-III criteria[a]

Non-affective disorders	Affective disorders
Schizophrenia	Manic disorder
Schizophreniform disorder	Bipolar disorder
	Atypical bipolar disorder (bipolar II)
Somatization disorder	Major depression
	Single episode
Alcohol abuse	Recurrent
Alcohol dependence	Dysthymic disorder
Drug abuse	
Drug dependence	
Barbiturates	
Opioids	
Cocaine	
Amphetamine	
Hallucinogen	
Cannabis	
Summary diagnosis	
Tobacco dependence	
Pathological gambling	
Psychosexual dysfunctions	
Transsexualism	
Ego-dystonic homosexuality	
Antisocial personality disorder	
Panic disorder	
Obsessive-compulsive disorder	
Simple phobia	
Social phobia	
Generalized anxiety disorder[b]	
Agoraphobia with and without panic attacks	
Anorexia nervosa	
Bulimia[b]	
Organic brain syndromes	

[a] Diagnoses also available by RDC and Feighner Criteria; contact Dr Lee Robins at Washington University for further details.
[b] Available from version III-A of the DIS.

expands on the Renard interview by making diagnostic assessments according to Feighner, RDC and DSM-III criteria.

When administering the DIS, interviewers read the items to subjects exactly as they are worded in the interview booklet. Clinical exploration of subjects' responses is neither required nor allowed. If a subject does not understand a question, it (or part of it) may be re-read to the subject, perhaps emphasizing the part that has been misunderstood. The interviewer, however, is discouraged from rewording any of the questions.

In place of the clinical exploration of whether or not a symptom is sufficiently severe to be considered positive, or caused by drugs or physical illness, interviewers use a standard set of questions, represented by a probe flow chart (Fig. 2). Any positive response to the questions in box A indicate that the symptom was severe enough to be considered clinically relevant. The other boxes attempt to ascertain the symptom's aetiology. If possible, a doctor's diagnosis is used, as determined by the questions from box D. Physical illness, injury, and the use of alcohol, street drugs or prescribed medication are organic causes of symptoms which the probe flow chart routinely attempts to rule out. If a doctor was not consulted, the subject's opinion on the cause of the symptom is obtained (boxes B and C). Symptoms unlikely to have an organic cause do not require use of the entire probe flow chart.

Fig. 3 displays the insomnia item from the depression section of the DIS. When the interviewer arrives at this point, somatization and several anxiety disorders have already been covered, and a question has been asked about whether the subject has ever had a period of 2 weeks of dysphoric mood. Each of the depression symptoms, however, is initially asked about on a lifetime basis. The interviewer asks the question as shown in the figure and, if the subject gives a positive response, then uses the probe flow chart to determine the final lifetime rating of this symptom. Since there is no '2' rating possible for this item, box A of the probe flow chart is skipped; the symptom is considered of clinically significant severity if it occurred as described in the initial question. If, according to the probe flow chart, neither the subject nor a doctor has attributed the symptom to physical illness (a rating of '4') or alcohol, drugs or medication (a rating of '3'), then the symptom is scored as positive ('5') and included in the symptom count towards the diagnosis. The interviewer makes notes by the lines marked 'MD' or 'Self' to specify in more detail what the cause of the symptom was.

If enough symptoms have been rated positive, the interviewer then asks a number of other questions about episodes of depression, such as time of onset, recency, treatment received and number of prior episodes. At the end of the depression section, he or she then returns to the symptoms, and asks if each one originally scored '5' on a lifetime basis occurred during the worst episode (or during the only episode if the subject only had one). The probe flow chart is not used at this point.

The DIS takes a minimum of about 40 minutes to administer, and can take a few hours with a talkative psychiatric patient who has experienced psychopathology in numerous areas. Information from sources other than

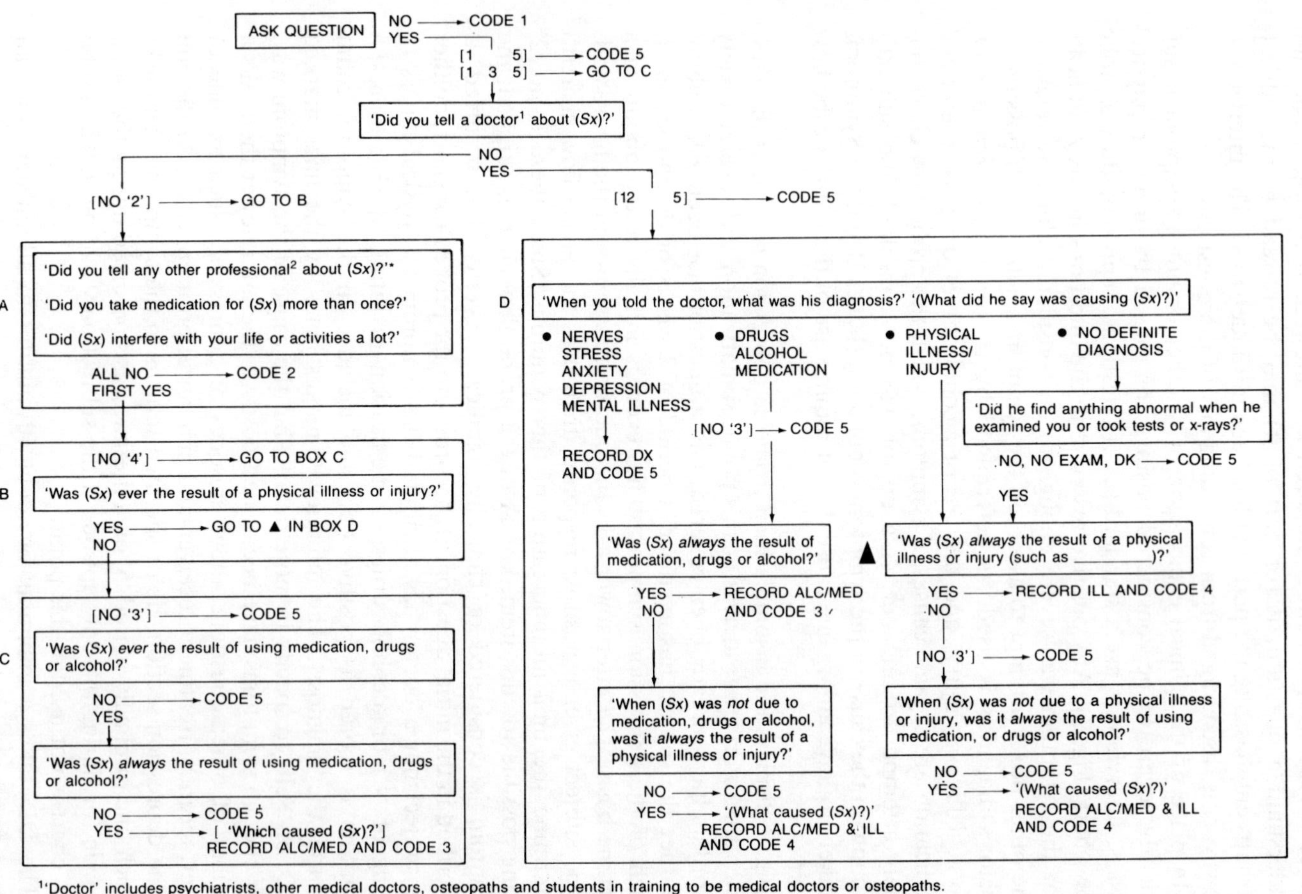

[1]'Doctor' includes psychiatrists, other medical doctors, osteopaths and students in training to be medical doctors or osteopaths.

[2]'Other professionals' include social workers, nurses, clergy, psychologists, counsellors, dentists, chiropractors and podiatrists.

Fig. 2. Probe flow chart for the Diagnostic Interview Schedule (DIS)

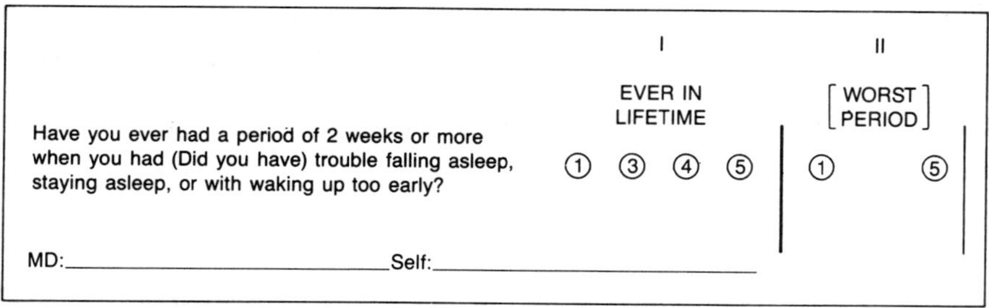

	I	II
	EVER IN LIFETIME	[WORST PERIOD]
Have you ever had a period of 2 weeks or more when you had (Did you have) trouble falling asleep, staying asleep, or with waking up too early?	① ③ ④ ⑤	① ⑤

MD:__________ Self:__________

Fig. 3. Example of an item from the DIS: insomnia. The item is initially asked about on a lifetime basis (I), using the probe flow chart. If sufficient symptoms are rated as positive and a 2 week period of dysphoria is also acknowledged, the interviewer goes over all symptoms considered psychiatrically determined under I, and asks if they were present during the (worst) spell of depression (II)

the subject is not ordinarily obtained, although occasionally in community surveys a significant other may give responses for a subject when the subject is completely unable to participate in the interview.

Once interviewers have completed a DIS interview and have checked it over for completeness and accuracy, their tasks are finished, since the diagnoses are generated by computer. The extensive computer programs for the diagnoses are written using the SAS package. These algorithms are, for the most part, quite straightforward and comprehensible, even to those without programming experience. Hard (paper) copies of the program are available, and potential users of the DIS should probably examine these algorithms since they are an important part of the procedures by which the DIS operationalizes diagnostic criteria. Translating the diagnostic programs into another statistical package such as SPSS-X or BMDP would be possible, but would involve an enormous amount of work and a high risk of programming error.

The programs provide for the output of the psychiatric diagnoses by the three different sets of diagnostic criteria (Feighner, DSM-III and RDC), with or without exclusion criteria. They also give the most recent occurrence of any aspect of the disorder (as indicated by the subject's response to a question) and the age at first occurrence. Hand-scoring instructions are also available for generating diagnoses using the DIS. The computer is much more efficient once the number of subjects in a study goes above 10 or 15, and is more likely to be accurate.

Interviewer Qualifications

Since the DIS was designed for use by non-clinicians, DIS interviewers are not required to have previous experience with psychiatric patients. The ability to read aloud, maintain a pleasant rapport with a wide variety of people, follow instructions carefully and code accurately are the main requirements for DIS interviewers (Munson *et al.*, 1985). Many studies have used clinicians as DIS interviewers, although the added cost of such a design may not be offset by any particular advantage (Hasin and Grant, 1987; Hesselbrock *et al.*, 1982).

Interviewer Training

Training for the DIS must be taken at Washington University in a week-long course, or from someone who has personally attended this course. The Washington University course consists of a general introduction to the interview, its conventions and the probe flow chart. Next, trainers conduct large-group practice with the probe flow chart. The large group then breaks up into smaller groups with numerous trainers, so that trainees may receive individual attention as they work toward mastering the probe flow chart. Once this introductory stage is complete, trainers then proceed through the DIS interview, explaining each diagnostic section in turn. Explanations and large-group practice are augmented by brief videotaped practice questions and numerous small group sessions. At the end of the week, research subjects are brought into each small group and trainees administer the DIS to these subjects.

Trainers who have attended the St Louis training should follow the same general format. While the videotapes are not currently available for distribution, trainers who are familiar with the type of subject intended for a particular study can present their own useful clinical examples for training new raters. All trainees who attend the St Louis training receive copies of the written training materials, which can then be used in training others.

Reliability

Oddly, we know of no studies on the test–retest or joint-rating reliability of the DIS with English-speaking lay interviewers, for whom the interview was designed. A German study with psychiatrists or psychologists as DIS raters found test–retest reliability at an acceptable or good level for most diagnoses and items (Wittchen *et al.*, 1985).

Validity

Much of the research on the validity of the DIS has taken the form of comparing DIS diagnoses to diagnoses made by some type of clinical evaluation. A large number of such studies have been carried out. Table 3 summarizes this research. These studies show mixed results, with many different clinical procedures used as standards of comparison. Taken as a group, the

Table 3. Agreement (kappa coefficient) between DIS interview and alternative clinical diagnostic procedure

Diagnosis	Robins *et al.* (1982)[a]	Hesselbrock *et al.* (1982)[b]	Burnam *et al.* (1983)[c]	Helzer *et al.* (1985)[d]	Wittchen *et al.* (1985)[e]		Anthony *et al.* (1985)[f]	Canino *et al.* (1987)[g]	Hasin and Grant (1987)[h]
Schizophrenia	0.60	–	0.56	–	0.44	−0.06	0.19	0.29	–
Major depression	0.63	0.72	0.36	0.41	0.84	0.78	0.25	0.26	0.13
Mania	0.65	–	0.23	–	0.86	−0.03	0.09	0.37	0.00
Panic disorder	0.40	–	0.14	0.34	0.45	0.30	−0.02	0.49	0.46
Alcoholism	0.86	1.00	0.62	0.68	–	–	0.35	0.61	0.66
Drug abuse/dependence	0.73	0.66	0.49	0.52	0.84	0.84	0.08	0.52	0.67
Phobia	0.67	–	0.32	0.49	0.91	0.88	0.24	0.52	0.31
Obsessive-compulsive	0.60	–	0.05	0.24	0.90	0.88	0.05	0.23	0.10
Antisocial personality	0.63	0.79	0.30	0.56	–	–	0.38	0.56	0.04

Key to footnotes: sample (*n*); types of DIS interviewer; type of alternative clinical procedure.

[a] Psychiatric patients, gamblers, health plan members (216); lay; psychiatrist's DIS with extra questions.
[b] Hospitalized alcoholics (42); lay/psychologist/psychiatrist; psychologist/psychiatrist's SADS-L.
[c] Hispanic psychiatric patients (151); lay; non-MD therapists administering DSM-III checklist interview.
[d] Community residents (370); lay; psychiatrist DIS + DSM-III checklist.
[e] Left: German psychiatric patients, community residents (262); right: German community residents (130) with DSM-III-like disorders; psychiatrists and psychologists; psychiatrist semi-structured ICD-8 interview.
[f] Community residents (810); lay; modified and expanded PSE administered by psychiatrists.
[g] Puerto Rican psychiatric patients and community residents (189); lay; psychiatrist DIS + extra questions.
[h] Hospitalized alcoholics (120); lay and masters-level clinicians; 1 SADS-L trainer and 1 psychologist.

DIS alcohol and drug diagnoses generally show the best agreement with clinical diagnoses. The agreement on other disorders varied considerably between studies. Some studies that showed good agreement between DIS diagnoses and clinical diagnoses either used the DIS idiosyncratically (as in Hesselbrock *et al.*, 1982, who used clinician consensus for DIS diagnoses, rather than computer-generated diagnoses) or only included subjects whose type of psychopathology was clear (Wittchen *et al.*, 1985). For clinical researchers, it is worth noting that agreement between DIS and clinical diagnoses was generally better with psychiatric patients than with community samples.

Affiliated Procedures and Future Directions

The Composite International Diagnostic Interview (CIDI) consists of the DIS interview with considerably increased diagnostic coverage (Robins, 1985, 1987; Cottler and Wittchen, 1987). The CIDI maintains the fully structured non-clinician approach of the DIS, along with the probe flow chart. In addition, it incorporates aspects of the Present State Examination (see below). It also includes onset and recency questions for each symptom (as compared to the DIS, which asks about onset and recency globally for each disorder). The CIDI-C (Core) is an instrument currently being field-tested by the World Health Organization. It differs from the CIDI by the omission of questions to assess RDC and Feighner Criteria, omission of the onset and recency questions for each symptom, and inclusion of questions to make diagnoses of alcohol and drug dependence by DSM-III-R and ICD-10 criteria. Further modifications of the CIDI to make DSM-III-R and ICD-10 diagnoses for other diagnostic categories are planned, but not completed at the time of writing. Also available from the developers of the DIS is the CIDI–SAM (Substance Abuse Module) (Cottler, 1987). This module elicits information to make alcohol, drug and tobacco dependence diagnoses by all diagnostic systems (including DSM-III-R and ICD-10), and obtains more detailed quantity and frequency information about substance use than that obtained in either the DIS or the two current versions of the CIDI.

Further Information

For further information about the DIS and related procedures, contact Dr Lee Robins, Washington University School of Medicine, Department of Psychiatry, 4940 Audubon Avenue, St Louis, Missouri 63110, USA; telephone (314) 362–2469.

STRUCTURED CLINICAL INTERVIEW FOR DSM-III-R

Considerable controversy attended the introduction and use of the DIS in the USA. Few argued that an inexpensive diagnostic procedure for use in both clinical and epidemiological samples would constitute an extremely important research tool. Many investigators, however, had concerns about whether valid psychiatric diagnoses could be made by a fully structured survey instrument administered by non-clinicians.

While the debate about the DIS unfolded, one developer of the SADS, Robert Spitzer MD, served as Chairperson of the American Psychiatric Association Task Force to produce DSM-III and DSM-III-R. Dr Spitzer had concluded that clinicians were necessary to the diagnostic process (Spitzer, 1983) and, therefore, began development of the Structured Clinical Interview for DSM-III-R (SCID) to ascertain diagnoses by the newer American criteria. Given the differences that evolved between DSM-III and DSM-III-R in several diagnostic categories, the decision was finally made to orient the SCID specifically to DSM-III-R (American Psychiatric Association, 1987).

The need for a clinician-administered procedure which could produce diagnoses according to the newest diagnostic criteria seemed clear. The developers of the SCID, however, hoped to achieve some additional goals. They wished to produce an instrument that:

1. Required less training time than the SADS.
2. Took less time to administer and code.
3. Made the diagnostic process simpler than the SADS, once the information was collected.

Hence, nearly all items in the SCID are specifically designed to assess DSM-III-R diagnostic criteria, and detailed dimensional information on current status is not obtained.

At the time of writing, the SCID comes in two major sections (SCID-I and SCID-II) and three versions (patient, out-patient, and non-patient). The SCID-I consists of probes for the diagnostic criteria for DSM-III-R Axis I disorders, organized by general areas (i.e. mood, anxiety, psychoactive substance use). Raters must begin the questioning on a specific symptom with the written probe that is given in the interview schedule. It is expected, however, that once subjects respond positively or doubtfully to any items, the interviewer will need to conduct a thorough exploration of the symptom. This exploration is needed to determine how the symptom should be rated by the SCID scoring scheme, which consists of three levels:

1. Present and of clinically significant severity.

2. Present but of subthreshold severity (not counted towards the diagnosis).
3. Absent.

The diagnoses covered by the SCID-I are shown in Table 4.

Fig. 4(a) provides the SCID item on sleep disturbance. (In the SCID, for economy of time, both hypersomnia and insomnia are combined in the same item.) This item occurs in the section on mood syndromes, the first in the interview after the introductory material on basic demographics, treatment and a brief clinical overview of current condition. If the subject has been depressed or anhedonic in the month prior to the interview, the insomnia items and other items covering depressive symptomatology are asked. Otherwise, the interviewer skips to a section on past depression, in which the same symptom items are included for a time of previous depression, if such a period occurred. Subjects who do not acknowledge a current or past period of dysphoria are not asked the insomnia item.

The interviewer actually introduces and explores sleep disturbance very similarly to the way the corresponding item in the SADS is approached. However, the ratings and criteria for the ratings are somewhat different. In the SCID, the sleep and other items are rated as absent, subthreshold, or present and clinically significant. If the symptom was not present nearly every day for at least 2 weeks (12 out of 14 days) then the symptom is not rated as positive. A symptom which is present about half of the time for at least 2 weeks would be rated as '2' or subthreshold, and not counted as positive toward a diagnosis.

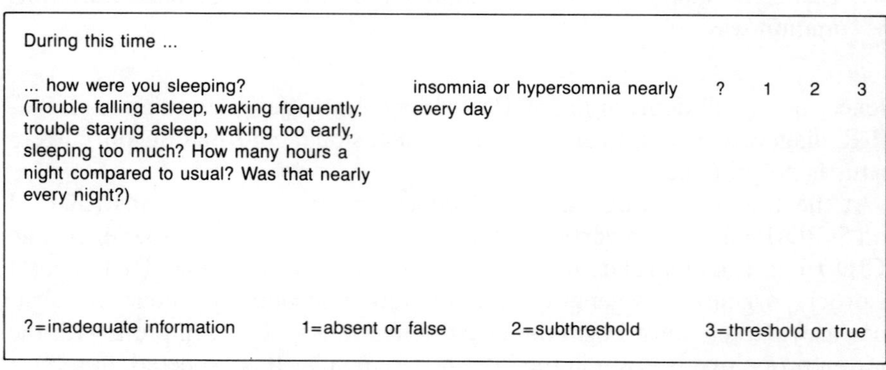
During this time ...

... how were you sleeping? (Trouble falling asleep, waking frequently, trouble staying asleep, waking too early, sleeping too much? How many hours a night compared to usual? Was that nearly every night?)	insomnia or hypersomnia nearly every day	?	1	2	3

?=inadequate information 1=absent or false 2=subthreshold 3=threshold or true

Fig. 4a. Example of an item from the SCID-I: sleep disturbance. If the subject has previously acknowledged dysphoric mood or anhedonia in the month prior to the interview, then this question is asked. If not, then the interviewer skips to a section on past depression and, if such a period occurred, the time frame for the same insomnia item is during the past episode. (Reproduced by permission of Dr R. Spitzer)

Table 4. Diagnoses and subtypes covered by the SCID-I interview, patient version (the most comprehensive version of the SCID). All diagnoses made according to DSM-III-R Criteria

Non-affective disorders	Affective disorders
Schizophrenia	Bipolar disorder
Schizophreniform disorder	if current, i.e. last month:
With good prognostic features	Manic
Without good prognostic features	Depressed
Schizoaffective disorder	Mixed
Bipolar type	Mild
Depressed type	Moderate
Delusional disorder	Severe, no psychotic features
Brief reactive psychosis	Mood-congruent psychotic features
Psychotic disorder NOS[a]	Mood-incongruent psychotic features
	Other bipolar disorder
Somatization disorder	
Hypochondriasis	Major depression
Undifferentiated somatoform disorder	If current, i.e. last month:
	Mild
Alcohol abuse	Moderate
Alcohol dependence	Severe, no psychotic features
	Mood-congruent psychotic features
Drug abuse	Mood-incongruent psychotic features
Drug dependence	
Sedative/hypnotic/anxiolytic	Dysthymia
Opioid	Primary
Cocaine	Secondary
Stimulant	
Hallucinogen/PCP	Depressive Disorder NOS[a]
Cannabis	
Poly-drug	
Other	
Panic disorder	
With agoraphobia	
Without agoraphobia	
Obsessive-compulsive disorder	
Simple phobia	
Social phobia	
Generalized anxiety disorder	
Agoraphobia without panic attacks	
Anorexia nervosa	
Bulimia	
Adjustment disorder	
Other DSM-III-R	
Axis I disorder	

[a] NOS = not otherwise specified.

The SCID-II represents something of a departure for a general diagnostic instrument, both in structure and in content. The SCID-II was designed to evaluate the adult personality disorders of DSM-III-R. It is probably best used in conjunction with the SCID-I, although it can be used alone.

Since the number of DSM-III-R personality disorders is large and each has numerous diagnostic criteria, the SCID-II interview is preceded by a paper-and-pencil screening questionnaire completed by the subject. The questionnaire covers all personality traits embodied in the diagnostic criteria for each personality disorder, although at a lower level of severity. After the subject completes the screening questionnaire, the interviewer introduces the SCID-II by explaining that the questions cover the subject's 'usual self', excluding episodes of Axis I disorders covered in the SCID-I.

The interviewer then carries out a brief general exploration of the subject's personality, including relationships with important others at home and work, usual ways of reacting to things that have caused problems, and how free time is spent. After this, the interviewer then explores all traits checked positive by the subject to determine whether the trait was persistent and severe enough to be considered symptomatic. The interviewer also covers items which he or she has reason to suspect may be positive from other sources of information, such as material from the SCID-I. If, after following this procedure, a subject is just below the number of symptoms required for a given personality disorder, the interviewer explores all symptoms of that disorder with the subject, even if the subject initially marked them negative on the screening questionnaire.

Fig. 4(b) displays the introduction to the self-administered screening questionnaire and the first item rated by the subject. In addition, Fig. 4(b) shows the corresponding item from the SCID-II. (The item covers an aspect of personality included in DSM-III-R's definitions of avoidant and dependent personality disorders.) The emphasis is on avoiding false positives; the subject must provide clear elaboration or examples of the symptoms, either verbally or by interview behaviour. Some probes that are used to encourage elaboration of the symptoms include: 'Give me the most extreme example'; 'Does that happen in a lot of different situations?'; 'Have you always been this way?'; and 'Do you regard this as a problem for you?'

In all sections of the SCID, directions are marked very clearly for making the DSM-III-R diagnoses as the interviewer proceeds through the interview, although earlier ratings may be changed if later discussion indicates that different ratings would be more accurate. The severity of each current disorder is scored as either mild, moderate or severe, according to the level of symptomatology and associated impairment in social or occupational functioning. Full or partial remission is also scored for each disorder. Onset and the proportion of time in the last 5 years when symptoms of each disorder were present are also scored.

Self-administered screening questionnaire instructions and question:

THESE QUESTIONS ARE ABOUT THE KIND OF PERSON YOU GENERALLY ARE, THAT IS, HOW YOU USUALLY HAVE FELT OR BEHAVED OVER THE PAST SEVERAL YEARS. CIRCLE 'YES' OR 'NO'. IF YOU DO NOT UNDERSTAND A QUESTION, LEAVE IT BLANK.

1.	Are your feelings more easily hurt than most people's if someone criticizes you or disapproves of something you say or do?	NO	YES

SCID-II interview item:

1.	You've said that your feelings are more easily hurt than most people's if someone criticizes you or disapproves of something you say or do. Most people feel 'bad' when they're criticized—do you feel it upsets you more than most people?	is easily hurt by criticism or disapproval	?	1	2	3

?=inadequate information 1=absent or false 2=subthreshold 3=threshold or true

Fig. 4b. Example of an item from the SCID-II: excessive sensitivity to criticism or disapproval (for avoidant and dependent personality disorders). (Reproduced by permission of Dr R. Spitzer)

The patient, out-patient and non-patient versions of the SCID are primarily distinguished by their introductions and the amount of detail recorded on psychotic symptoms and disorders. The introductions to each version differ in how the interviewer orients the subject to the interview. The patient version of the SCID contains considerable detail on the types of psychotic symptoms experienced by subjects, which allows for the differential diagnosis of the many types of DSM-III-R psychotic disorders. The out-patient and non-patient versions contain a psychotic screening section which elicits enough information to indicate that a psychotic disorder has probably been present, although not enough detail to determine its precise type. As indicated by the versions of the SCID, this instrument may be used with subjects who are in treatment, or non-patients selected for various purposes.

Interviewer Qualifications

As noted, the SCID was designed to be administered by clinicians. Psychiatrists, clinical psychologists and psychiatric social workers should all be able to become good SCID interviewers. For non-physicians, previous experience with psychiatric diagnosis according to specified criteria should shorten and simplify training.

Interviewer Training

The procedures for training interviewers to adminster the SCID are still under development to some extent, since this is a new interview. Trainees read the different versions of the interview and a brief instruction manual. They are given a general didactic explanation of the interview, and then more specific instructions, section by section. They then view videotapes of SCID interviews (a library of such videotapes is under development). Finally, they administer the interview under the observation of an experienced SCID rater (by audiotape or videotape, if convenient). After administration of practice interviews, the trainees' scoring and interviewing techniques are reviewed.

Reliability

Because the SCID is new, little reliability data are available. The only published study of the reliability of diagnoses made using the SCID (Riskind *et al.*, 1987) showed that the SCID can be employed reliably to differentiate major depression from generalized anxiety disorder in out-patients; the respective kappa values were 0.72 and 0.79.

An extensive, five-site test–retest reliability study of the SCID has recently been completed, however, and the data from this study are currently being analysed. It is expected that a report based on these data will be forthcoming soon.

Validity

The only published study addressing the validity of SCID diagnoses investigates SCID-II (Skodol *et al.*, 1988). SCID diagnoses of schizotypal, antisocial and dependent personality disorders were found to be significantly associated with longitudinal diagnoses made by a group of clinical experts who observed patients over several months of in-patient hospitalization.

Further Information

For further information on the SCID, contact Dr Robert Spitzer, Columbia University College of Physicians and Surgeons, 722 W 168th Street, Box 74, New York, New York 10032, USA; telephone (212) 960–5524.

PRESENT STATE EXAMINATION

The Present State Examination (PSE) (Wing *et al.*, 1974) was developed by clinical researchers at the Maudsley Hospital, London. The PSE was developed in the UK for reasons similar to those that stimulated development of structured assessment procedures in the USA: to achieve some degree of standardization of content and form in the diagnostic process in order to increase reproducibility. Earlier phases of the development of the PSE were done in conjunction with the US–UK diagnostic project (Cooper *et al.*, 1972), an important milestone in the international standardization of diagnostic practices. Earlier versions of the PSE also formed an important part of the World Health Organization's (WHO) International Pilot Study of Schizophrenia (World Health Organization, 1973).

The PSE was intended as a clinical interview, not 'a questionnaire' (Luria and McHugh, 1974). The major focus of the interview is on symptomatology and functioning during the month prior to the interview. Psychotic and major affective disorders are covered in considerable detail. The PSE includes items covering many varieties of psychotic experience. Over 15 separate types of delusions may be rated, as well as numerous types of hallucinations, subthreshold distortions in reality testing, and disturbances in affect and behaviour associated with psychotic states. Depressive symptoms are those most commonly associated with the concept of endogenous depression; atypical depressive symptomatology (overeating, oversleeping) is not covered. Numerous other items in the PSE cover non-specific distress, anxiety, obsessional features and aspects of observed behaviour and affect during the interview. The process of 'cross-examination' is used to evaluate whether symptoms are present: when subjects respond positively to initial probes from the interview schedule, interviewers use their own questions to carefully examine whether any occurrence of a symptom warrants a positive rating. Only information stated by the subject or observed by the interviewer during the interview can be used to score items in the PSE. In most studies, interviewers are encouraged to read any available case records and other relevant materials prior to conducting the interview. However, case material is used only to guide enquiry in the interview itself; it is not used for rating items. The PSE is expected to take about an hour to administer. In the PSE, many items are required for all subjects, but some are skipped if certain aspects of psychopathology have not occurred. Items are grouped loosely by diagnostic content.

Along with the interview schedule itself, PSE raters are given the Glossary of Definitions. The Glossary of Definitions includes 140 definitions, each one corresponding to one of the 140 items in the PSE. Examples of PSE items for assessing sleep disturbance and the corresponding symptom definitions from the glossary are presented in Fig. 5. Prior to reaching this point in the

PSE item:

** Have you had any trouble getting off to sleep during the past month?
(How long do you lie awake?)
(What happens if you take sleeping tablets?)
(How often does it happen?)

RATE DELAYED SLEEP

1 = 1 hour or more delay (irrespective of sleeping tablets).
2 = 2 hours or more delay (irrespective of sleeping tablets).
(In either case, ten or more nights during month.) ☐ (35)

Glossary definition:

35. DELAYED SLEEP

Rate delay in getting off to sleep after the subject has gone to bed. Rate 1 hour's delay as (1) and 2 hours' delay as (2), irrespective of whether the patient is taking sleeping tablets. (Such medication should be noted on the front page of the schedule.) In either case, the sleeplessness must be fairly frequent, during the past month, say, or ten or more nights (unless fewer were more or less consecutive, i.e. constituting an episode).

This symptom can co-exist with 'early waking' (symptom no. 37).

PSE item:

Do you wake early in the morning?

RATE EARLY WAKING *(one hour before usual).*

1 = 1 hour or more before ordinary time.
2 = 2 hours or more before ordinary time.
(In either case, ten or more nights during month.) ☐ (37)

Glossary definition:

37. EARLY WAKING

Rate waking 1 hour before usual time as (1) and 2 hours before usual time as (2), irrespective of whether subject is taking sleeping tablets (record this on front sheet of schedule). In either case, the early waking must be fairly frequent during the month, say on ten or more occasions (unless fewer were fairly consecutive, i.e. constituting an episode).

This symptom can co-exist with 'delayed sleep' (symptom no. 35).

Fig. 5. Examples of items for delayed sleep and early waking from the Present State Examination (PSE) and the corresponding symptom definitions from the Glossary of Definitions. The starred (**) question referring to trouble getting to sleep is asked of every subject; the question about waking early in the morning is only asked if the subject has been rated as having sleep disturbance (i.e. item 35 is rated '1' or '2') or depression from a previous question

interview, the interviewer has covered six of the 20 major subsections of the interview:

1. Introduction (an overview of the subject's difficulty and a rating of the adequacy of the information about possible problems he or she has been having).
2. Health, worry or tension.
3. Autonomic anxiety.
4. Thinking and concentration.
5. Depressed mood.
6. Self and others (relationship of the self to others).

The items for delayed sleep and early awakening are part of Section 7: appetite, sleep, retardation, libido.

The question assessing trouble getting to sleep is a 'starred' (**), or obligatory, question. It is one of 54 such questions in the ninth edition of the PSE that must be asked of every subject. The questions in parentheses or brackets that follow the main question are intended to help define the nature and extent of a symptom and are to be asked if the subject's reply to the obligatory question is at all ambiguous. The question referring to early morning awakening is asked only if the subject has been rated as having sleep disturbance (i.e. a rating on item 35 of '1' or '2') or depression from the questions under Section 5, depressed mood.

The definitions of the symptoms 'delayed sleep' and 'early waking' emphasize that the interviewer rate the sleep disturbances irrespective of the use of hypnotics and clarify the minimum frequency of occurrence of sleep problems in the past month (ten or more nights, unless fewer were consecutive) necessary for rating the symptoms as present.

Classification of the information collected in the PSE interview is made by computer. A computer program, CATEGO, allows for output from the interview on a number of levels of complexity. On the simplest level, information can be obtained on scores on individual symptoms. CATEGO also summarizes the symptom data into 38 syndromes, some corresponding to diagnostic entities, some covering aspects of non-specific psychopathology, and others covering aspects of functioning. Examples of the syndromes include nuclear syndrome (corresponding to Schneiderian first-rank symptoms of schizophrenia), simple depression, self-neglect and social unease.

CATEGO also provides for a set of classifications indicating the likelihood of 'caseness'. This categorization, the Index of Definition (Wing, 1976), is probably most useful when subjects have been selected from a source other than a treatment facility (Wing *et al.*, 1977b, 1978). Its eight levels are defined by the number, type and severity of symptoms. Level 5, the threshold level, provides for a minimum degree of symptomatology necessary for a subject to be considered a case. A number of moderately severe affective symptoms occurring together would be sufficient. Levels 6, 7 and 8 provide increasing degrees of certainty that the disturbance can be classified as a functional psychosis or neurosis, by clinical judgement or the CATEGO program, according to the International Classification of Diseases (World Health Organization, 1977). The diagnoses generated by the PSE/CATEGO system are indicated in Table 5.

The PSE was originally developed for use with psychiatric patients. However, it has also been used in community epidemiological research (Bebbington *et al.*, 1981; Surtees *et al.*, 1983). Since its primary focus is on current status rather than lifetime diagnoses, it is probably not useful for family/genetic studies unless the information on current status is supplemented with additional material.

The PSE has undergone numerous revisions since its introduction in 1967. While earlier versions contained 500–600 items, these were reduced to 140 for the ninth revision, for which the Glossary of Definitions was provided. While symptoms scores between the different versions are not compatible, Wing *et al.* (1974) state that all versions of the PSE become comparable at the syndrome level (the 38 syndromes which are produced by combining symptoms).

Interviewer Qualifications

For clinical research, investigators will probably require interviewers with clinical experience, although non-clinician interviewers have been used in epidemiological research. Non-physicians must be trained carefully to avoid 'over-rating' items and 'over-diagnosing' subjects; research has shown that non-physician raters tend to produce ratings which lead to diagnoses more often than physicians (Wing *et al.*, 1977a).

Interviewer Training

Wing *et al.* (1974) describe an optimal training process extending over several weeks, during which learner and teacher take turns in conducting interviews with successive patients. A detailed discussion of each interview follows, covering interviewing technique and discrepancies in ratings between the experienced PSE interviewer and the trainee. Ten to twenty such sessions are considered the minimum to bring a trainee up to the standard of an experienced interviewer. Detailed descriptions of PSE training programs in Europe (Cooper *et al.*, 1977) and the USA (Luria and Berry, 1980) have been described elsewhere.

Table 5. Categorization of cases by PSE/CATEGO/ICD-9 system

PSE constituent subscores	Syndromes	Class	ICD-9 diagnoses
Delusional and hallucinatory syndromes (DAH)	Nuclear syndrome (NS) Depressive delusions and hallucinations (DD) Auditory hallucinations (AH) Delusions of persecution (PE) Delusions of reference (RE) Grandiose and religious delusions (GR) Sexual and fantastic delusions (SF) Visual hallucinations (VH) Olfactory hallucinations (OH) Subcultural delusions and hallucinations (SC)	Schizophrenic psychoses (S+) Manic and mixed affective psychoses (M+) Depressive psychoses (D+)	Schizophrenic psychoses Simple type Hebephrenic type Catatonic type Paranoid type Acute schizophrenic episode Latent schizophrenia Residual schizophrenia Schizoaffective type Other Unspecified
Behaviour, speech and other syndromes (BSO)	Catatonic syndrome (CS) Incoherence of speech (IS) Residual syndrome (RS) Affective flattening (AF) Hypomania (HM) Overactivity (OV) Motor slowness (SL) Non-specific psychotic syndrome (NP) Agitation (AG) Self-neglect (NG)	Paranoid psychoses (P+) Other psychoses (O+) Uncertain psychotic classes (S?, P?, M?, D?)	Affective psychoses Manic-depressive psychosis, manic type Manic-depressive psychosis, depressed type Manic-depressive psychosis, circular types Paranoid states Paranoid state, simple Paranoia Paraphrenia

(*Continued*)

Table 5 (*Continued*)

PSE constituent subscores	Syndromes	Class	ICD-9 diagnoses
			Other non-organic psychoses Depressive type Excitative type Reactive confusion Acute paranoid reaction Psychogenic paranoid psychosis Other and unspecified reactive psychosis Unspecified psychosis
Specific neurotic syndromes (SNR)	Depressed mood (SD) Obsessional syndrome (ON) General anxiety (GA) Situational anxiety (SA) Hysteria (HT) Special features of depression (ED)	Retarded depression (R) Neurotic depression (N)	Neurotic disorders Anxiety states Hysteria Phobic state Obsessive-compulsive disorders Neurotic depression Neurasthenia Depersonalization syndrome Hypochondriasis Other neurotic disorders Unspecified

Non-specific neurotic syndromes (NSN)	Depersonalization (DE) Ideas of reference (IR) Tension (TE) Lack of energy (LE) Worrying (WO) Irritability (IT) Social unease (SU) Loss of interest and concentration (IC) Hypochondriasis (HY) Somatic symptoms of depression (OD)	Anxiety states (A) Residual states (X)
	Organic impairment (OR) Doubtful interview (DI)	

Reliability

Several series of patients have been included in reliability studies of the PSE in its several editions. In one series (Wing *et al.*, 1967), percentage agreement on diagnoses (uncorrected for chance agreement) was 84%. This series included both jointly rated interviews and test–retest examinations. Product–moment correlations (rather than intraclass correlations, the preferred and more conservative measure of agreement on quantitative measures) between symptom scores assigned by two raters were generally high when the raters were experienced, and were quite high when the second rater made his or her ratings based on audiotapes of the interview administered by the first rater. In general, ratings of behaviour, affect and speech observed during the interview were less reliable than ratings of subjective symptoms described to the interviewer.

Comparisons of agreement between joint and test–retest ratings on a series of in-patients showed that the mean kappa for items decreased from 0.71 when items had been jointly rated to 0.41 when a test–retest procedure was used, and the mean kappa for sections fell from 0.84 for joint ratings to 0.64 for test–retest ratings (Kendell *et al.*, 1968). Cooper *et al.* (1977) reported a mean kappa of 0.74 for inter-rater reliability and 0.54 for test–retest reliability in a study of out-patients. While generally poor agreement on test–retest reliability could indicate serious problems in the PSE, joint-rating reliability may provide more useful information on the PSE than on diagnostic procedures which assess lifetime diagnoses. The PSE focuses on the month prior to the interview, and acutely ill patients' statuses can change considerably within days during such a short time. Therefore, a test–retest design may show lower reliability coefficients due to occasion variance—a true source of variance, rather than criterion or information variance—sources of error variance which are produced by problems in the interview process or diagnostic criteria. Luria and Berry (1979) found high reliability for the 20 PSE symptoms of most diagnostic importance and 19 psychopathological profiles constructed from symptom data. As in previous work, they found that symptom sections were more reliably rated than behavioural sections. When classifying the profiles into eight major psychiatric syndromes to describe the diagnoses of their in-patient sample, these authors obtained generalized kappas of 0.92 for videotaped interviews and 0.96 for live interviews.

In the community, the PSE has also been reported to be reliable. Wing *et al.* (1977b) trained non-medical interviewers to administer the PSE to 237 randomly selected women. A subsample of women were re-interviewed by psychiatrists. Agreement between the two interviewers on symptoms, syndromes, total PSE score and index of psychiatric disorder was judged acceptable by the authors, although kappa levels of agreement, corrected for chance, were generally considerably lower than were the figures for percentage agreement. Strictly speaking, the comparison of a lay-administered interview to a psychiatrist's interview is not a study of reliability, but rather procedural validity, since the procedures are not identical, even though the instrument is administered a second time.

Validity

The PSE has been used to describe patients and measure change in a wide range of research studies on the epidemiology, causes and treatment of mental disorders (e.g. Leff and Wing, 1971; Vaughn and Leff, 1976; Orley and Wing, 1979; Leff *et al.*, 1982; Bebbington *et al.*, 1981). The newly developed Composite International Diagnostic Interview (CIDI) (see above) has recently been validated using the PSE as the standard (Farmer *et al.*, 1987). Agreement on individual items was disappointing, but on syndrome classification, diagnostic class, and severity, agreement attained statistical significance.

Associated Procedures

Since the only source of information for the PSE is the subject's report of symptoms in the previous month and the interviewer's ratings of interview behaviour, the PSE may lack crucial information for making a valid diagnosis (for example, a manic episode occurring more than a month prior to the interview followed immediately by a severe, unremitting depression). The Syndrome Check-list (SCL) allows for the introduction of other information into the diagnostic process. Data to rate the SCL can be obtained from clinical case records or from an informant.

The use of the SCL helps complete the clinical picture. The interviewer rates the presence of a set of syndromes as defined by the Glossary of Definitions. Raters are instructed to rate these conservatively, requiring good evidence of their presence before assigning a positive rating.

The Aetiology Schedule allows for the recording of a number of factors which may be needed to interpret the results of the PSE. Such factors include recent psychological or social conflicts, alcohol/drug abuse, cerebral disease and intelligence, to name a few. This schedule (rated by the interviewer as accurately as possible from any available information) was not intended as more than a 'guide' to clinicians and research workers. Preliminary research showed, however, that the use of this schedule might be more beneficial than originally thought, and further work in the development of the Aetiology Schedule was considered warranted.

Recently, a new psychiatric symptom change scale, based on the PSE, has been introduced (Tress *et al.*, 1987). This scale preserves the advantages of the PSE while improving on its sensitivity to change. It is highly reliable and can be used, for example, in drug trials for a variety of mental disorders.

Future Directions

At the time of writing, a draft version of ICD-10 is currently being tested in field trials. This newest international nomenclature differs in many ways from the older ICD revisions, including ICD-8, the diagnostic system assessed by the PSE. To assess psychiatric diagnoses according to ICD-10, a new instrument based on the PSE is in its final stages of development by Wing and his colleagues. This instrument, the Schedules for Clinical Assessment in Neuropsychiatry (SCAN), will also include items to assess components of DSM-III-R. It is currently being field tested, and therefore not in final form at the time of writing.

The SCAN is characterized as a 'network' of instruments. It includes the tenth revision of the PSE (currently in development) which represents an expansion of PSE-9 with some alterations in the scoring system. The Glossary of Definitions will be expanded to cover the additions to PSE-10. Additional schedules provide information for rating past and lifetime episodes. Since coverage for the great variety of conditions of interest in psychiatry in one interview schedule is not considered practical, modules are currently being developed to cover additional areas in more detail. The CATEGO computer programs are being updated to accommodate the changes in the PSE and associated schedules included in the SCAN. If studies show the SCAN to be reliable and valid in diverse research settings, this instrument should be of considerable interest to researchers on a variety of topics in psychiatry. The instrument must be completed and tested, however, before its utility can be evaluated.

Further Information

For more information on the PSE, contact Dr John Wing, MRC Social Psychiatry Unit, Institute of Psychiatry, De Crespigny Park, London SE5 8AF; telephone 01–703 5411.

SUMMARY

In this chapter we have attempted to provide researchers with descriptions of the four major standardized diagnostic interviews in use in psychiatry today, throughout the world. We have summarized those features, such as diagnostic coverage, interviewer qualifications and training, reliability, validity and associated procedures, which we believe will guide researchers in selecting the interview most suited to their needs.

REFERENCES

American Psychiatric Association (1980) *Diagnostic and Statistical Manual of Mental Disorders* (3rd edn), Washington, DC.

American Psychiatric Association (1987). *Diagnostic and Statistical Manual of Mental Disorders* (3rd edn, revised), Washington, DC.

Andreasen, N. C., Endicott, J., Spitzer, R. L. and Winokur, G. (1977). The family history method using diagnostic criteria; reliability and validity. *Arch. Gen. Psychiatry* **34**, 1229–1235.

Andreasen, N. C., Grove, W. M., Shapiro, R. W., Keller, M. B., Hirschfeld, R. M. A. and McDonald-Scott, P. (1981). Reliability of lifetime diagnoses. *Arch. Gen. Psychiatry* **38**, 400–405.

Andreasen, N. C., McDonald-Scott, P., Grove, W. M., Keller, M. B., Shapiro, R. W. and Hirschfeld, R. M. A. (1982). Assessment of reliability in multicenter collaborative research with a videotape approach. *Am. J. Psychiatry* **139**, 876–882.

Andreasen, N. C., Scheftner, W., Reich, T., Hirschfeld, R. M., Endicott, J. and Keller, M. B. (1986). The validation of the concept of endogenous depression: a family study approach. *Arch. Gen. Psychiatry* **43**, 246–251.

Andreasen, N. C., Rice, J., Endicott, J., Coryell, W., Grove, W. M. and Reich, T. (1987). Familial rates of affective disorder: a report from the NIMH Collaborative Depression Study. *Arch. Gen. Psychiatry* **44**, 461–469.

Anthony, J. C., Folstein, M., Romanoski, A. J., Von Korff, M. R., Nestadt, G. R., Chahal, R., Merchant, A., Brown, C. H., Shapiro, S., Kramer, M. and Gruenberg, E. M. (1985). Comparison of the lay Diagnostic Interview Schedule and a standardized psychiatric diagnosis. *Arch. Gen. Psychiatry* **42**, 667–675.

Asberg, M., Perris, C., Schalling, D. and Sedvall, G. (1978). The CPRS—development and applications of a psychiatric rating scale. *Acta Psychiatr. Scand.* (Suppl.), 271.

Bebbington, P., Hurry, J., Tennant, C., Sturt, E. and Wing, J. K. (1981). Epidemiology of mental disorders in Camberwell. *Psychol. Med.* **11**, 561–579.

Bromet, E. J., Dunn, L. O., Connell, M. M., Dew, M. A. and Schulberg, H. (1986). Long-term reliability of diagnosing lifetime major depression in a community sample. *Arch. Gen. Psychiatry* **43**, 435–440.

Burnam, M. A., Karno, M., Hough, R. L., Escobar, J. I. and Forsythe, A. B. (1983). The Spanish Diagnostic Interview Schedule. *Arch. Gen. Psychiatry* **40**, 1189–1196.

Canino, G. J., Bird, H. R., Shrout, P. E., Rubio-Stipec, M., Bravo, M., Martinez, R., Sesman, M., Guzman, A., Guevara, L. M. and Costas, H. (1987). The Spanish Diagnostic Interview Schedule: reliability and concordance with clinical diagnoses in Puerto Rico. *Arch. Gen. Psychiatry* **44**, 720–726.

Cohen, J. (1960). A coefficient of agreement for nominal scales. *Educational Psychol. Measurement* **20**, 37–46.

Cooper, J. E., Kendell, R. E., Gurland, B. J., Sharpe, L., Copeland, J. R. M. and Simon, R. (1972). *Psychiatric Diagnosis in New York and London*, Oxford University Press, London.

Cooper, J. E., Copeland, J. R. M., Brown, G. W., Harris, T. and Gourlay, A. J. (1977). Further studies on interview training and inter-rater reliability of the Present State Examination (PSE). *Psychol. Med.* **7**, 517–523.

Coryell, W., Endicott, J., Reich, T., Andreasen, N. and Keller, M. (1984a). A family study of bipolar II disorder. *Br. J. Psychiatry* **145**, 49–54.

Coryell, W., Lavori, P., Endicott, J., Keller, M. and Van Eerdewegh, M. (1984b).

Outcome in schizoaffective, psychotic, and nonpsychotic depression: course during a six- to 24-month follow-up. *Arch. Gen. Psychiatry* **41**, 787–791.

Coryell, W., Andreasen, N. C., Endicott, J. and Keller, M. (1987). The significance of past mania or hypomania in the course and outcome of major depression. *Am. J. Psychiatry* **144**, 309–315.

Cottler, L. B. (1987). The reliability of the CIDI-SAM. *DIS Newsletter* Spring, 2–4; DIS Training Faculty and Staff, Washington University School of Medicine, St Louis, Missouri.

Cottler, L. B. and Wittchen, H. U. (1987). A report on the CIDI field trials. *DIS Newsletter* Fall, 3–4; DIS Training Faculty and Staff, Washington University School of Medicine, St Louis, Missouri.

Derogatis, L., Lipman, R., Rickels, K., Uhlenhuth, E. H. and Covi L. (1974). The Hopkins Symptom Checklist (HSCL): a self-report symptom inventory. *Behav. Sci.* **19**, 1–15.

Endicott, J. and Spitzer, R. L. (1972a). What! Another rating scale? The Psychiatric Evaluation Form. *J. Nerv. Ment. Dis.* **154**, 88–104.

Endicott, J. and Spitzer, R. L. (1972b). Current and Past Psychopathology Scales (CAPPS): rationale, reliability and validity. *Arch. Gen. Psychiatry* **27**, 678–687.

Endicott, J. and Spitzer, R. L. (1978). A diagnostic interview: the Schedule for Affective Disorders and Schizophrenia. *Arch. Gen. Psychiatry* **35**, 837–844.

Endicott, J., Nee, J., Cohen, J., Fleiss, J. L. and Sarantakos, S. (1981). Hamilton Depression Rating Scale extracted from Schedule for Affective Disorders and Schizophrenia and SADS-C. *Arch. Gen. Psychiatry* **38**, 98–103.

Endicott, J., Nee, J., Cohen, J., Fleiss, J. L. and Simon, R. (1986a). Diagnosis of schizophrenia: prediction of short-term outcome. *Arch. Gen. Psychiatry* **43**, 13–19.

Endicott, J., Nee, J., Coryell, W., Keller, M., Andreasen, N. and Croughan, J. (1986b). Schizoaffective, psychotic and nonpsychotic depression: differential familial association. *Compr. Psychiatry* **27**, 1–13.

Farmer, A. E., Katz, R., McGuffin, P. and Bebbington, P. (1987). A comparison between the Present State Examination and the Composite International Diagnostic Interview. *Arch. Gen. Psychiatry* **44**, 1064–1968.

Feighner, J. P., Robins, E., Guze, S. B., Woodruff, R. A., Winokur, G. and Munoz, R. (1972). Diagnostic criteria for use in psychiatric research. *Arch. Gen. Psychiatry* **26**, 57–63.

Foulds, G. A. (1976). *The Hierarchical Nature of Personal Illness*, Academic Press, London.

Foulds, G. A. and Bedford, A. (1975). Hierarchy of classes of personal illness. *Psychol. Med.* **5**, 181–192.

Gibbon, M., McDonald-Scott, P. and Endicott, J. (1981). Mastering the art of research interviewing. *Arch. Gen. Psychiatry* **38**, 1259–1262.

Hasin, D. S. and Grant, B. F. (1987). Diagnosing depressive disorders in patients with alcohol and drug problems: a comparison of the SADS-L and the DIS. *J. Psychiatr. Res.* **21**, 301–311.

Hasin, D. S., Endicott, J. and Keller, M. B. (1989) RDC alcoholism in patients with affective syndromes: 2-year course. *Am. J. Psychiatry*, in Press.

Helzer, J. E., Robins, L. N., Croughan, J. L. and Weiner, A. (1981). Renard diagnostic interview; its reliability and procedural validity with physicians and lay interviewers. *Arch. Gen. Psychiatry* **38**, 393–398.

Helzer, J. E., Robins, L. N., McEvoy, M. A., Spitznagle, E. L., Stoltzman, R. K., Farmer, A. and Brockington, I. F. (1985). A comparison of clinical and diagnostic interview schedule diagnoses: physician reexamination of lay-interviewed cases in the general population. *Arch. Gen. Psychiatry* **42**, 657–666.

Hesselbrock, V., Stabenau, J., Hesselbrock, M., Mirkin, P. and Meyer, R. (1982). A comparison of two interview schedules: the Schedule for Affective Disorders and Schizophrenia–Lifetime version and the National Institute of Mental Health Diagnostic Interview Schedule. *Arch. Gen. Psychiatry* **39**, 674–677.

Katz, M. M., Secunda, S. K., Hirschfeld, R. M. A. and Koslow, S. H. (1979). NIMH Clinical Research Branch Collaborative Program on the psychobiology of depression. *Arch. Gen. Psychiatry* **36**, 765–771.

Keller, M. B., Lavori, P. W., McDonald-Scott, P., Scheftner, W. A., Andreasen, N. C., Shapiro, R. W. and Croughan, J. (1981). Reliability of lifetime diagnoses and symptoms in patients with a current psychiatric disorder. *J. Psychiatr. Res.* **16**, 229–240.

Keller, M. B., Lavori, P. W., Coryell, W., Andreasen, N., Endicott, J., Clayton, P. J., Klerman, G. L. and Hirschfeld, R. M. A. (1986). Differential outcome of pure manic, mixed/cycling and pure depressive episodes in patients with bipolar illness. *J. Am. Med. Assoc.* **255**, 3138–3141.

Keller, M. B., Lavori, P. W., Friedman, B., Nielsen, E., Endicott, J., McDonald-Scott, P. and Andreasen, N. C. (1987). Longitudinal interval follow-up evaluation. *Arch. Gen. Psychiatry* **44**, 540–548.

Kendell, R. E., Everitt, B., Cooper, J. E., Sartorius, N. and David, M. E. (1968). Reliability of the Present State Examination. *Soc. Psychiatry* **3**, 123–129.

Leff, J. P. and Wing, J. K. (1971). Trial of maintenance therapy in schizophrenia. *Br. Med. J.* **3**, 599–604.

Leff, J. P., Kuipers, L., Berkowitz, R., Eberlein-Vries, R. and Sturgeon, D. (1982). A controlled trial of social intervention in the families of schizophrenic patients. *Br. J. Psychiatry* **141**, 121–134.

Luria, R. E. and Berry, R. (1979). Reliability and descriptive validity of PSE syndromes. *Arch. Gen. Psychiatry* **36**, 1187–1195.

Luria, R. E. and Berry, R. (1980). Teaching the Present State Examination in America. *Am. J. Psychiatry* **137**, 26–31.

Luria, R. E. and McHugh, P. R. (1974). Reliability and clinical utility of the 'Wing' Present State Examination. *Arch. Gen. Psychiatry* **30**, 866–871.

Manuzza, S., Fyer, A., Klein, D. and Endicott, J. (1986). Schedule for Affective Disorders and Schizophrenia–Lifetime Version modified for the study of anxiety disorders (SADS–LA): rationale and conceptual development. *J. Psychiatr. Res.* **20**, 317–325.

Munson, M. L., Orvashel, H., Skinner, E. A., Goldring, E., Pennybacker, M. and Timbers, D. M. (1985). Interviewers: characteristics, training and field work. In *Epidemiologic Field Methods in Psychiatry: The NIMH Epidemiologic Catchment Area Program* (W. W. Eaton and L. G. Kessler, eds), Orlando, Florida, Academic Press, Orlando, Florida, pp. 69–84.

Orley, J. and Wing, J. K. (1979). Psychiatric disorders in two African villages. *Arch. Gen. Psychiatry* **36**, 513–520.

Orvashel, H., Thompson, W. D., Belanger, A., Prussoff, B. A. and Kidd, K. K. (1982). Comparison of the family history method to direct interview; factors affecting the diagnosis of depression. *J. Affect. Disord.* **4**, 49–59.

Regier, D. A., Myers, J. K., Kramer, M., Robins, L. N., Blazer, D. G., Hough, R. L., Eaton, W. W. and Locke, B. Z. (1984). The NIMH epidemiological catchment area program. *Arch. Gen. Psychiatry* **41**, 934–941.

Rice, J., Endicott, J., Knesevich, M. A. and Rochberg, N. (1987a). Estimation of diagnostic sensitivity using stability data: an application to major depressive disorder. *J. Psychiatr. Res* **21**, 337–345.

Rice, J., Reich, T., Andreasen, N., Endicott, J., Van Eerdewegh, M., Fishman, R., Hirschfeld, R. and Klerman, G. (1987b). Familial transmission of bipolar illness. *Arch. Gen. Psychiatry* 441–447.

Riskind, J. H., Beck, A. T., Berchick, R. J., Brown, G. and Steer, R. A. (1987). Reliability of DSM-III diagnoses for major depression and generalized anxiety disorder using the Structured Clinical Interview for DSM-III. *Arch. Gen. Psychiatry* **44**, 817–820.

Robins, L. N. (1985). The Composite International Diagnostic Interview. *DIS Newsletter* Spring, pp. 1–2; DIS Training Faculty and Staff, Washington University School of Medicine, St Louis, Missouri.

Robins, L. N. (1987). CIDI field trials. *DIS Newsletter* Spring, pp. 1–2; DIS Training Faculty and Staff, Washington University School of Medicine, St Louis, Missouri.

Robins, L. N., Helzer, J. E., Croughan, J. and Ratcliff, K. S. (1981). National Institute of Mental Health Diagnostic Interview Schedule. *Arch. Gen. Psychiatry* **38**, 381–389.

Robins, L. N., Helzer, J. E., Ratcliff, K. S. and Seyfried, W. (1982). Validity of the Diagnostic Interview Schedule, version II: DSM-III diagnoses. *Psychol. Med.* **12**, 855–870.

Shrout, P. E. and Fleiss, J. L. (1979). Intraclass correlations: uses in assessing rater reliability. *Psychol. Bull.* **86**, 420–428.

Skodol, A. E., Rosnick, L., Kellman, D., Oldham, J. M. and Hyler, S. E. (1988). Validating structured DSM-III-R personality disorder assessments with longitudinal data. *Am. J. Psychiatry* **145**, 1297–1299.

Spitzer, R. L. (1983). Psychiatric diagnoses: are clinicians still necessary? *Compr. Psychiatry* **24**, 399–411.

Spitzer, R. L., Fleiss, J. L., Endicott, J. and Cohen, J. (1967). Mental Status Schedule: properties of factor-analytically derived scales. *Arch. Gen. Psychiatry* **16**, 479–493.

Spitzer, R. L., Fleiss, J. L., Endicott, J. and Cohen, J. (1970). The Psychiatric Status Schedule: a technique for evaluating psychopathology and impairment in role functioning. *Arch. Gen. Psychiatry* **23**, 41–55.

Spitzer, R. L., Endicott, J., Cohen, J. and Fleiss, J. L. (1974). Constraints on the validity of computer diagnosis. *Arch. Gen. Psychiatry* **31**, 197–203.

Spitzer, R. L., Endicott, J. and Robins, E. (1978). Research Diagnostic Criteria: rationale and reliability. *Arch. Gen. Psychiatry* **35**, 773–782.

Surtees, P. G., Dean, C., Ingham, J. G., Kreitman, N. B., Miller, P. McC. and Sashidharan, S. P. (1983). Psychiatric disorder in women from an Edinburgh community: association with demographic factors. *Br. J. Psychiatry* **142**, 238–246.

Thompson, W. D., Orvashel, H., Prusoff, B. A. and Kidd, K. K. (1982). An evaluation of the family history method for ascertaining psychiatric disorders. *Arch Gen. Psychiatry* **39**, 53–58.

Tress, K. H., Bellenis, C., Brownlow, J. M., Livingston, G. and Leff, J. P. (1987). The Present State Examination Change Rating Scale. *Br. J. Psychiatry* **150**, 201–207.

Vaughn, C. E. and Leff, J. P. (1976). The influence of family and social factors on the course of psychiatric illness. *Br. J. Psychiatry* **129**, 125–137.

Weissman, M. M., Gershon, E. S., Kidd, K. K., Prusoff, B. A., Leckman, J. F., Dibble, E., Hamovit, J., Thompson, W. D., Pauls, D. L. and Guroff, J. J. (1984).

Psychiatric disorders in the relatives of probands with affective disorders. *Arch. Gen. Psychiatry* **41**, 13–21.

Wing, J. K. (1976). A technique for studying psychiatric morbidity in in-patient and out-patient series and in general population samples. *Psychol. Med.* **6**, 665–671.

Wing, J. K., Birley, J. L. T., Cooper, J. E., Graham, P. and Isaacs, A. (1967). Reliability of a procedure for measuring and classifying 'present psychiatric state'. *Br. J. Psychiatry* **113**, 499–515.

Wing, J. K., Cooper, J. E. and Sartorius, N. (1974). *The Measurement and Classification of Psychiatric Symptoms*, Cambridge University Press, New York.

Wing, J. K., Henderson, A. S. and Winckle, M. (1977a). The rating of symptoms by a psychiatrist and a non-psychiatrist: a study of patients referred from general practice. *Psychol. Med.* **7**, 713–715.

Wing, J. K., Nixon, J. M., Mann, S. A. and Leff, J. P. (1977b). Reliability of the PSE (ninth edition) used in a population survey. *Psychol. Med.* **7**, 505–516.

Wing, J. K., Mann, S. A., Leff, J. P. and Nixon, J. M. (1978). The concept of a 'case' in psychiatric population surveys. *Psychol. Med.* **8**, 203–217.

Wittchen, H. U., Semler, G. and von Zerssen, D. (1985). A comparison of two diagnostic methods. Clinical ICD diagnoses vs. DMS-III and Research Diagnostic Criteria using the Diagnostic Interview Schedule (version 2). *Arch. Gen. Psychiatry* **42**, 677–684.

Woody, G. E., McLellan, A. T., Luborsky, L. and O'Brien, C. P. (1985). Sociopathy and psychotherapy outcome. *Arch. Gen. Psychiatry* **42**, 1081–1086.

World Health Organization (1973). *Report of the International Pilot Study of Schizophrenia*, World Health Organization, Geneva.

World Health Organization (1977). *International Classification of Diseases,* 9th Revision, World Health Organization, Geneva.

The Instruments of Psychiatric Research
Edited by C. Thompson

CHAPTER 3

A review of rating scales for measuring symptom changes in schizophrenia research

RAHUL MANCHANDA,[1] STEVEN R. HIRSCH[2] and THOMAS R. E. BARNES[2]

[1]*Department of Psychiatry, St Thomas Psychiatric Hospital, University of Western Ontario, St Thomas, Ontario, Canada*

[2]*Department of Psychiatry, Charing Cross and Westminster Medical School, London, UK*

INTRODUCTION

Rating scales are commonly used in research in schizophrenia. Their main advantages over the free interview are that phenomena are rated according to defined criteria and thus the effects of conceptual divergence between psychiatrists using these scales is minimized. Information is collected in a standard manner and this allows meaningful comparison between different patients and between groups of patients. Change in the nature and severity of a patient's condition may be assessed systematically; this is a critical consideration in studies of the effectiveness of treatment since the interpretation and generalization of the results are generally derived from the change in scores measured by these instruments. In order to determine which rating scales are most commonly employed to assess schizophrenic phenomena, we surveyed the treatment studies on the schizophrenic patients published over a six-year period (1979–1985) in five widely read psychiatric journals (see Table 1). Of the established scales used, the Inpatient Multidimensional Psychiatric Scale (IMPS) (Lorr *et al.*, 1962), the Present State Examination

Table 1. Rating scales for measuring change in schizophrenia (1979–1985)*

	N	%
Brief Psychiatric Rating Scale (BPRS)	73	(59.8)
Clinical Global Impression Scale (CGIS)	29	(23.7)
Other global scales	9	(7.4)
Present State Examination (PSE)	9	(7.4)
Manchester Scale (MS)	8	(6.5)
Comprehensive Psychopathological Rating Scale (CPRS) inc. subscales	8	(6.5)
Inpatient Multidimensional Psychiatric Rating Scale (IMPS)	4	(3.3)
Self-structured scale	9	(7.4)
Others	15	(12.3)
No scales	4	(3.3)
Total number of studies reported = 122		

* Journals reviewed: *Acta Psychiatrica Scandinavica, American Journal of Psychiatry, Archives of General Psychiatry, British Journal of Psychiatry, Psychological medicine*

(PSE) (Wing *et al.*, 1974) and the Comprehensive Psychopathological Rating Scale (CPRS) (Asberg *et al.*, 1978) are relatively long scales, while the Brief Psychiatric Rating Scale (BPRS) (Overall and Gorham, 1962), the Schizophrenia Change Scale (SCS) (Montgomery *et al.*, 1978) and the Manchester Scale (MS) (Krawiecka *et al.*, 1977) are shorter scales. The Manchester Scale is also known as the Krawiecka, or Krawiecka and Goldberg, scale. In this Chapter we describe these six scales in order of chronological development and mention the recently introduced Comprehensive Assessment of History and Symptoms (CASH) including the Scale for the Assessment of Positive Symptoms (SAPS) and the Scale for the Assessment of Negative Symptoms (SANS) (Andreasen, 1981). In addition, we describe the Global Assessment Scale (GAS) (Endicott *et al.*, 1976), which may be a useful adjunct to a specific symptom related rating scale, and some of the scales recently introduced for rating negative symptoms.

The spectrum of psychopathology covered by each scale is considered, and the usefulness of the scales in current psychopharmacological research in schizophrenia is critically reviewed. First, we will discuss the concepts which underlie the differences in the way the scales are structured and scored.

IMPLICIT RATIONALE IN THE STRUCTURE OF RATING SCALES

The Rating of Severity

In order to assess the relative merits of these rating scales it is useful to examine the assumptions on which they have been based and the similarities and differences in their construction. All the scales, except the GAS, are constructed so that a higher score corresponds to a greater degree of disturbance or deviation from normal, i.e. a greater severity.

This approach provides a quantitative measure of the characteristics under scrutiny. However, the severity of a symptom can be rated on a number of different criteria, such as frequency, intensity, duration or degree of incapacitation or tolerability. Where descriptive cues for scoring degree of severity are provided, these may incorporate qualitative changes and the introduction of additional criteria for rating severity. For example, to be rated as pathological on the CPRS, Other auditory hallucinations need to be 'definite hallucinations which may be persistent but not intrusive', while to qualify as the extreme degree of the symptom they need to be 'loud' or 'unpleasant', or 'forceful commands'. Similarly, when rating Coherently expressed delusions on the MS, a rating of 1 or 2 can refer to eccentric beliefs or over-valued ideas which may be considered normal phenomena, while a rating of 3 or 4 denotes delusions, as a psychotic symptom. Whether or not such shifts in emphasis are considered a valid reflection of increased severity depends upon one's conceptual and clinical view of the phenomenon.

However, if researchers wish to investigate the nature and associations of a specific symptom, they will need to identify the relevant item on the rating scale they plan to use, and be aware of the criteria used to rate severity, and any other assumptions inherent in the scoring system.

Definition of Scale Items

Scale items are usually defined in terms of observable behaviour, or depend on the verbal reports of patients. A difference between rating scales is whether they are meant to rate clinically defined phenomena or whether they are based on descriptive items not closely linked with clinical concepts. In either case, the descriptive statement should be specific enough to identify a distinct symptom. For example, items such as Rapid speech or Third person hallucinations may be clearly defined and delimited. However, the item Suspiciousness on the BPRS covers a wide range of different symptoms such as vague suspiciousness, over-valued ideas, ideas of reference and delusions of reference. Specific symptoms such as Third person persecutory hallucinations would not be rated as such, but would be rated as Suspiciousness *and* Unusual thought content. Thus, Suspiciousness on the BPRS is used as a general heading which encompasses a whole range of different behaviours. The problem with this approach is that the items are not mutually exclusive, so a particular behaviour may warrant a score on more than one item. This devalues the scale as either a qualitative or quantitative measure of specific phenomena, although scales like the BPRS are successful in providing an overall quantitative rating of the severity of the illness. Absence of clinical specificity characterizes scales that depend on general terms to describe behaviour, rather than ratings of the presence or absence of well-established clinical signs and symptoms.

It can be argued that a scale which rates well-defined clinical symptoms has a sounder conceptual basis, particularly with regard to the psychoses, which are believed to have their roots in abnormalities of biological function. Scales which simply rate the behavioural expressions of these abnormalities are not as likely to yield a useful clinical profile of ratings, but may be more sensitive in identifying non-specific changes in behaviour and be more suitable for studies of personality disorder and neurotic conditions.

Qualitative versus Quantitative Approach

Scales differ in the number of response categories. A numerical scale is usually used to reflect severity in terms of frequency of occurrence, or intensity, or duration of the symptom. The hard-minded approach is that a clearly defined symptom, such as a delusion or an hallucination, is rated as either present or not, an approach which is most relevant to psychotic illness. Neurotic symptoms vary from mild experiences which occur in normal individuals to severe, incapacitating symptoms; the argument for rating severity on a quantitative scale from normal to severely abnormal has force for such symptoms as anxiety, tension or depressed mood. The problem here is that psychiatric observations are partly based on the qualitative changes, most notably in the psychoses, and partly based on quantitative variations from the normal, which characterize neuroses.

Sensitivity, Specificity and Reliability

The 'sensitivity' of a scale refers to its ability to detect the presence of symptoms when they are truly present, while 'specificity' is the ability of the scale to avoid rating symptoms as present when they are not. A scale can be made more sensitive by broadening the criteria for rating symptoms, or lowering the threshold for rating. However, this could result in poor specificity, i.e. falsely detecting a symptom. In fact, sensitivity and specificity are terms which have generally been used in the context of diagnostic decisions, and not with reference to the ability of scales to detect a symptom. Hence it is not surprising that the sensitivity and specificity of the scales used for measuring change in schizophrenia have not been determined, although this can be inferred from an inspection of the scales (see Table 2). All the scales described, except for the PSE, should have a high sensitivity as they allow a low threshold for rating symptoms as present, or use very broad criteria (e.g. the BPRS) which enable a rating to be made if any of a wide variety of different symptoms or signs are present. Some researchers may feel that this is an advantage, because it allows the rater to rate some of the unspecified aspects of behaviour which more specific scales avoid. In contrast, because the PSE requires a symptom to be moderately severe before it qualifies for

Table 2. Comparison of scales used for rating schizophrenic symptomatology

	Long Scales			Short Scales			
	PSE	IMPS	CPRS	BPRS	SCS	MS	GAS
Diagnosis	+++	+	−	+	−	−	−
Sensitivity	++	++++	++++	+++	+++	++	++++
Specificity	++++	++	++	+	++	+++	−
Positive Symptoms	++++	++	++	++	+++	++	overall functioning
Negative Symptoms	++	++	++	+	+	++	
Neurotic Symptoms	++	++	++	++	+	+	
Glossary and Guidelines	++++	++	+++	+	+++	++++	++
Standardised interview	yes	no	no	no	no	yes	no
Scoring	0–2	8*	0–3	0–6 (1–7)	0–3+	0–4	0–100 (units of 10)
Approx. time taken (min.)	45–90	30–45	30–45	15–30	10–15	10–15	<5

The strength of each scale is rated + to ++++
* 9 points, 5 points and 2 points of severity
\+ use of half scores recommended.

rating, it can be argued that treatment effects could be missed. The counter argument is that if the rater is uncertain whether or not a symptom is present, or a change has occurred, it is unlikely to be of clinical relevance and is better not scored. Nevertheless, results of a recently published study of benzodiazepines and counselling for stress disorder by the World Health Organization suggested that the PSE was very sensitive to treatment effects on minor neurotic disorders (World Health Organization, 1988).

For most of the scales discussed here, evidence for the reliability of symptom rating has been presented in terms of a correlation coefficient, *r*, for inter-rater reliability. This measure can be misleading; it suffers from the drawback that it will indicate high inter-rater agreement if the raters have consistently scored a symptom as absent. When a specific symptom is rare in the patient sample being studied, the correlation coefficient may be a poor reflection of reliability.

Further, Cairns *et al.* (1982) argue that psychiatric practice is characterized by independent interviews and hence inter-rater variance should be taken into consideration when calculating inter-rater reliability. For example, Klett and McNair (1966) found high intraclass correlation coefficients for IMPS items, but these were based on scores by raters who observed the interview together, and hence do not fully measure the inter-rater variance. However, when patients are interviewed separately, other sources of variance (namely, time effect, order effect, practice effect and change in clinical condition) come into play.

A danger with all scales is the tendency of the rater to rate improvement over time and for more aberrant items to become less so. This tendency of regression to the mean is perhaps exaggerated with longer scales with many items and high total scores for abnormality. The problem is partly mitigated by scales which provide precise operational criteria for each item, and by using trained raters to administer the scales. In this respect, the PSE and MS, and perhaps to a lesser extent the CPRS and SCS, are the better instruments. But the most effective safeguard is the use of a control group to measure the non-specific influences on ratings over time.

AN EXAMINATION OF SIX COMMONLY USED RATING SCALES

The In-patient Multidimensional Psychiatric Scale (IMPS)

The IMPS is one of the oldest scales for assessing psychotic behaviour still in use. The scale was developed from Lorr's Multidimensional Scale for Rating Psychiatric Patients (MSRPP) (Lorr *et al.*, 1953) and includes observable and reported behavioural characteristics of major psychiatric syndromes. The items were identified by systematic observation of psychiatric patients and reference to symptom descriptions in psychiatric texts at the time, with special attention to psychotic behaviour and thinking. The scale is designed and recommended for use with patients with functional psychoses and severe neuroses.

In its revised form (Lorr and Klett, 1967) the IMPS consists of 89 items, each with a short behavioural description. The information is recorded by means of a semi-structured interview. While the social history, case notes and ward behaviour reports may be used to structure the interview, abnormal behaviour and thinking not evident at the time of rating are ignored. Of the 89 items, 51 are recorded on a nine-point scale of severity, 21 on a five-point scale and the remainder are two-valued (yes–no) items. Factor analysis of these items resulted in 12 syndromes as follows: Excitement; Hostile belligerence; Paranoid projection; Grandiose expansiveness; Perceptual distortions; Obsessional-phobic; Anxious-depression; Impaired functioning; Retardation and apathy; Disorientation; Motor disturbance; and Conceptual disorganization. The syndromes are conceptualized as unipolar variables present to a greater or lesser extent in most people: the more severe the disturbance, the higher the score. Factor analysis of these 12 syndromes results in four major factors which have been labelled Schizophrenic disorganization, Paranoid process, Psychotic depression and Disorganized hyperactivity. These correspond to the, now outdated, ICD-8 major classes of Schizophrenia, Paranoid states, Depression and Mania, respectively (Lorr and Klett, 1968). Schizophrenic disorganization in the IMPS is derived from ratings on Psychomotor retardation, Functional disorientation, Motor disturbance and Conceptual disorganization. Paranoid process is derived from Paranoid projection, Perceptual distortion, Grandiosity and Obsessive thinking. According to von Zerssen and Cording (1978) factor analysis of IMPS ratings on 127 psychiatric patients results in five syndromes. Two of these refer to positive symptoms of schizophrenia, while another relates to negative symptoms. The two remaining factors reflect depressive symptomatology.

The reliability of individual items was tested in the early stages of development of the IMPS and high intraclass correlation coefficients of 0.9 or higher were found for all syndromes except Motor disturbance (Klett and McNair, 1966). Mariotto and Farrell (1979) also found very good reliabilities for ranked scores, but their raters differed in their tendency to score high or low across the instrument. The formulation of psychiatric symptoms in everyday language facilitates the understanding and use of the IMPS by lay raters. An obvious advantage are the operational definitions provided for the items, a particular superiority at the time it was introduced. The scale is comprehensive with respect to the behavioural manifestations of functional psychoses. The scale values are sensitive to change and can be used successfully in longitudinal investigations in schizophrenia (von Zerssen, personal communication).

The scoring procedure is, unfortunately, rather inconsistent. Some items are rated 0–8 while others are rated 0–4 or on a two-point (yes–no) scale. The broadest nine-point scale allows the rater to score suspected or questionable symptoms. This may be seen as an advantage in that abnormality is detected sensitively, but this might tempt raters to guess at the lower level of severity.

Further problems arise from the use of different rating scores. Any single syndrome may consist of items with different types of scores. For example, Grandiosity consists of five items, three of which are scored as present or absent, one of which is scored on the nine-point scale (0–8), and the last is scored on a five-point scale (0, 2, 4, 6, or 8). This confused procedure can lead to undesirable syndrome scale distribution with distortions in change scores. Cairns *et al.*, (1982) suggests that these distortions could be eliminated by the use of a four-point scale throughout.

The biggest limitation of the IMPS may be that it relies on the rating of behavioural manifestations of psychosis expressed in lay terms, rather than rating symptoms. As discussed earlier, various behaviours may result from a single core symptom, thus an improvement or deterioration in one symptom could affect the rating on several IMPS items, resulting in an exaggerated change in total score. Similarly, a rating may be affected by a number of symptoms, one or many of which would give rise to the same degree of change on a single rating.

Brief Psychiatric Rating Scale (BPRS)

The primary purpose in developing the BPRS was to have a comprehensive but rapid evaluation procedure for use in assessing response to treatment. The original scale consisted of 16 symptom constructs, 14 of which were derived from factor analysis of psychiatric rating data. Unusual thought content and Blunted affect were added before the original scale was published, and Excitement and Disorganization items were subsequently added to aid the classification of hypomania (Overall and Gorham, 1963). The ratings consist of a seven-point severity scale, ranging from 'absent' to 'extremely severe'. These are made on the basis of patients' verbal reports and observation of patients during a brief interview lasting between 15 and 30 minutes. Items which predominately reflect observed behaviour include Mannerisms and posturing, Motor retardation and Uncooperativeness. Items based on information from interview include Conceptual disorganization, Unusual thought content, Anxiety, Depressive mood, and Blunted affect.

For evaluating patient change during treatment, the authors recommend the use of a 'total score', which is the sum of the 16 ratings. However, when using the scale for a particular diagnostic group, such as schizophrenic or depressed patients, it was thought appropriate to weight certain scores more than others in order to reflect the symptoms most relevant for that condition. In a subsequent paper, Overall (1974) points out that the objectives of clinical research in psychopharmacology have changed since the introduction of antipsychotic drugs; the research emphasis has shifted from whether a new drug has *any* therapeutic effect to whether it has a *superior* (and perhaps specific) effect compared to those currently available. In this regard, the BPRS contains four higher-order factors (clusters of symptoms that tend to occur together). Each of these higher-order factors can be scored by simply combining ratings on three of the most relevant scales, as follows:

1. *Thinking disturbance:* comprises Conceptual disorganization, Hallucinatory behaviour and Unusual thought content.
2. *Withdrawal retardation:* comprises Emotional withdrawal, Motor retardation and Blunted affect.
3. *Anxious-depression:* comprises Anxiety, Guilt feelings and Depressive mood.
4. *Hostile suspiciousness:* comprises Hostility, Suspiciousness and Uncooperativeness.

The BPRS has been subjected to minor modifications to extend the range of symptoms scored and to improve definitions for specific ratings. Yorkston *et al.* (1974) modified the scoring so that the absence of a symptom is designated by a 0 rather than 1. They reclassified the items into three groupings: a 'thought disorder' sub-scale and a 'non-thought disorder' subscale (together constituting the schizophrenia scale), and a 'non-schizophrenia' subscale. The BPRS in this form has been used for measuring change in several British studies (Yorkston *et al.*, 1974, 1981; Manchanda and Hirsch, 1981, 1986).

The BPRS has obvious advantages as a brief scale covering both florid and deficit symptoms of schizophrenia. Its wide use all over the world yields comparable data from a large number of studies on a variety of patient populations. However, there are several flaws in this scale which are apparent when it is employed in the study of schizophrenia.

The BPRS was not designed specifically for assessing schizophrenia, although it is widely used for this purpose. Only six items (Conceptual disorganization, Hallucinatory behaviour, Unusual thought content, Emotional withdrawal, Motor retardation, and Blunted affect), and possibly three further items (Suspiciousness, Grandiosity, and Mannerisms and posturing), reflect psychotic phenomena in schizophrenia, and none of these correspond closely to specific symptoms or symptom groupings. Yet, in more than a third of the 73 studies conducted employing the BPRS, the total score was the only measure used for analysis (Table 3). As a result, it is unclear whether the reported treatment effects reflect changes in psychotic, neurotic or affective symptomatology. Like the IMPS, the BPRS is not able to identify the specific areas of psychopathology that have changed; a drug's global

Table 3. Use of brief psychiatric rating scale (1979–85)

Total number of studies using BPRS = 73		
Measures used:		
Total score only	27	(37%)
Total score + individual item/s	13	(17.8%)
	—	54.8%
Subscores only	7	(9.6%)
Total score + subscores	26	(35.6%)

effects such as sedation or a reduction in suspiciousness, could be misinterpreted as a specific antipsychotic action even when the patient is not psychotic.

The BPRS was established in the USA when there was less interest in rating specified symptoms in relation to diagnosis and improvement. The scale is particularly liable to the halo effect between items and a confusion of rating because of the lack of correspondence to well-differentiated observable behaviour and recognized clinical symptoms.

This is the problem commented on previously with regard to the IMPS, because items overlap and are only broadly and indistinctly defined. For example, the item Conceptual disorganization can cover nearly all forms of speech disorder, vague thinking and delusions. On the BPRS, a patient who is only suspicious is not easily differentiated from a patient with paranoid delusions. Delusions are rated as Suspiciousness unless they are unusual, when they may qualify for rating on the Suspiciousness *and* Unusual thought content items, the latter being used to rate both odd or over-valued ideas and bizarre delusions, which differ in their diagnostic implications. Similarly, non-paranoid psychotic symptoms, such as erotic delusions or the Capgras syndrome, can only be rated under the Conceptual disorganization or Unusual thought content items or both.

Although high inter-rater reliability can be achieved within centres, the lack of cues for rating severity is likely to be a problem when interpreting results between centres, and provides less of a check against the trial bias toward improvement in successive ratings than scales with well-defined glossaries and rating points. The rater is expected to have extensive psychiatric experience, being asked to compare the degree of severity of symptoms in the patient to the population of patients who do not have the symptoms in question. Thus, ratings can be highly idiosyncratic and subjective, giving rise to marked differences in the level of rating between centres. The problem is illustrated by the fact that Turner's (1963) guidelines for moderate and extremely severe ratings are incompatible with the instructions of Wiles *et al.* (1976) for rating levels of severity. These differences between the various interpretations of the scale serve to reflect its inherent weakness. Although the BPRS has been used successfully to rate improvement in affective and schizophrenic psychoses, we consider that the construct validity of this scale is incompatible with current concepts of psychopathology.

The Present State Examination (PSE)

The development of the PSE began in the late 1960s, but since then it has been revised a number of times through to a tenth edition which is currently in press. The PSE consists of a structured clinical interview for ascertaining the presence of symptoms of functional psychoses and neuroses. The clinical phenomena elicited can be used to derive syndromes and scores suitable for use in clinical research. A computer program, CATEGO, classifies patients according to CATEGO class, which is highly concordant with clinical diagnosis. However, the scale was not designed around specific diagnostic criteria and should rather be considered as providing a comprehensive picture of psychiatric symptomatology. Luria and Guziec (1981) describe it as 'a crystallisation of Anglo-European clinical methods and concepts, much influenced by the phenomenological approach of Jaspers and Schneider.'

The PSE consists of 140 items which systematically cover all the phenomena likely to be relevant when conducting a mental state examination. An important feature is that, although certain initial questions are compulsory, the onus is on the interviewer to carry out clinical cross-examination to establish the presence or absence of a symptom according to the criteria listed in the glossary for each symptom. There is a system of cut-off points following obligatory probe questions so that the interviewer can move on to another group of symptoms if he feels that there are no symptoms in a particular area. The score sheet needs to be completed during the interview as the rater would be unwise to trust his memory for such a comprehensive scale. Attendance to the various cut-off points and familiarity with the score sheet are required if erroneous ratings are to be avoided. Experienced raters are expected to divert from the strict order of questions in the PSE in order to track down a particular symptom and follow the patient's line of thought. A practised rater can avoid presenting the scale like a structured interview, but it is hard to disguise from patients the formal nature of the procedure. Exploration of sensitive issues, which is possible in an open interview, are likely to be limited when administering the PSE.

The inter-rater reliability was studied extensively during the USA–UK diagnostic project (Cooper *et al.*, 1972) and the International Pilot Study of Schizophrenia (WHO, 1973). Wing and associates (1967) and Kendell and co-workers (1968) reported higher reliability for earlier versions of the PSE, and found that ratings based on verbal reports were generally more reliable than ratings based on observations of behaviour. Two subsequent studies have demonstrated high levels of rater agreement for the instrument within a single centre, between centres and between psychiatrists and non-medical interviewers (World Health Organization, 1979; Wing *et al.*, 1977). A test of intracentre reliability revealed a high correlation coefficient of more than 0.93 from the same interview. Using lay interviewers and psychiatrists, the product–moment correlation for sets of total PSE scores was 0.73 (n = 123), for repeated interviews $r = 0.67$ (n = 95) and for tape-recorded interviews $r = 0.96$ (n = 28) (Wing *et al.*, 1977).

As a measure of change, the PSE has some concurrent validity, as it correlates well with change on the General Health Questionnaire (GHQ) (Goldberg, 1972), which is regarded as a sensitive but non-specific instrument for detecting psychiatric disorder in the general population. Newsom-Smith and Hirsch (1979) evaluated hospitalized self-poisoning patients with psychiatric symptoms on three occasions with the GHQ and the PSE. For all three interviews, highly significant correlations of 0.78, 0.81 and 0.77, respectively (significance $P < 0.0001$), were obtained. Similar results were obtained in a large multicentre trial carried out by the World Health Organization (1988). Further, Hirsch *et al.* (1973) carried out a controlled trial of maintenance therapy in schizophrenia using a single criterion for relapse, namely a decision by the clinical team that the patient had so deteriorated that he or she must be taken out of the trial and given a known treatment. For PSE ratings done at the same time, deterioration was defined as the appearance of new psychotic symptoms or an increase in severity of two or more symptoms. The investigators observed 85% agreement between the clinical and PSE criteria for relapse.

One of the shortcomings in using the PSE criteria is that patients who are uncommunicative can only be rated on behavioural items that are less reliable and may not show a rateable change. Scales which are less specific in the rating criteria for particular symptoms could allow for guessing that the patient is deluded or hallucinated, but provision could be made for rating 'appears hallucinated' to adapt the PSE in a similar way. Knights *et al.* (1980) showed how the PSE could be used to measure change in a heterogeneous sample of all psychiatric admissions from a catchment area population of 90 000. Over 20% of the sample were schizophrenic. The measures used were the total score, and four sub-scores, which are combinations of PSE syndromes which relate to specific areas of psychopathology: DAH (Delusional and Hallucinatory syndromes); BSO (Behavioural, Speech and other syndromes); SNR (Specific Neurotic syndromes) and NSN (Non-specific Neurotic syndromes) (Wing *et al.*, 1977). Knights and her colleagues combined DAH and BSO to derive a psychotic subscore and SNR and NSN to derive a neurotic sub-score, and found these sensitive to change over two weeks. Contrary to general belief, the PSE can effectively detect changes in minor neurotic symptoms. In a recent collaborative study covering more than 600 patients, the PSE detected a superior effect with low doses of benzodiazepine compared with placebo and this difference was not detected with the General Health Questionnaire (World Health Organization, 1988).

When schizophrenics improve, symptoms may diminish in the conviction with which they are held, the degree to which they disturb the patient (as reflected by the neurotic symptoms) and the number of psychotic symptoms present. Each of these dimensions can be scored separately on the PSE by specific ratings for most symptoms, although the degree of conviction in a false belief can only be reflected by a rating of either 'full' or 'partial' delusion.

The reliability of the PSE depends upon the expertise of the raters as well as the instrument itself. Before embarking upon the PSE, raters should have attended an approved training session, lasting one week; Wing (1983) recommends at least 20 interviews under proper supervision before use of the technique.

The main practical limitation of the PSE is the difficulty in completing the full scale with patients who are disturbed, uncooperative or uncommunicative. It is, therefore, advisable in any formal research study to use a short scale in addition to the PSE. Also, minor psychopathology at assessment may be missed because of the high threshold for rating the PSE, especially in the observed items in the Behaviour, Affect and Speech section at the end of the schedule. To remedy this, the ratings may be modified, by using either half scores or the amendments suggested by Myers *et al.* (1981). Further, the Behaviour, Affect and Speech section of the PSE has been expanded into the Psychological Impairments Rating Scale (PIRS) (see below), designed to serve as a supplement to the PSE.

Comprehensive Psychopathological Ratings Scale (CPRS)

In 1971 an interdisciplinary group of psychiatrists, psychologists and clinical pharmacologists from Sweden and England was formed to construct a new scale consisting of items sensitive to change with treatment. The result was the CPRS, which was first published in 1978.

The scale consists of 65 items covering a wide range of reported (1–40) and observed (41–65) psychopathology, as well as 'global rating of illness' (66) and 'assumed reliability of the rating' (67) items. Each item is described in simple, non-technical terms. For each variable, the scale steps from 0 to 3 have been operationally defined, and the use of half steps is recommended. The following general rules have been used in their construction: 0 = absent; 1 = pathological although it may even be a normal variation; 2 = clearly pathological; and 3 = an extreme degree of psychopathology. The dimensions used for defining and arranging the individual items are intensity, frequency and duration of the symptoms. The scale is recommended for use by trained mental health workers from various professions.

An interview technique that is as close to the clinical psychiatric interview as possible is recommended, although it is also possible to use the scale as a questionnaire, asking about each item separately.

Generally, correlations for inter-rater reliability for the reported psychopathology have been higher than those recorded for observed psychopathology (Jacobsson *et al.*, 1978; Kasa and Hitomi, 1985). Jacobsson *et al.* (1978) conducted an inter-rater reliability study of the CPRS, covering 39 items relevant to patients with schizophrenia and paranoid syndromes. Between the doctors involved, the inter-rater reliability of the 16 reported symptoms was greater than 0.9 for all items except Inability to feel and Reduced sleep. Sixteen out of the 23 observed items had high inter-rater reliability (r = 0.78–0.97). Low values were obtained for Mood disturbance, Incontinence of affect, Incongruous affect, Labile emotional response, Hostility, Distractibility and Speech defects.

Montgomery and Asberg (1978) have derived a depression sub-scale from the CPRS. Seventeen items were chosen on the basis of their frequency of occurrence in depressive illness. These authors also constructed a schizophrenia scale (see below). Although no specific scale for mania has been extracted, there are several relevant items in the CPRS, such as Elation, Increased sexual interest, Ideas of grandeur, Pressure of speech, Flight of ideas and Overactivity. Organic symptoms (including failing memory, labile emotional response, disorientation, perseveration and involuntary movements) are also represented. Neurotic symptoms (including those for anxiety) which may be present on their own, or as part of a depressive, manic or schizophrenic illness, are also adequately covered by this scale.

The merits of the scale are the clear descriptions of items with appropriate guidelines for rating severity. The items are familiar to those in current psychiatric practice. As with the PSE, the rater is asked to differentiate symptoms which may appear superficially to convey similar psychopathology, such as Worrying and Muscular tension, Worrying and Pessimistic thoughts, Hypochondriasis and Compulsive thoughts, and Phobias and Indecision. However, the explicit definitions provided should allow discrimination between these items.

In terms of the amount of psychopathology encompassed by the CPRS, it falls between more detailed scales such as the PSE or IMPS and shorter scales such as the BPRS and the MS. There is considerably less differentiation of schizophrenic symptomatology compared with the PSE, although both positive and negative symptoms are reasonably well covered. As ratings are made on a seven-point scale, the CPRS is potentially a more sensitive instrument for rating change than the PSE and may be particularly useful in the evaluation of new psychotropic compounds. The range of items of the scale enables a comprehensive evaluation of treatment effects, perhaps detecting specific changes that could be missed by the more restricted assessment of a briefer scale. The advantage claimed by the authors, of excluding items rating a pronounced character trait, or a particular psychiatric syndrome, or items influenced by socio-cultural differences, is also shared by other scales like the PSE, BPRS and MS. In the development of the CPRS, emphasis was put on selecting items which were considered likely to change over time, rather than those possessing diagnostic specificity. The CPRS is thus a sensitive scale but perhaps less specific for a particular disorder.

Schizophrenia Change Scale (SCS)

This is a short scale for schizophrenia derived from the full CPRS described above. Scores on individual CPRS items were examined to see which were the most sensitive to change in response to antipsychotic drug treatment. Thirty-six schizophrenic patients were assessed by clinicians after four weeks treatment with antipsychotic medication and judged as 'responders' or 'non-responders'. The 12 items which discriminated most powerfully between the two groups were included in the schizophrenia scale. Listed in order of sensitivity to change they are: Feeling controlled, Lack of appropriate emotion, Disrupted thoughts, Commenting voices, Depersonalization, Perplexity, Inability to feel, Sadness, Pessimistic thoughts, Other delusions, Ideas of persecution, and Delusional mood. Note that there is no specific place to score hallucinations or paranoid delusions. According to the authors, the change in scores on the new scale discriminated between treatments significantly better than the BPRS did, but as yet there is no published confirmation by other researchers.

When examined, the scale provides only limited description of the schizophrenic symptomatology to be scored, and hallucinations (other than 'commenting voices') and rare or unusual symptoms are not included. The negative or deficit symptoms of schizophrenia, considered unresponsive to currently available antipsychotic medication, are not adequately represented. Improvement in the acute symptomatology will be detected by the scale but this does not necessarily imply recovery from the illness. Failure to rate negative symptoms in treatment trials of schizophrenia excludes a critical aspect of the condition from the assessment. However, if the full CPRS is used, response to treatment in negative symptoms may be gauged on the basis of change in items such as Poverty of speech, Indecision, Lassitude, Withdrawal, and Reduced speech.

Some items are relatively non-specific; for example, Lack of appropriate emotion could include both blunting and incongruity of affect, and Disrupted thoughts as a general item covers thought blocking, thought insertion and thought withdrawal. The 12 items in the sub-scale are not mutually exclusive and several items are subject to the error of proximity, which can have too great an effect on results when using a short scale. For example, it may be difficult to differentiate between Perplexity and Delusional mood, so that they will tend to be scored similarly. The same might be true for the Lack of appropriate emotion and Inability to feel items, although the former is rated on the basis of observed behaviour, while the latter is rated according to the patient's subjective report. Hallucinations, other than 'commenting voices' are not included in the subscale, so one must resort to either rating these under Other delusions or leave them out. When the patient is either uncooperative or unresponsive, the rater is allowed to use his judgement to arrive at a score. However, this pragmatic manoeuvre may reduce the level of inter-rater and intercentre agreement. In other respects, the SCS has the same characteristics and merits outlined above for the full CPRS.

Manchester Scale (MS)

This scale, also referred to as the Krawiecka, or Krawiecka and Goldberg scale, was designed for the brief rating of chronic psychotic patients by doctors who know them well. The items are, however, relevant to both acute and chronic psychotic illness and are sensitive to change with treatment. The scale consists of eight items based on both reported and observed psychopathology. The items rated on the basis of replies to questions are Depression, Anxiety, Delusions and Hallucinations, while the ratings based on observation are Incoherence and irrelevance of speech, Poverty of speech, Muteness, Flattened or incongruous affect, and Psychomotor retardation.

A new rater can partially train himself by using available video training tapes (from the Department of Psychiatry, University of Manchester) and establish his reliability by using additional video tapes especially prepared for this purpose. A manual offers probe questions and guidelines for rating. The scale is not intended to be used blindly, and the rater is expected to be familiar with the patient's case records and aware of areas in which the patient has previously experienced symptoms. Such background information might be considered essential when assessing chronic patients who have encapsulated delusions and hallucinations which are only likely to be elicited by relatively direct questioning. Manchanda and Hirsch (unpublished 1979) modified the manual by introducing a series of questions derived from the PSE in order to facilitate interviewing and provide adequate coverage of symptoms seen in acute patients.

The ratings are made on a five-point scale of severity, detailed as follows: 0 represents the absence of an item; a rating of 1 suggests some evidence of the presence of the symptom in question, but it is not considered pathological; a rating of 2 refers to a degree just sufficient to be pathological; and ratings of 3 and 4 refer to marked and severe psychopathology, respectively. The ratings are made for presence or absence of symptoms during the preceding week. A rating of 3 for delusions describes the abnormal experiences having occurred in the past month. This period should be modified according to the frequency of assessment. For anxiety and depression, the degree of distress to the patient is a variable incorporated within the rating.

Krawiecka *et al.* (1977) carried out reliability testing of the scale and produced satisfactory levels of inter-rater reliability with five psychiatrists rating from video tapes and patient interviews. Ratings based on a verbal report had a correlation coefficient ranging from 0.75 to 0.87, except for Anxiety for which the figure was around 0.65. The corresponding range for items based on observation was 0.62–0.73, except for Flattened or incongruous affect where the figures were between 0.50 and 0.58. Further, there were no differences between the raters in their mean severity scores except for the Flattened or incongruous affect item. In another study (Manchanda *et al.*, 1986) the BPRS and MS were used by two raters from different cultures and different educational backgrounds (Indian psychiatrist and German psychologist/medical student) without any previous experience in the use of the two scales. The correlation coefficients for the majority of the items on the MS were higher than those for the BPRS. A higher inter-rater reliability for items on the MS was seen whether patients were rated at the same or different points in time by the two raters.

The MS has been used not only in the assessment of chronic psychotics (Owens and Johnstone, 1980) but also as a measure of change in acute treatment trials (Johnstone *et al.*, 1978). The investigators have found it brief, simple to use and sensitive to change. Johnstone and her colleagues (1978) subdivided the scale into positive, negative and non-specific subscales of schizophrenia. The negative symptom sub-scale consists of only two items—Flattening (but not incongruity) of affect, and Poverty of speech—and thus provides a limited measure of the 'Type II' syndrome (Crow, 1980). In our study (Manchanda and Hirsch, 1981) improvement in the non-specific symptoms of the scale correlated well with an improvement in the neurotic sub-score of the PSE but not with the non-schizophrenia score of the BPRS.

The Manchester Scale can be a reliable substitute for brief scales like the BPRS provided that one does not need to rate neurotic symptoms or a wider range of pathology. Its advantage over the SCS would seem to be that it covers both positive and negative symptoms of schizophrenia, and the ratings more closely correspond to well-recognized clinical symptoms and syndromes. One major disadvantage is the lack of items covering affective symptoms other than depression, such as elated mood, pressure of speech and overactivity, which are seen in schizophrenia.

EXAMINATION OF TWO FURTHER SCALES

Global Assessment Scale (GAS)

In 1962, Luborsky reported the development of the Health–Sickness Rating Scale (HSRS) as a means by which global assessments of overall mental health could be rated on an anchored 100-point scale. Although useful as a criterion for measuring change, the diagnostic constraints in the HSRS, as well as the need to consult a series of 34 case vignettes, made it a rather cumbersome instrument. Also, the case descriptions were of patients on admission, invalidating other evaluations during the course of the illness. Endicott *et al.* (1976) carried out extensive modifications and hence the new name, GAS, although it retains the basic idea and structure of the HSRS.

The GAS utilizes a different strategy compared with other scales. It is designed on the principle of using the broadest rating possible that is also sensitive to change that can be regarded as clinically advantageous. Therefore, it relies on a 'gestalt' approach to the measurement of change, based on the rater's general clinical experience. It evaluates the overall functioning of a subject on a continuum from psychological sickness to health (scoring 1–100, respectively). The scale is divided into 10 intervals, each a 10-point scale of global severity. Each level of severity is operationally defined. The two highest intervals (81–100) are used for individuals without significant psychopathology who also exhibit traits of a positive mental health (e.g. superior functioning, wide range of interests, social effectiveness, warmth and integrity). The next interval, 71–80, is for individuals where psychopathology is minimal or absent. The majority of patients in treatment will be rated between 1 and 70. In making a rating, one selects the lowest interval that describes the patient's overall functioning. The final rating within the scale interview (for example 21–30) is done on the basis of the proximity of overall psychopathology to the higher rating (31–40) or the lower one (11–20). The time period assessed is generally the week prior to the evaluation. It is recommended that the rating should be based on an individual's overall functioning and the severity of symptoms, but not influenced by the nature of the psychiatric disorder.

The GAS can be used for measuring change in affective and neurotic disorders as well as schizophrenia. It provides a clinical impression of overall functioning, allowing the rater to take into account unspecified nuances of behaviour, such as social responsiveness and deportment, which cannot be easily defined in the rating scale but contribute to a clinician's overall assessment of improvement or deterioration. The GAS is simple, quick and easy to use. According to Endicott and his co-workers (1976) the intraclass correlation of inter-rater reliability varies from 0.69 to 0.91, and there was 95% confidence for the ratings to be within 10 or 11 points of each other. They claim that the validity of the GAS is supported by its sensitivity to change, and the relationship of scores with re-admission to hospital.

The GAS has been used as a measure of change in several recent studies and can be recommended as a useful summary statement, complementary to a multidimensional rating scale. It should not be used entirely on its own because it does not distinguish between the clinical and social aspects of a patient's functioning, or reflect any specific aspect of functioning which may be affected by pharmacological treatment.

Scale for Assessment of Positive Symptoms (SAPS) and Scale for the Assessment of Negative Symptoms (SANS)

The Comprehensive Assessment of Symptoms and History (CASH) covers medical history, neurological examination and social data. This assessment package was introduced relatively recently and reliability data are scarce. Thus, it is a relatively untried scale which is included here because it focuses particularly on negative symptoms. The main components of interest are a Scale for Assessment of Positive Symptoms (SAPS) and the Scale for Assessment of Negative Symptoms (SANS) (Andreasen, 1981, 1982) which rates negative symptoms, and was developed from two earlier scales, the scale to assess Thought, Language and Communication (TLC) (Andreasen, 1979a) and the Affect Rating Scale (Andreasen, 1979b). The CASH does not cover a fixed period, but, like the PSE, is appropriate for assessment of the previous month. The positive and negative symptom ratings were designed as instruments to measure change, and are suitable for use in treatment and outcome studies in both in-patient and out-patients samples.

For the positive symptom ratings, detailed definitions are provided for rating on five- or six-point scales. Where appropriate, severity is based on frequency of occurrence during the interview, while for other items it is a clinical judgement, rating from 'questionable' through to 'severe'. Most of the positive symptoms are phenomena elicited by direct questioning of the patient, while the negative symptoms are primarily observational items, although patient reports are necessary for rating items such as Subjective complaints of emotional emptiness or loss of feeling, and Subjective complaints of inattentiveness.

The refined rating of positive formal thought disorder in the positive symptoms scale reflects Andreasen's interest in this area. Raters are asked to distinguish between Tangentiality, Derailment, Incoherence, Illogicality, Circumstantiality, Pressure of speech, Distractible speech, and Clanging, which are rated as separate items. Detailed descriptions and examples of these phenomena are provided.

The sections on delusions and hallucinations contain items referring to specific types of these phenomena and, in addition, items designed to further define the nature of these symptoms. These extra items refer to the persistence, mood congruity, bizarreness, fragmentary nature and number of the hallucinations or delusions that have already been rated. Although an admirable device, the definitions provided, especially for multiple delusions and fragmentary delusions, may not be precise enough to allow confident rating.

For the SAPS and, to a lesser extent, the SANS, raters would need to be very familiar with the symptom definitions if they hoped to ask sufficiently detailed and systematic questions during the interview to allow the scales to be completed afterwards. Therefore, like the PSE, the administration of these scales requires a semi-structured, relatively formal, interview. As discussed above, the possible disadvantage of such an approach may be that it discourages the patient from confiding in the interviewer, and the more subtle interrogation of the free interview may be lost.

The SANS is based upon a particular conceptual view of negative symptoms, a group of schizophrenic features for which operational definitions have proved difficult to produce. Andreasen recognizes five sub-groups of negative features: Alogia, comprising poverty of speech, poverty of content of speech, blocking and increased speech latency; Affective flattening, including unchanging facial expression, decreased spontaneous movements, paucity of expressive gestures, affective non-responsivity and inappropriate affect; Avolition-Apathy, including impersistence at work and school, physical anergia and subjective complaints of avolition and apathy; Anhedonia-Asociality, including ratings of sexual interest and activity and ability to feel intimacy and closeness; and Attention, which includes social inattentiveness and subjective complaints of inattentiveness. Whether the items within each of these five categories constitute valid symptom groupings is open to debate. For example, the combination of poverty of content of speech, blocking and increased speech latency is less than convincing as a logical and clinically valid sub-syndrome. However, the individual items constitute a comprehensive assessment of negative symptoms, such as flattening of affect and poverty of speech, and the inclusion of items addressing the patient's subjective awareness of deficits revives a potentially valuable phenomenological approach to these symptoms which has been relatively ignored in the USA and the UK, despite consistent emphasis in the German literature (Huber, 1966; Koehler and Sauer, 1984).

The elements of anhedonia and social functioning referred to in the scale may comprise its specificity for schizophrenia. To qualify for a rating on the Subjective awareness of Anhedonia-Asociality item the patient must describe himself as having 'lost the ability to enjoy himself . . . to experience pleasure, or a loss of interest in relationships with others.' Many would consider such a phenomenon as a non-specific symptom, and it can certainly be a mark of depressive illness. Further, the Global Assessment Scale at the end of the

SANS seems to consider that the severity of negative schizophrenia is closely related to the level of social functioning, an assumption that remains largely untested.

OTHER SCALES INCLUDING THE ASSESSMENT OF NEGATIVE SYMPTOMS

Recent reviews conclude that the negative, or deficit, symptoms of schizophrenia do respond to antipsychotic drug treatment (Goldberg, 1985; Kane and Mayerhoff, 1989). These symptoms require reliable assessment in treatment studies and, in addition to the SANS already described, several scales designed for this purpose have been introduced in the last few years.

Positive and Negative Syndrome Scale (PANSS)

The use of the PANSS involves a 30–40-minute formalized psychiatric interview. A detailed rating manual is available (Kay *et al.*, 1986) which contains guidelines for the interview, including suggested questions for probing particular areas of psychopathology. For each item, a definition of the symptom is provided as well as detailed criteria for each rating level, from 1 (absent) to 7 (extreme).

As reflected in the title of this scale, the originators of this scale subscribe to the notion of two phenomenologically distinct syndromes within schizophrenia (Kay *et al.*, 1987; Kay *et al.*, 1988). Of the 30 items included in the PANSS, seven constitute a negative sub-scale: Blunted affect; Emotional withdrawal; Poor rapport; Passive/apathetic social withdrawal; Difficulty in abstract thinking; Lack of spontaneity and flow of conversation; and Stereotyped thinking. Seven items comprise a positive sub-scale and the remaining 16 items a general psychopathology sub-scale.

High inter-rater reliability and test–retest reliability have been demonstrated for the scale (Kay *et al.*, 1987, 1988). In addition, the PANSS shows a close correspondence with the Andreasen scales, SAPS and SANS, which Kay *et al.* (1988) present as a demonstration of criterion-related validity for the scale. Particularly, the negative syndrome of the PANSS was found to be highly correlated with the SANS. Further, the positive and negative syndrome sub-scales were found to be significantly inversely related, after adjustment for the overall level of severity of the illness, as measured by the general psychopathology sub-scale. The authors took this finding as an illustration of the mutually exclusive nature of the positive and negative syndrome ratings, and evidence for the construct validity of the sub-scales.

The Psychological Impairments Rating Scale (PIRS) and the Behavioural Observation Schedule (BOS)

The PIRS was originally designed to serve as a supplement to the PSE in a number of collaborative studies by the World Health Organization. It rates observed behaviour, and represents an elaboration of the final sections of the PSE covering behaviour, affect and speech (Jablensky *et al.*, 1980; Biehl *et al.*, 1989).

The total schedule contains 97 items divided into 10 sections. Four of these sections (Slowness/'psychic tempo', Attention/withdrawal, Fatiguability, and Initiative) are grouped under the title Activity/withdrawal, while the other six sections (Communication by facial expression, Communication by body language, Affect display, Conversation skills, Self-presentation, and Cooperation) are grouped as ratings of social skills. Each section has an Overall impression item rated from 0 (no disturbance) to 5 (maximum disturbance). Extensive training, involving both clinical interviews and prepared video tapes may be necessary to achieve an adequate level of inter-rater reliability (Biehl *et al.*, 1989).

Over the last decade, the scale has been used in many studies, particularly in the context of the World Health Organization Mental Health Programme. For example, Biehl *et al.* (1986) used the PIRS to assess impairment in a prospective, five-year study of a cohort of 70 first-onset schizophrenic patients. In this, as in most studies, the scale was employed in combination with a semi-structured interview such as the PSE.

Recently, the PIRS has been revised in response to a number of perceived problems (Atakan and Cooper, 1989). First, there was apparently a need for more detailed rating instructions and more precise definitions for many of the scale items. Secondly, there was possibly some overlap between some of the items, in that they might be rating the same behaviour. Thirdly, certain common aspects of observed behaviour were thought to be missing from the schedule. Lastly, the scale was considered to require reorganization so that the general order of the items corresponded more closely to the routine, clinical examination of the mental state. The authors claim that the new version, named the Behavioural Observation Schedule (BOS), includes observed behaviours seen in a wider range of psychiatric disorder than just the functional psychoses.

The High Royds Evaluation of Negativity (HEN)

This new scale (Mortimer *et al.*, 1989) was designed to be quick and easy to use, without the need for an informant. It places particular emphasis on the objective rating of disturbance of affect, with items for Constricted affect, Emotional withdrawnness and Shallow/coarsened affect. The description of this last symptom includes a caution to raters not to confuse it with inappropriate affect.

The scale essentially comprises 18 symptom ratings divided into six categories: Appearance; Behaviour; Speech; Thought, Affect; and Functioning. Each symptom is rated from 0 (absent) to 4 (severe). In addition, there is a global score item for each category and a summary score consisting of the sum of the six global scores. Good inter-rater reliability has been demonstrated (Mortimer *et al.*, 1989) and the 'face validity' of the scale established by showing a significant positive correlation with the ratings related to negative symptoms but not positive symptoms in the Social Behaviour Scale (SBS) of Wykes and Sturt (1986).

The Negative Symptom Rating Scale (NSRS)

The NSRS is a relatively short scale for rating negative symptoms in schizophrenia (Iager *et al.*, 1985). Each item is rated on a seven-point scale from 0 (normal) to 6 (severely impaired). While the scale covers symptoms included in other scales for negative symptoms, such as a lack of emotional response and amount of coherent speech, it also addresses less usual features such as the patient's ability to make decisions and judgements, and expressive relatedness, described as 'the spontaneity, amount and sincerity of interactions between the patient and others . . .' Also included in the scale are tests of cognitive functioning, with items for rating memory impairment, attention and orientation. Volition and motivation are assessed with items for grooming and self-care, degree of supervision and help required for tasks of daily living and the amount and speed of voluntary body movement.

Inter-rater reliability was found to vary between the items, with the best level of agreement being achieved with the cognitive items and speech content, and the poorest levels with the items for decision and judgement, grooming and expressive relatedness.

Subjective Experience of Deficits in Schizophrenia (SEDS)

This scale was designed principally to measure the subjective experience of negative symptoms, i.e. to evaluate patients' awareness of the disorganization or impoverishment of mental activity in schizophrenia which is more usually inferred from observation of behaviour (Liddle and Barnes, 1988). The SEDS consists of 21 items covering awareness of impairments and disturbances of thinking, emotion, drive and energy, perception, strain and voluntary movement. In a sample of chronic schizophrenic in-patients it proved possible to rate the various experiences with satisfactory inter-rater reliability.

CONCLUSION

The long scales described are not required if the aim is merely to identify improvement in the positive symptoms of schizophrenia. Brief scales are a practical and satisfactory alternative for this purpose, but have the disadvantage that they may miss other phenomena. It is the authors' view that the BPRS is perhaps the least satisfactory brief scale when compared with the Manchester Scale (MS), particularly because of the overlap of items, the lack of clear operational definitions and the lack of correspondence between items and the symptoms of schizophrenia. The SCS is good for evaluating change in florid psychotic symptoms but cannot be recommended in its present form because it omits hallucinatory and other acute phenomena, and negative symptoms, and thus important treatment effects may be missed. The MS provides perhaps the best compromise between brevity, specificity of schizophrenic symptoms, and sensitivity to change. It relies heavily on objective ratings of observable behaviour, and is therefore suitable for established schizophrenic patients for whom prolonged questioning is stressful and very often not particularly informative.

If the researcher has broader aims than just measuring change, or wishes to detect a treatment effect over as wide a range of well-defined symptoms as possible, a longer scale should be administered at the onset and completion of the trial. The IMPS is probably outmoded because of the inconsistency of the rating method and the lack of correspondence with clinically defined symptoms. The CPRS was designed specifically for clinical trials, and should be a sensitive and suitable scale to use in the early stages of assessment of a new psychotropic drug, looking at the range of treatment effects. Both the CASH (SAPS and SANS) and the PSE provide ratings of a comprehensive range of psychiatric symptoms, and both allow items to be condensed into syndromes of varying clinical relevance and validity. Because of its high threshold for rating symptoms the PSE would be appropriate for controlled trials of a putative antipsychotic drug in replication and confirmatory studies, and in studies where a precise description or profile of symptoms affected by the therapy is required.

In order to provide a record of the overall effect of treatment, including non-specific changes, comprehensive scales such as the GAS and the SAPS and SANS are worthy of consideration. Otherwise, the use of more than one scale is advisable.

In practice, all of the scales mentioned appear to have reasonable reliability and validity as measures of change, between raters at the same centre. The information yielded by the scales which involve more specific and discrete ratings should provide more accurate and comprehensive descriptions of patient samples. This is essential if the effects of treatment on psychopathology are to be investigated in a progressively more refined and accurate manner.

REFERENCES

Andreasen, N. C. (1979). Thought, language and communication disorders: I. Clinical assessment, definition of terms and evaluation of their reliability. *Arch. Gen. Psychiatry* **36**, 1315–1321.

Andreasen, N. C. (1979b). Affective flattening and the criteria for schizophrenia. *Am. J. Psychiatry* **136**, 944–947.

Andreasen, N. C. (1981). *Scale for the Assessment of Negative Symptoms (SANS)*, University of Iowa, Iowa. City.

Andreasen, N. C. (1982). Negative symptoms in schizophrenia: Definition and reliability. *Arch. Gen. Psychiatry* **39**, 784–788.

Asberg, M., Montgomery, S. A., Perris, C., Shalling, D. and Sedvall, G. (1978). The comprehensive psychopathological rating scale, *Acta Psychiatr. Scand. Suppl.* **271**, 5–27.

Atakan, Z. and Cooper, J. E. (1989). Behavioural Observation Schedule (BOS), PIRS 2nd Edition. *Br. J. Psychiatry* (supple.), in press.

Biehl, H., Maurer, K., Schubart, C., Krumm, B. and Jung, E. (1986). Prediction of outcome and utilization of medical services in a prospective study of first onset schizophrenics. *Eur. Arch. Psychiatry Neurol. Sci.* **236**, 139–147.

Biehl, H., Maurer, K., Jablensky, J. E., Cooper, J. E. and Tomov, T. (1989). The PIRS/WHO: I. Introducing a new instrument for rating observed behaviour and the rationale of the psychological impairment concept. *Br. Psychiatry* (supple.), in press.

Cairns, V., Faltermaier, T., Wittchen, H., Dilling, H., Mombour, W. and von Zerssen, D. (1982). Some problems concerning the reliability and structure of the scales in the Inpatient Multidimensional Psychiatric Scale (IMPS) *Arch. Psychiatr. Nervenkr.* **232**, 395–406.

Cooper, J. E., Kendell, R. E., Gurland, B. J., Sharpe, L., Copeland, J. R. M. and Simon, R. (1972). *Psychiatric Diagnosis in New York and London*, Oxford University Press, London.

Crow, T. J. (1980). Molecular pathology of schizophrenia: more than one disease process? *Br. Med. J.* **280**, 66–68.

Endicott, J., Spitzer, R. L., Fleiss, J. L. and Cohen, J. (1976). The global assessment scale, a procedure for measuring overall severity of psychiatric disturbance. *Arch. Gen. Psychiatry* **33**, 766–771.

Goldberg, D. P. (1972). *The Detection of Psychiatric Illness by Questionnaire*, Oxford University Press, London.

Goldberg, S. C. (1985). Negative and deficit symptoms in schizophrenia do respond to neuroleptics. *Schizophrenia Bull.* **11**, 453–456.

Hirsch, S. R., Gaind, R., Rhode, P. D., Stevens, B. C. and Wing, J. K. (1973). Outpatient maintenance of chronic schizophrenic patients with long acting phenothiazine: double-blind placebo trial. *Br. Med. J.* **i**, 633–637.

Huber, G. (1966). Reine Defectsyndrome und Basisstadien endogener Psychosen. *Fortschr. Neurol. Psychiatr.* **34**, 409–426.

Iager, A.-C., Kirch, D. G. and Wyatt, R. J. (1985). A negative symptom rating scale. *Psychiatry Res.* **16**, 27–36.

Jablensky, A., Schwartz, R. and Tomov, T. (1980). WHO collaborative study on impairments and disabilities associated with schizophrenic disorders. A preliminary communication: objectives and methods *Acta Psychiatr. Scand.* **62** (suppl. 285), 152–163.

Jacobsson, L., von Knorring, L., Mattsson, B., Perris, C., Edenius, B., Kettner, B.,

Magnusson, K. E. and Villemoes, P. (1978). The comprehensive psychopathological rating scale—CPRS—in patients with schizophrenic syndromes. Inter-rater reliability and in relation to Martens' S-scale. *Acta Psychiatr. Scand.* (suppl) **271**, 39–44.

Johnstone, E. C., Crow, T. J., Frith, C. D., Carney, M. W. P. and Price, J. S. (1978). Mechanism of the antipsychotic effect in the treatment of acute schizophrenia. *Lancet*, **i**, 848–851.

Kane, J. M. and Mayerhoff, D. (1989). Do negative symptoms respond to pharmacologic treatment? *Br. J. Psychiatry* (supple.), in press.

Kasa, M. and Hitomi, K. (1985). Inter-rater reliability of the Comprehensive Psychopathological Rating scale in Japan. *Acta Psychiatr. Scand.* **71**, 388–391.

Kay, S. R., Opler, L. A. and Fiszbein, A. (1986). *Positive and Negative Syndrome scale (PANSS) Rating Manual*, Department of Psychiatry, Albert Einstein College of Medicine Montefiore Medical Center, and Schizophrenia Research Unit, New York.

Kay, S. R., Fiszbein, A. and Opler, L. A. (1987). The Positive and Negative Syndrome Scale (PANSS) for schizophrenia. *Schizophrenia Bull.* **13**, 261.

Kay, S. R., Opler, L. A. and Lindenmayer, J.-P. (1988). Reliability and validity of the positive and negative syndrome scale for schizophrenics. *Psychiatry Res.* **23**, 99–110.

Kendell, R. E., Everitt, B., Cooper, J. E., Sartorius, N. and David, M. E. (1968). Reliability of the Present State Examination. *Soc. Psychiatry* **3**, 123.

Klett, C. J. and McNair, D. M. (1966). Reliability of the acute psychotic types. In *Explorations in Typing Psychotics* (M. Lorr, ed.), Pergamon Press, New York.

Knights, A., Hirsch, S. R. and Platt, S. D. (1980). Measurement of clinical change as a function of brief admission to hospital: a controlled study. *Br. J. Psychiatry* **137**, 170–180.

Koehler, K. and Sauer, H. (1984). Huber's basic symptoms: another approach to negative psychopathology in schizophrenia. *Comprehen. Psychiatry* **25**, 174–182.

Krawiecka, M., Goldberg, D. and Vaughan, M. (1977). A standardised psychiatric assessment scale for rating chronic psychotic patients. *Acta Psychiatr. Scand.* **55**, 299–308.

Liddle, P. F. and Barnes, T. R. E. (1988). The subjective experience of deficits in schizophrenia. *Comprehen. Psychiatry* **29**, 157–164.

Lorr, M. and Klett, C. J. (1967). *Inpatient Multidimensional Psychiatric Scale (IMPS)* (revised manual), Consulting Psychologists Press. Palo Alto, California.

Lorr, M. and Klett, C. J. (1968). Major psychotic disorders. A cross cultural study. *Arch. Gen. Psychiatry* **19**, 652–658.

Lorr, M., Klett, C. L., McNair, D. M. and Lasky, J. J. (1962). *Inpatient Multidimensional Psychiatric Scale. Psychiatric Scale Manual*, Consulting Psychologists Press, Palo Alto, California.

Lorr, M., Jenkins, R. L. and Holsopple, J. Q. (1953). Multidimensional scale for rating psychiatric patients. *VA Tech. Bull.* **10**, 507.

Luborsky, L. (1962). Clinicians' judgments of mental health. *Arch. Gen. Psychiatry* **7**, 407–417.

Luria, R. E. and Guziec, R. J. (1981). Comparative description of the SADS and PSE. *Schizophrenia Bull.* **7**, 248–257.

Manchanda, R. and Hirsch, S. R. (1981). (Des-Tyr-l)-gamma-endorphin in the treatment of schizophrenia. *Psychol. Med.* **11**, 401–404.

Manchanda, R. and Hirsch, S. R. (1986). Does propranolol have an antipsychotic

effect? A placebo controlled trial in acute schizophrenia. *Br. J. Psychiatry* **148**, 701–707.
Manchanda, R., Saupe, R. and Hirsch, S. R. (1986). Comparison between the Brief Psychiatric Rating Scale and the Manchester Scale for the rating of schizophrenic symptomatology. *Acta Psychiatr. Scand.* **74**, 563–568.
Mariotto, M. J. and Farrell, A. D. (1979). Comparability of the absolute level of ratings on the Inpatient Multidimensional Psychiatric Scale within a homogeneous group of raters. *J. Cons. Clin. Psychol.* **47**, 59–64.
Montgomery, S. A. and Asberg, M. (1978). A new depression scale designed to be sensitive to change. *Br. J. Psychiatry* **134**, 382–389.
Montgomery, S. A., Taylor, P. and Montgomery, D. (1978). Development of a schizophrenia scale sensitive to change. *Neuropharmacology* **17**, 1061–1063.
Mortimer, A., McKenna, P. J. and Lund, C. E. (1989). Rating of negative symptoms using the HEN scale. *Br. J. Psychiatry* (supple.), in press.
Myers, D. H., Campbell, P. L., Cocks, N. M., Flowerdew, J. A. and Muir, A. (1981). A trial of propranolol in chronic schizophrenia. *Br. J. Psychiatry* **139**, 118–121.
Newson-Smith, J. G. B. and Hirsch, S. R. (1979). Psychiatric symptoms in self-poisoning patients. *Psychol. Med.* **9**, 493–500.
Overall, J. E. (1974). The brief psychiatric rating scale in psychopharmacology research. In *Psychological Measurements in Psychopharmacology. Modern Problems in Pharmacopsychiatry* (P. Pichot, ed.), vol. 7, Karger, Basel, pp. 67–78.
Overall, J. E. and Gorham, D. R. (1962). The brief psychiatric rating scale. *Psychol. Rep.* **10**, 799–812.
Overall, J. E. and Gorham, D. R. (1963). A pattern probability model for classification of psychiatric patients. *Behav. Sci.* **8**, 108–116.
Owens, D. G. C. and Johnstone, E. C. (1980). The disabilities of chronic schizophrenia their nature and the factors contributing to their development. *Br. J. Psychiatry* **136**, 384–395.
Turner, W. J. (1963). *Glossaries for Use with the Overall and Gorham Brief Psychiatric Rating Scale and for a Modified Melamud-Sands Rating Scale*, Research Division Central Islip State Hospital, Central Islip, NY.
von Zerssen, D. and Cording, C. (1978). The measurement of change in endogenous affective disorders. *Arch. Psychiatry. Nervenkr.* **226**, 95–112.
Wiles, D. H., Kolakowska, T., McNeilly, A. S., Mandelbrote, B. M. and Gelder, M. G. (1976). Clinical significance of plasma chlorpromazine levels I. Plasma levels of the drugs, some of its metabolites and prolactin during treatment. *Psychol. Med.* **6**, 407–415.
Wing, J. K. (1983). Use and misuse of the Present State Examination. *Br. J. Psychiatry* **143**, 111–117.
Wing, J. K., Birley, J. L. T., Cooper, J. E., Graham, P. and Isaacs, A. (1967). Reliability of a procedure for measuring and classifying 'Present Psychiatric State'. *Br. J. Psychiatry* **113**, 499–575.
Wing, J. K., Cooper, J. E. and Sartorius, N. (1974). *The Measurement and Classification of Psychiatric Symptoms*, London, Cambridge University Press.
Wing, J. K., Nixon, J. M., Mann, S. A. and Leff, J. P. (1977). Reliability of the PSE (ninth edition) used in a population study. *Psychol.* **7**, 505–516.
World Health Organization (1973). *The International Pilot Study of Schizophrenia*, Geneva.
World Health Organization (1979). *Schizophrenia, An International Follow-up Study*. John Wiley, Chichester.

World Health Organization (1988). Benzodiazepines and therapeutic counselling: report from a WHO collaborative study. Berlin, Springer-Verlag.

Wykes, T. and Sturt, E. (1986). The measurement of social behaviour in psychiatric patients: an assessment of the reliability and validity of the SBS schedule. *Br. J. Psychiatry* **148**, 1–11.

Yorkston, N. J., Zaki, S. A., Malik, M. K. U., Morrison, R. C. and Havard, C. W. H. (1974). Propranolol in the control of schizophrenic symptoms. *Br. Med. J.* **iv**: 633–635.

Yorkston, N. J., Zaki, S. A., Weller, M. P., Gruzelier, J. H. and Hirsch, S. R. (1981). DL-propranolol and chlorpromazine following admission for schizophrenia. A controlled comparison. *Acta Psychiatr. Scand.* **63**, 13–27.

The Instruments of Psychiatric Research
Edited by C. Thompson

CHAPTER 4

Affective disorders

CHRIS THOMPSON
Southampton University,
Royal South Hants Hospital,
Southampton, UK

DEPRESSION RATING SCALES

Depression is a term which has a number of rather different meanings which must not be confused if sense is to be made of the literature on rating scales.

The first meaning is that of a mood, which may be normal. In this sense it is a synonym for plainer English terms such as sad, unhappy, miserable, low in spirits, blue or downhearted. Because there are a number of ways of describing the feeling it is possible to construct scales for the intensity of the mood using the various adjectives as items of the scale (e.g. Lubin, 1965). A number of such scales have been constructed for use in psychology rather than psychiatry but will not be covered in this volume as they do not relate to psychiatric conditions. Indeed their applicability to psychiatric populations in which there may be a quantitative difference in mood from the normal population is in itself dubious.

The second meaning of depression is a mood disorder which is a symptom, part of the syndrome of an affective disorder. In this case the words which have been used to describe the mood above may still be appropriate. However, as the disorder becomes more severe other aspects of the feeling may become more salient as descriptions. Thus patients may be 'near to tears' or weeping. They may go beyond weeping into a state of anhedonia, which many hold to be the core symptom of a depressive illness and one which predicts a good response to antidepressants. In this state nothing gives the patient any pleasure and nothing interests him or her.

Finally depression is also used as the name of a syndrome or syndromes of mental illness. In these syndromes the severe lowering of mood may be accompanied by a number of other features which can be categorised as follows:

1. Cognitive symptoms: negative thoughts about the self, the future and the state of the world (Beck, 1976). Patients feel themselves to be worthless, the future to be black and hopeless and the world to be in a parlous state. They feel that there is nothing they can do which would make any difference either to the world or to their own condition (helplessness). Sometimes these beliefs take on delusional proportions so that the patient becomes convinced that they are worthless, perhaps that their only hope is to die to make the world a better place. Other delusions which occur in depression are of poverty, guilt or physical illness.
2. Biological, vegetative or somatic symptoms: 'biological' is a poor term for these symptoms as presumably most psychiatrists would accept the premise that thought itself is a biological phenomenon. Although most of these symptoms relate to functions in which the hypothalamus or limbic system is probably involved it would undoubtedly be premature to call them hypothalamic symptoms. They include such things as reduced (or increased) appetite and weight, lowering of libido and energy, and poor sleep with both initial insomnia and early morning wakening (or sometimes hypersomnia). In females amenorrhoea occurs. Sometimes diurnal variation in mood is included with the vegetative symptoms as it tends to occur together with them. Somatic symptoms of excessive fatigue, muscular aches and pains and painful abdominal sensations might also be included.
3. Associated mood states: in 'neurotic' depression especially, the lowering of mood is accompanied by anxiety, sometimes to such a degree that it is difficult to know which is primary or more significant. Patients may describe a constant background of fear with somatic accompaniments, sudden and severe panic attacks apparently unrelated to external factors, or phobic disorders, especially agoraphobia.

   Irritability is also a frequent association of neurotic depression and anxiety, and can be described in rating scales as impatience, loss of temper or impending loss of control.
4. Psychomotor symptoms: two cardinal symptoms are agitation (inability to keep still—generally an observed phenomenon, although the patient may also be aware of it) and retardation (slowness to start and continue a movement or train of thought).

This list does not by any means exhaust the symptoms which accompany lowering of mood to form the various syndromes of depression. In general, studies have demonstrated the validity of separating out the syndrome of endogenous depression (e.g. Carney *et al.*, 1965) or Melancholia (American Psychiatric Association, 1980) from other types. It appears to have a greater loading in family pedigrees, an association with mania in some patients (bipolar disorder) and a better response to physical treatments than in non-endogenous syndromes (Raskin and Crook, 1976).

Hamilton (1976) has offered a typology of rating scales in depression in which they are divided into four categories:

1. For assessment of severity.
2. For making a diagnosis either of the presence of depression or of the subtypes, for example endogenous versus non-endogenous, major versus minor, primary versus secondary.
3. For assessing prognosis.
4. For selection of treatment.

Instruments which are designed for making a diagnosis of depression necessarily involve a more or less generalized psychiatric interview and therefore are dealt with in Ch. 2. However, some instruments are designed to diagnose particular syndromes of depression within a group, all of whom are depressed. These will be described here. Few scales have been devised to look specifically at prognosis or choice of treatment so most of the chapter will be concerned with rating scales of the severity of depression.

There are probably more scales available to carry out this task than for any other job in psychiatric research. Consequently there is a confusing array of eponymous and anonymous scales whose relative values and uses are debated. Many of them are developments of previously constructed and tested instruments which are claimed to be improvements in various ways. Sometimes it is impossible to tell why another scale should have been constructed. So much work has gone into constructing new scales and relatively little into validating them that Snaith (1981) has called for a moratorium on any further development until the value of the existing scales has been fully assessed. On the other hand Hamilton (1976) has stated that 'There can be no such thing as a best scale for all purposes in all circumstances and for use by all kinds of raters'. It is therefore important that the appropriate scale is selected from the variety available to do the job intended, and in the future more scales may become necessary to perform previously unthought of tasks. For example, the recent delineation of a putative syndrome of seasonal affective disorder (SAD) caused some difficulties with measurement of severity (Rosenthal *et al.*, 1984). This was because almost all patients with the syndrome suffered the so-called atypical vegetative symptoms of depression:

gain in appetite and weight, and hypersomnia. In order to measure change during treatment trials an addendum to the Hamilton Rating Scale had to be devised to take this into account, as the items for appetite, weight and sleep which make up a large proportion of the total score of the HDRS were keyed in the wrong direction (i.e. improvement of SAD symptoms would have been rated as worsening depression).

Rating scales for the severity of depression can be divided into those designed for self-rating and those to be completed by an observer.

Self-rated scales are not only concerned with depression but also frequently with anxiety and other neurotic symptoms. There is therefore some material in common with the chapter on anxiety (Ch. 5) and the chapter on self-rated scales of neurotic symptoms (Ch. 6). Self-rated scales for mixed mood disorder will be covered in Ch. 5.

Some instruments take into account both self-and observer-rated information on depression and these are included in a small separate section.

INSTRUMENTS FOR THE DIAGNOSIS OF DEPRESSION

We will start with a word about some diagnostic instruments. The main diagnostic systems and interview schedules which have been covered in Ch. 2 apply here, particularly Research Diagnostic Criteria, DSM-III, and the Present State Examination. However, there are some which are particularly applicable to depression. Where comparisons have been made between the systems generally fairly low concordances have been found because of differences in definition. For Example, Bech and Clemmesen (1983) found kappa coefficients of only 0.14–0.27 between the Newcastle scales and RDC or DSM-III.

It should also be noted that a threshold score from a severity scale is not the same as a diagnosis. For example, in 80 patients with a Hamilton Depression Score greater than 25 only 68% satisfied Feighner Criteria and 71% Research Diagnostic Criteria for major depressive disorder (Zisook *et al.*, 1980).

World Health Organization Schedule for Standardized Assessment of Depressive Disorders (WHO/SADD)

This assessment schedule aims to provide a single instrument for different uses—diagnosis, epidemiological studies, therapeutic trials, etc.—and to be reliable across a wide range of national and cultural boundaries. It is a partially standardized interview, training is not excessive and the administration is brief. The fifth revision is in four parts (Gastpar, 1983):

Part 1: identification and socio-demographic data.

Part 2: clinical description. This consists of 40 symptoms, each scored on a three-point scale (a) at the time of assessment and (b) for the entire episode. The psychiatric history, course of the illness, family and childhood history are also given. Particular attention is paid in this section to cross-cultural issues with the provision of a glossary.
Part 3: treatment in the present episode. As well as standard probes there is an open section to allow for culture-specific treatments.
Part 4: a severity score on a five-point scale. Diagnosis is given as a clinical one using local criteria and ICD-9.

Information from any available source may be used to complete the items.

The schedule has been used in the WHO collaborative study on the assessment of depressive disorders (Sartorius *et al.*, 1980). For part 2 the inter-rater reliabilities were high: between centres, 0.88 (including different languages and cultures), and within centres, 0.96.

A factor analysis of the results yielded two dominant factors of endogenous and psychogenic depression, but in all 15 factors could account for only 50% of the variance. Bech *et al.* (1980) have worked out a system of making Newcastle scores from the WHO/SADD instrument, either for the first Newcastle (Carney *et al.*, 1965) or the revision (Gurney, 1971). However, they did encounter some difficulties in the translation of one to the other, so that the two systems of diagnosis of endogenous depression cannot be regarded as equivalent.

Newcastle Scales

Several scales have been produced by the group around Roth in Newcastle (Roth *et al.*, 1983). It is therefore rather confusing to refer to any or all of them as the Newcastle scales. They are all concerned with making diagnostic distinctions between endogenous and reactive depression, or anxiety and depression, or with predicting treatment response. The first (Carney *et al.*, 1965) was a scale to separate endogenous from neurotic depression and was based on the results of a discriminant function analysis. Some items also related to ECT response, although sometimes with different loadings (Table 1). A score of 6 or more indicates endogenous depression. A similar severity score using the Hamilton Depression Rating Scale has been found for groups of both types, suggesting that the scale does not simply reflect severity of depression (Bech *et al.*, 1980). For the related ECT scale a score of 1 or more suggests a good response and 0 or less a poor response.

The second Newcastle scale (Gurney, 1971) contains fewer items but also separates endogenous from neurotic depression. There has been prolonged debate about the validity of this type of approach to classification, but the scale continues to be used and its validity appears to have been enhanced

Table 1. Weights for deriving diagnostic and ECT indices (Carney *et al.*, 1965)

Clinical features	Diagnostic index	ECT index
Adequate personality	+1	
No adequate psychogenesis	+2	
Distinct quality to mood	+1	
Previous episode	+1	
Depressive psychomotor activity	+2	
Nihilistic delusions	+2	
Guilt	+1	
Blame others	−1	
Weight loss	+2	+3
Anxiety	−1	−2
Pyknic build		+3
Early wakening		+2
Somatic delusions		+2
Paranoid delusions		+1
Worse in afternoon		−3
Self-pity		−1
Hypochondriacal		−3
Hysterical		−3

by studies showing a relationship between Newcastle scores and biological markers of depression such as the growth hormone response to clonidine (Checkley *et al.*, 1984) and the dexamethasone suppression test (DST; Holden, 1983). Inter-rater reliability is high, around 0.90 (Bech *et al.*, 1980). Both the indices tabulated above predict response to ECT, although the ECT index is the better (Carney *et al.*, 1965). The ECT scale also predicts the outcome with tricyclic antidepressants and predicts ECT outcome better than the DST (Katona and Aldridge, 1983).

Thus these scales appear to have some biological validity and predictive validity. Although the premise on which they were originally based (the idea that if a bimodal distribution of scores were to be found it would indicate that there were two distinct types of depression) may not have been sound the scales continue to be used, especially in studies of the biology of depression. Here it is particularly useful as it is a relatively strict criterion of endogenous depression in comparison with Research Diagnostic Criteria or DSM-III, identifying fewer patients as having endogenous depression.

Multi-Axial Classification of Affective Disorders (MULTICLAD)

This system was devised by Rafaelsen *et al.* (1983) to standardize assessment, particularly in psychopharmacological studies. There are three axes: (a) symptoms (inclusion and exclusion criteria); (b) course (from a representative selection of episodes the probability of manic-depression, the polarity of the illness and any atypical features are defined); and (c) the response to treatment. The aims were to identify a nuclear manic-depressive group, to differentiate unipolar and bipolar illnesses and to identify atypical, schizo-affective and possible manic-depressives; and melancholia, possible melancholia and non-melancholia. It has a glossary like the Present State Examination. For diagnosis of the episode it has an inter-rater agreement of about 80%.

While this system has been particularly used in Scandinavia there is no reason why it should not translate into psychiatry in other countries. The main problem for any of these systems is the variety of competing systems which are already 'on the market'.

AMDP Scales

The Association for Methodology and Documentation in Psychiatry (Pietzecker and Gebhart, 1983) came from German and Swiss groups aiming to develop a comprehensive system for data collection in the clinic and in research. Unlike the American ECDEU (Early Clinical Drug Evaluation Unit), which incorporated a variety of already existing instruments, the AMDP group set out to develop their own from scratch. The system covers all diagnoses and has a global reliability of approximately 0.86.

A factor analysis of large groups of unselected clinic attenders yielded eight syndromes, of which one was depressive. The authors claim that 67–88% of patients with depression can be accurately classified as endogenous or neurotic using a discriminant function. Correlations of 0.6–0.7 between HDRS scores and AMDP syndromes of retarded depression or manic-depression have been found. Similarly high correlations between the Comprehensive Psychopathological Rating Scale (CPRS) scores of depressive syndrome and the AMDP scales of apathy (0.81), somatic depression (0.84), retarded depression (0.89), hypochondriasis (0.83) and manic-depressive syndrome (0.94) have been found.

However, the depression diagnostic categories have been found to be no more valid than those of the ICD-9 (which is only intended as a classifactory system, not a diagnostic one). In addition, it is difficult to see why a researcher who wishes to measure, say, recent life event incidence and the symptoms of depression, should tie themselves to the AMDP for both, when there may be better validation information about other instruments. In other words the goal of *comprehensive* assessment may be neither desirable nor, in the end, achievable.

OBSERVER-RATED SCALES OF SEVERITY OF DEPRESSION

Hamilton Depression Rating Scale (HDRS)

Hamilton first described his rating scale for depression in 1960. Although there had been a number of rating scales devised before this time Hamilton's was the first to be widely accepted and put to use. The Cronholme–Ottosson scale had been devised for a study of the efficacy and mode of action of ECT (Cronholme and Ottosson, 1960) and had achieved some popularity, but unlike Hamilton's scale it was not designed primarily to assess a wide range of depressive symptoms in a wide range of contexts. Other scales were aimed at normal mood (Costello and Comfrey, 1967) and still others were aimed at personality traits (e.g. the MMPI-D scale).

The original description (Hamilton, 1960) was of a 17-item scale to be completed by a skilled psychiatrist. It is unsuitable for use by non-psychiatrically trained personnel, as its completion requires a considerable exercise of clinical skill. Information about the patient may be acquired from any number of sources and used to make the ratings, in addition to information obtained at interview. The state of the patient over the previous few days is taken into account. It should only be used with already diagnosed depressive illness and hence can be regarded as squarely within the medical tradition, i.e. no continuity between normal and depressive mood is assumed.

The Hamilton scale is not accompanied by standardized interview questions, so that the 'information variance' (see Ch. 1) is uncontrolled and depends upon the interviewer's skill. The criterion variance is controlled as far as possible by the provision of a rough glossary of terms, and a description of the meaning of each level of severity. Where possible each grade of severity is tied to an objective criterion but for some items this is not possible and the rater has to decide for himself the meaning of 'mild, moderate or severe'. The time needed for completion varies from 10 to 30 minutes.

The item bias (i.e. those aspects of the syndrome which are best sampled by the items) is somatic (see Ch. 1, Table 1). Thus there is a maximum score of 4 for depressed mood plus a further 4 for psychic anxiety. Depressive thought content items (guilt, suicide and hypochondriasis) together make up a maximum score of 12, while vegetative symptoms (insomnia, appetite, weight, libido, fatigue and somatic anxiety symptoms) make up a maximum score of 18, and psychomotor symptoms a further 6. A total failure to continue with work or interests scores 4, and lack of insight scores 2.

Hamilton (1960) recommends that two raters see each patient and that the sum of the two scores be used. When only one rater is available the score should be doubled. This latter procedure seems rather pointless, and the former appears unnecessary in view of the high inter-rater reliability which has been found in several studies. Many studies when reporting Hamilton scores do not specify whether they have been doubled, are the sum of two raters or are single-rater raw scores. This can be crucial to the interpretation of the study. The maximum total score for a single rater is 50 and for two raters 100.

As well as these 17 items which together make up the severity score, Hamilton (1969) provides four more. Diurnal variation is included here because it is a feature which helps to make a diagnosis of endogeneous depression but does not contribute to severity. One might also question the validity of loss of insight (17) as a severity item. Symptoms which are sometimes present in association with depression but also do not give any information of severity, or occur infrequently, are included for interest. These are depersonalization (19), paranoid thinking (20) and obsessionality (21).

Many modifications exist of Hamilton's scale. Sometimes the modifications have been made for one study only and these are often poorly described. Other modifications offer clear advantages in particular respects and have become established instruments in their own right (e.g. Paykel, 1985). Hamilton's scale is still probably the most used in depression research for describing levels of severity in different groups of subjects, to ensure adequate matching (e.g. Checkley *et al.*, 1984), or to measure improvements during treatment trials. The adequacy of the Hamilton scale for these purposes will now be assessed on the relevant criteria.

Validity

To be a valid measure of severity of depression the score should accurately reflect different grades of severity of illness. This has been examined in two ways. The crudest way is to look at the mean scores of several different populations of depressed patients who are assumed on a priori grounds to have different levels of severity. Thus, patients seen in general practice, in out-patients, and as in-patients might be assumed to have ascending levels of severity. There are of course several problems with an assumption of this kind but it suffices as one of several validiating criteria. Schwab *et al.* (1967a) found in a group of 163 patients with either medical or depressive diagnoses that the two groups were clearly separable on the basis of the Hamilton scores. Carroll *et al.* (1973) looked at three groups of depressed patients, drawn from general practice, day-patient care and in-patient wards. The total sample was 67 patients and the HDRS was found to distinguish significantly between each group of patients. This result was in contrast to the failure on the same task of the Zung self-rating depression scale.

The second and potentially more sophisticated measure of validity is to compare the scores on the scale against psychiatrists' global ratings of severity. A high correlation between the two scores shows that the HDRS is a fairly true reflection of clinical judgements. This procedure has been used many times to validate the HDRS, with generally good results. Zealley and Aitken (1969) found a pretreatment correlation with global severity of 0.90, falling to 0.55 after treatment. However, Welner (1972) obtained a correlation of only 0.48 with a five-point global severity scale. Bech *et al.* (1975a) in a thorough piece of work found the correlation to be 0.84, and Knesevich *et al.* (1977) found 0.89 using a ten-point global scale. Montgomery and Asberg (1979) found a low correlation of only 0.59, although the sample size was comparatively small ($N = 35$), and Feinberg *et al.* (1981) obtained a correlation of 0.77. The generally good results lead to the question of the possibility of error in the global judgements in those studies obtaining lower correlations. This interpretation is strengthened when one considers the high face validity of the Hamilton, and the uncertainty surrounding the criteria on which psychiatrists make global judgements.

Concurrent validity can be assessed by correlating the HDRS scores with other rating scales on the same patients. Many comparisons are available. However, in the majority of cases the HDRS was being used as a validating criterion for the newer often self-rating scale, and clearly it would be inadmissible to claim these figures as evidence for the validity of the HDRS. It suffices to say that against other observer rating scales the concurrent validity is high (e.g. Kearns *et al.*, 1982) and against self-rating scales somewhat lower, although this may be due to the relative unreliability of the latter (Hedlund and Vieweg, 1979a).

The inter-rater *reliability* of the Hamilton scale is also consistently high. The first reported value was 0.90 (Hamilton, 1960). This result used the procedure of two raters independently scoring the same interview and probably maximizes the similarity of the ratings by making the same information available to each rater, a fact of importance for a scale like the Hamilton which has no interview schedule attached. Knesevich *et al.* (1977) obtained a similar result of 0.94 using the same procedure. Bech *et al.* (1975a) reported inter-rater correlations varying from 0.88 to 0.98. Hedlund and Vieweg (1979a) in a review of studies to that date found reported inter-rater reliabilities of 0.87–0.98, but criticized most of the available studies on methodological grounds.

A type of validity which is of some importance for rating scales of severity is their *sensitivity to change*. How accurately are changes in the patient's clinical state reflected by changes in rating scale scores? This can be examined by correlating change in global scores during treatment with change in scale scores. Knesevich *et al.* (1977) found the Hamilton scores to correlate 0.68 with change in global rating on a ten-point scale. This was slightly worse than the Bech six-item melancholia subscale of the Hamilton (see below), which correlated 0.72. Bech *et al.* (1975a) obtained a figure of 0.73 using a similar tequnique with an 11-point scale. Montgomery and Asberg (1979) in the construction and validation of their own scale, which was specifically intended to be sensitive to change, found the HDRS to be less sensitive to change than their own scale (MADRS), especially at the severe end of the range. This lack of sensitivity at the upper end of the range was also found by Knesevich *et al.* (1977). Correlation with change in global rating within each severity range was 0.49 for mild depression (median score 10), 0.52 for moderate (median score 13.5) and only 0.38 for severe (median score 23.5). Bailey and Coppen (1976) found it to be more sensitive to change than Beck's self-rating depression inventory, although other studies have found them to be roughly equivalent (see Hedlund and Vieweg, 1979a).

How *internally consistent* is the Hamilton rating scale? In other words how valid is the operation of summing the separate item scores to give a single score for severity? This can be approached in a number of ways: (1) factor analysis; (2) item total correlations; and (3) Rasch modelling (Rasch, 1960).

1. Factor analysis is a way of apportioning the variance in scores along dimensions. The first dimension or factor found by Hamilton (1960) appeared to be tapping the variance due to retardation and items associated with it. The second factor had loadings on agitation but depressed mood did not contribute to this factor. Two other factors were isolated but did not appear to have a great deal of clinical relevance. On the basis of these results it would appear that the factor structure of the scale bears little relationship to clinical practice. However, a subsequent study by Hamilton (1967) gave more satisfactory results. Separating males and females into two groups, he found both genders to have two major factors which accounted for almost all the variance. The first appeared to be a factor of general severity, as all items loaded positively, confirming the validity of summing scores by showing a predominantly unidimensional structure. It correlated 0.93 with the total 17-item score. The second factor was bipolar, with anxiety and agitation at one pole and retardation and suicidal ideation at the other.

   Mowbray's (1972b) factor analysis produced a similar result, with the first factor in both sexes being one of general severity. However, only males showed the bipolar second factor which was isolated by Hamilton, while females had different, and clinically uninterpretable, factors of low saturation. Feinberg *et al.* (1981) confirmed the severity dimension as the first factor and showed that the Carroll Rating Scale which was designed to be a direct self-rating equivalent of the Hamilton had a similar structure. Bech (1981) in a review of these factor studies commented that they shed little light on the dimensions of depression because of the divergent results and the different populations used. However, it can be stated that, using factor analysis, most studies (seven were found by Hedlund and Vieweg in their review, 1979a) isolate a dominant factor of general severity, which enhances the credibility of the scale as a unidimensional measure of severity. In fact factor scores themselves have not been found to be useful over and above the total score.

2. Item total correlations: in this technique each item score is correlated with the total score. If a large number of items fail to correlate significantly it suggests that the scale may be measuring more than one dimension of illness. In this case the meaning of a moderate score is uncertain as it may be caused by illness in one of the several different dimensions which are tapped by the scale. Schwab *et al.* (1967a) found the item total correlations to vary from 0.45 to 0.78 in his group of depressed medical patients. This is higher than for the Beck Depression Inventory (0.32–0.61) but the effect of using medical rather than psychiatric patients is unknown.
3. Bech *et al.* (1981) has carried out some of the most sophisticated testing of the Hamilton scale using the Rasch statistical models of objectivity. These models examine the question of how (a) homogeneous and (b) transferable a scale is. Homogeneity refers to internal consistency, i.e. does the scale measure only one variable? Application of the Rasch models produced poor results for homogeneity, while the six-item subscale derived by Bech *et al.* (1975a) in a previous study fared better.

   Transferability refers to the ability of a scale to measure the severity of the variable in any situation or population, regardless of, for example, diagnosis or severity. Initial data on this question were encouraging. Carney and Sheffield (1972) showed that in a large group of depressed patients the severity scores of Newcastle endogenous and non-endogenous depressed patients (see Newcastle scale) were equal. This was initially confirmed by Bech *et al.* (1980). However, using the Rasch models Bech *et al.* (1981) showed poor transferability across categories of age, sex, diagnosis and severity. Once again the six-item Bech subscale performed better.

Montgomery–Asberg Depression Rating Scale (MADRS)

This scale was specifically designed for use in treatment studies, to be sensitive to change (Montgomery and Asberg, 1979). The items were drawn from the Comprehensive Psychopathological Rating Scale (CPRS) as used in a number of antidepressant drug trials (Asberg *et al.*, 1978).

The 17 most commonly occurring items from the CPRS were entered into the pilot scale. The score on these items correlated 0.89 with global ratings (seven-point scale) and 0.94 with the HDRS, thus confirming a high validity. Each item was then assessed further on two criteria:

1. Mean change in score during the treatment trials of a variety of antidepressants.
2. Correlation of the change in item score with the total change in 17-item CPRS score.

The items were ranked on each criterion and the two ranks were summed for each item. The ten items with the highest sum of ranks were then entered into the final version. This technique attempts to balance sensitivity and validity as a measure of depression (rather than of side effects).

The inter-rater reliabilities for various groups (psychiatrists versus GPs, English versus Swedish) ranged from 0.89 to 0.97, suggesting that it may be useful in cross-national studies and usable by non-expert raters. With only seven items it is relatively brief and quick (Montgomery *et al.*, 1978).

Change scores for the ten-item and 17-item versions and the HDRS all distinguished the responders from the non-responders in a drug trial. However, a power calculation showed that in order to find a difference between placebo and active drug conditions at a given level of significance 28 patients would have been required using the HDRS but only 19 using the MADRS. It is therefore about half as sensitive again as the HDRS. This has implications not only for economy in trials but also for their ethics—the fewer patients required in a study the better. All items are core symptoms of depression, so the construction of the scale succeeded in ensuring high face validity.

Kearns *et al.* (1982) found the MADRS to distinguish significantly between all levels of severity on a five- and six-point global rating scale and to perform this task as well as the HDRS. It was better than the HDRS for distinguishing moderate from severe depression. However, the information access or item bias is different. The MADRS contains no items for somatic or psychomotor symptoms. This lack of somatic bias also suggests the use of the MADRS in studies of physically unwell depressed patients (see also Hospital Anxiety and Depression Inventory, Ch. 5).

Snaith and Taylor (1985) found a high correlation between the MADRS, the depression scales of the self-rated Hospital Anxiety and Depression Inventory (HAD, 0.81) and the Irritability Depression Anxiety Questionnaire (IDA, 0.72). The corresponding correlations with the anxiety scales of these instruments were low (HAD = 0.37, IDA = 0.36), thus confirming the specificity of the scale and its validity as a measure of the severity of depression. These authors demonstrated that the validity and specificity could be further enhanced by the removal of two items. However, the effect of this on the main function for which the scale was devised, i.e. to be sensitive to change, was not examined.

The MADRS is becoming a regular inclusion in antidepressant studies and appears to deserve its more prominent position on methodological and ethical grounds. The cross-cultural genesis of the scale has led to its increasing use further afield and Dratcu *et al.* (1987) have reported its satisfactory use in Brazil.

Bech–Rafaelsen Melancholia Scale (BRMS)

This scale was initially derived by an examination of each item of the HDRS on three criteria (Bech *et al.* 1981):

1. Calibration: each item should occur sufficiently often in the populations being tested to warrant inclusion. An arbitrary cut-off of 10% was adopted.
2. Ascending monotonicity: each item should correlate significantly with the global clinical assessment.
3. Dispersion: each item should have little dispersion about the regression line with the global clinical assessment. This is a test of reliability.

Only six individual items from the HDRS survived these tests, although it must be emphasized that the results are very dependent upon the population observed. This is not so much the case with the Rasch models, which were used to confirm the adequacy of this six-item subscale, described below.

The six items selected in this way were:

1. Depressed mood
2. Suicidal thoughts
3. Loss of interest and inability to work
4. Retardation
5. Psychic anxiety
6. General somatic symptoms

These are the six items which correlate best with the global score and together make up an extremely homogeneous scale. Knesevich *et al.* (1977) found the scores on these items to correlate 0.89 with global ratings and the change in score to correlate 0.72 with the change in global score. However, in this study, the same workers may have made both sets of assessments (Snaith, 1977). Knesevich *et al.* (1977) also found that the six-item scale had no greater validity than a scale made up of the 11 items which had been taken out. However, Bech criticizes this study because of the high scores obtained by the group as a whole, which was composed of out-patients. He argues that such severity in out-patients means that the group had a high number of non-specific symptoms and were therefore unusual or atypical depressives.

Kearns *et al.* (1982) compared the six-item scale with the full HDRS for sensitivity against various global rating scales, utilizing different numbers of grades of severity. Using five grades the six-item scale distinguished moderate and severe depression better than did the full scale. However, this advantage was lost when six grades were used in the global rating. In further development Bech *et al.* (1981) applied the Rasch models to the scale and found that the item for general somatic symptoms was inadequate. However, within the mild to moderate range of severity this item did appear to be satisfactory, so it was retained. The inter-rater reliability of the scale is similar to the full HDRS.

Bech then wished to create two companion scales of similar content to measure symptoms of both melancholia and mania, which together would be useful for following changes in symptoms during manic-depressive illness, or for quantifying severity in mixed affective disorder, a condition in which the patient has symptoms of both mania and depression at the same time, or in rapid succession. The mania scale had already been developed and had 11 items, six of which matched, but were the opposite of, the corresponding items of the melancholia scale. The missing five items were added to form an 11-item melancholia scale which now is referred to as the Bech–Rafaelson Melancholia Scale (BRMS; Bech, 1981; Bech and Rafaelsen, 1980).

The BRMS has been used in a number of antidepressant studies. Like the HDRS it requires psychiatrically trained raters to give adequate results. Results using this newer scale correlate 0.96 with the older six-item scale derived from the Hamilton. The Rasch models have been applied to the 11-item scale and it does appear to fulfil the criteria, as the smaller six-item scale did (Maier and Phillip, 1985). A score of 15 or more indicates severity in the region of major depressive disorder (Bech and Clemmesen, 1983). Bech *et al.* (1986) provided a glossary for the items and included both the BRMS and the HDRS items side by side, making it simple to obtain scores on both scales.

Clinical Interview for Depression

A review of the development and use of this scale has been given by Paykel (1985) and will be followed in the present description.

The scale consists of items covering the range of symptoms of depression and anxiety and was developed from a modification of the Hamilton scale. It is in the format of a semi-structured interview, and contains 36 items, each rated on a seven-point scale. Seven points were chosen because the failure of raters to use the end points causes constriction of values when ratings are to be used to assess change. When seven items are included five of them may be used regularly. Each point is anchored with a definition. One item is rated on a four-point scale (Depressive delusions). Most ratings are made on the basis of the average intensity in the previous week, but some are rated on maximal intensity as reported by the patient. Other items are rated on observable behaviour only.

It takes 30–40 minutes to complete, although a short form is available which takes only 20 minutes. A Hamilton Rating Scale score can be derived from the same interview with the addition of a few extra questions. Some training is needed but this only involves interviewing about ten patients.

The reliability for trained raters is good. Mean item correlations are around 0.81, and 95% of ratings are within one point of the other rater. Two subscores can be derived, one for anxiety and the other for depression, in addition to the overall total score. The item–total correlations for the two subscales are comparable with the Hamilton Rating Scale. Factor analysis yields a general factor of severity, with a second factor discriminating endogenous and neurotic symptoms. A third factor contrasts depressive and anxiety symptoms.

The interview has been used in a number of outcome studies and has shown itself able to detect changes, although it has not been compared with other scales in the same study, unlike the MADRS (Montgomery and Asberg, 1979). The concurrent validity is high. The depression scale correlates 0.53–0.70 with the HDRS, 0.54–0.73 with the Raskin Three-area Depression Scale, and 0.62–0.71 with a global severity score of depression. The anxiety scale correlations with these scores are lower, indicating satisfactory independence of scores. The correlations between items and the corresponding items of the HDRS range from 0.52 to 0.92.

The instrument has been used in a wide range of studies. It has the advantage of a broad spread of items, for use in descriptive studies, and a seven-point scoring for each item, making it sensitive to change. It is argued, with some justification by the scale's architects, that no other instrument combines these properties. On the other hand an instrument of this length may be thought to be too comprehensive for the measurement of change during an antidepressant trial in many centres.

Miller Modification of the HDRS

Hamilton specified that the HDRS was for use by trained psychiatrists; however, in many cases this requires an expenditure of time beyond the resources of the department carrying out the research. Apart from using self-rating scales, with their attendant disadvantages, the only alternative would be to use partially trained raters. Miller *et al.* (1985) modified the HDRS in three ways to make it suitable for use by para-professional staff. First, they modified the rating points to make more specific the criteria for making each level of rating. Second, they provided standard prompt questions for each item, thus turning it into an interview (and inevitably removing some information on which ratings would be made using the HDRS). Third, they added some items to take into account symptoms now thought to be important and appearing in other scales or diagnostic manuals (e.g. DSM-III; American Psychiatric Association, 1980).

The reliability of this new scale in the hands of para-professional users was 0.94 for the 25-item version and 0.93 for a 17-item version containing the same items as the original HDRS (Miller *et al.*, 1985). The 17 items had individually excellent reliability (0.75–1.0), seven had good reliability (0.60–0.74) and one was fair (psychic anxiety 0.40–0.59).

Against expert raters the para-professionals also fared well. With agitation and retardation removed, because of the use of audiotapes for rating, the correlations were 0.93 for 23 items and 0.80 for the 15 remaining items of the original HDRS. The correlation with the original HDRS, performed in the usual way by expert raters, was 0.84 for the relevant 17 items. Correlation with Beck's Depression Inventory was 0.62 for the full 25-item scale and 0.58 for the 17 items from the original HDRS. These figures are similar to the correlation with the HDRS itself (0.51–0.74).

Thus it appears that this interview version of the HDRS is valid and reliable as a measure of depression severity when used by non-psychiatrists. It has been little tested as yet in the field and further validation and reliability studies are necessary before it can be recommended for use as the sole measure of depression severity in any study. In addition it is in direct competition with Paykel's Clinical Interview for Depression (CID), which is also a modification of the HRS, and has been regularly and successfully used by non-psychiatric raters (Paykel, 1985). The sensitivity to change of the Miller version is unknown.

Bunney–Hamburg Mood Check-list

This is an observer-rated scale of several mood states, not just depression, which was designed for use by ward nurses to show day to day changes in mood during in-patient trials, and for studies of the natural history of cyclic disorders in particular. There are 24 items, which are rated on 15-point scales from absent to very high (Bunney and Hamburg, 1963). Some items have the grading points objectively specified while others constitute global ratings. Six areas of behaviour are dealt with: depression, anger, anxiety, psychotic behaviour, somatic complaints and pacing behaviour. A glossary of definitions and instructions for rating were constructed.

Inter-rater reliability was found to be variable and was quite low at the extremes of the scales. Agreement on the 24 items varied from 0.11 to 0.83. Anger was particularly poorly agreed upon. The most prominent example of its use was a paper by Goodwin *et al.* (1970) and it remains poorly validated against work in other centres. The reliability data are not encouraging.

Cronholme–Ottosson Scale

The Cronholme–Ottosson Scale was developed to measure change in a trial of ECT (Cronholme and Ottosson, 1960). It was used in several investigations in the 1960s and has a satisfactory reliability in the hands of trained raters as reported by d'Elia *et al.* (1969) in Asberg *et al.* (1973). It was modified (Asberg *et al.*, 1973; Cronholme *et al.*, 1974) with a view to designing a scale for use across several different nationalities. Behind this attempt was the need to reduce the number of cross-national replications of pharmacological studies which failed for technical psychometric reasons.

The original scale of eight items was translated into English and Danish from its original Swedish. The original range of rating for each item from 0 to 3 was retained but half points were inserted, and a glossary was provided to indicate how ratings should be made. The eight items were:

Depressed mood
Anxiety
Death wish–suicidal intent
Depressive thought content
Hypochondriacal ideas
Sleep disturbance
Intellectual retardation (inefficient thinking)
Emotional retardation (anhedonia)
Psychomotor retardation

Two raters of different nationalities rated each patient at the same interview. Seventy-one patients of the three nationalities were interviewed. Inter-rater reliabilities varied for each item from 0.51 to 1.0, a result which was not improved by further training of raters. The reliability of the summed score was 0.86–0.97. The total score correlated 0.87 with nurses' ratings of depression, and 0.63 with the Beck Depression Inventory. Thus, this scale appears to be well transferred across these particular national and linguistic boundaries.

However, it must be remembered that this was not a stringent test of the scale's potential, for several reasons. The ratings were done at the same interview; the raters were presumably bilingual in order to understand the patients' responses; and these three languages and cultures are not so dissimilar as has been the case in other cross-cultural studies of rating instruments, such as the PSE. Nevertheless for the specific task of supplying results which can be interpreted easily in other countries it is a promising result.

This scale has, however, been somewhat overtaken by the development of a WHO scale designed for the same purpose (Sartorius *et al.*, 1980).

MIXED OBSERVER–SELF-RATING SCALES

Raskin Three-Area Depression Rating Scale

This instrument, consisting of three parts, was developed for a factor analytical study of the symptoms of depression (Raskin *et al.*, 1969, 1970) but has been used as a comprehensive measure of change (e.g. Raskin *et al.*, 1969). The three areas referred to are interview ratings, self-ratings and behavioural ratings of depressive signs.

The interview scale was developed from the Hopkins symptom check-list (Frank *et al.*, 1957). It consisted of 43 items, each rated on a seven-point discomfort scale, and called the Inventory of Psychic and Somatic Complaints (IPSC).

Fifteen extra items were added to this for the self-rating instrument, and the responses were put into an appropriate form. The extra items all related to specific somatic complaints. Another part of the self-rating procedure was a 52-item mood adjective check-list. The items in this section were gleaned from a variety of sources, but particularly those in which the adjectives had been shown to be sensitive to change.

The behaviour rating scale was a 141-item version of the Ward Behaviour Rating Scale (Burdock *et al.*, 1960). Each item was rated on a four-point frequency of occurrence scale.

Clearly this scale is a most appropriate instrument for studies of the factor structure of depressive symptoms, and the results have proved to be highly replicable. However, as a measure of change in a therapeutic trial it is a hammer to crack a walnut when the reliability and validity of simpler instruments is good.

Wechsler Depression Rating Scale

This scale was devised in 1963 and hardly appears to have been used in practice or further developed. The HDRS allows the information on which ratings are made to come from observations, reports of the patient, reports of the nursing staff or anywhere else. Wechsler *et al.* (1963) made an attempt to control this by creating a scale in which, for each item, the source of the information would be specified.

It is a 28-item scale, each item being rated on a three- to six-point scale. Fourteen items deal with the patient's attitudes and feelings, and five with the patient's reports of physiological function, e.g. sleep. Nine are observer-rated. The maximum score is 131 and the minimum 28. In the initial study Wechsler obtained inter-rater reliabilities of 0.88 with simultaneous ratings ($N = 22$) and 0.78 when ratings were made one week apart. In another sample, mean inter-rater reliability was 0.67, although ratings made on the same day only achieved 0.52. This may have been due to diurnal variation in mood, although it is impossible to tell as no item is included for diurnal variation. Giving normative data, Wechsler found that 80% of non-depressives scored below 69, while 80% of depressives scored above 70. Median figures of grades of severity were: mild = 67, moderate = 79, and severe = 93.

Mowbray has commented (1972a) that the scale does not include diurnal variation or reduced libido, and does not differentiate between agitation and retardation. In addition, a large number of items deal with failure to cope socially, which is not specific for depression. Furthermore, the distinction between observer- and self-rated items produces some interesting anomalies which are not suffered by the permissive system of the HDRS. For example, in the item on self-reported physiological change, a patient sometimes may report difficulty sleeping while the staff have definitely observed a good night's sleep. In spite of the possession of objective data to the contrary the patient's account would prevail.

SELF-RATING SCALES OF DEPRESSION

Self-rating scales have several disadvantages when compared with observer rating scales. However, they have a single obvious advantage, which in some cases may outweigh the disadvantages, and that is the economic one of saving experimenter's time so more patients can be assessed or studies can be carried out with fewer resources of manpower.

What are the disadvantages? The most severe is that reliability is often unknown and virtually inaccessible to study. Of the types of reliability used to examine observer-rated scales none is applicable to self-rated scales. Thus inter-rater reliability is by definition inapplicable and this is the most important statistic available for observer ratings. Split half reliability is feasible but requires the construction of a scale in two equivalent parts. It will be seen that some workers have achieved this to a limited degree. Test–retest reliability has only limited value as in most cases it is expected that severity *will* change with time, i.e. the scales are not designed to measure enduring characteristics.

The validity of self-rated scales is also more open to doubt than observer ratings, although it is more open to testing than is reliability. Patients themselves may not use words descriptive of emotion in the same way as psychiatrists. For example, depression and anxiety are not differentiated by a large proportion of the population. Hence, only commonly used words with obvious meaning to the layman can be used in self-rating scales (e.g. sadness, misery). Even so there is no guarantee that patients are using these words in the way intended. When the patient is trying to decide how to rate a particular item, say sadness, the standards they will use depend upon their own experience, which may be very different from that of a qualified psychiatrist. In particular, items requiring judgements of intensity of emotion may well be over-rated by the patient compared with the psychiatrist, as the psychiatrist will in most cases have seen patients more depressed than the patient herself.

Obvious disadvantages are that severely ill patients are usually unable to complete the form either through retardation or agitation or because of indecision or lack of concentration. Literacy is a prerequisite. Unlike the situation in a clinical interview it is very easy for the patient who is so inclined to conceal illness during completion of a rating form. There may be many reasons for this. For example, the anorexic or the non-compliant patient may not want the doctor to know the severity of their illness in order to be discharged.

In addition there is the well-described problem of social desirability set, the tendency to answer in a way which is thought by the patient to be socially acceptable. Indeed in depression the situation is even more complicated since the desirability set may be reversed, becoming a social undesirability set. This is because depressed patients with low self-esteem frequently assume that they are worthless and would answer accordingly (Langevin and Stancer, 1979). There is also contamination of the answers by overall agreement sets, i.e. the tendency to say 'yes' to more questions than 'no'. When answers are in the form of a scale, either numerical or visual analogue, other sets come in to play. Some people have a tendency to overuse the middle rating while others (more rare) overuse the extremes of the scale. Self-rating scales are unable to tap information about important aspects of the syndrome such as psychomotor disturbances or insight. A critical review of these issues is provided in Ch. 1 and by Boyle (1985).

These criticisms are supported by empirical data. Prusoff *et al.* (1972) found low concordance rates between self- and observer ratings, especially in the acute phases of the illness. At follow-up concordance improved. The individual scales described below all have a tendency to correlate less well between themselves than do observer ratings, and to correlate less well with global severity ratings, the usual criterion for validation.

Zung Self-rating Depression Scale (SDS)

Zung (1965) constructed the SDS as a rapid means to assess severity of depression in trials and in clinics. There are 20 items, each rated on a scale of 0–4, giving a theoretical maximum of 80. It was recommended that scores be expressed as a decimal of this maximum score, but usually raw scores are reported. Each item is rated according to frequency of occurrence rather than intensity of the symptom, i.e. 'a little of the time, some of the time, good part of the time, most of the time'. Thus, a symptom which was infrequent but very severe would be rated low. Diurnal variation is included as a severity item. Half of the items are worded positively and half negatively, for example 'I eat as much as I used to' is a positive wording, while 'I feel downhearted and blue' is a negative item. This was done to overcome response bias (Cronbach, 1946).

In practice the validity and sensitivity to change of the SDS is in doubt. The initial validation (Zung, 1965) was performed using three groups, diagnosed depressed patients, other psychiatric patients and normal subjects. The scores were respectively 0.74, 0.53 and 0.33. This was thought to be a satisfactory separation of groups, with all three scores being significantly different from each other. After treatment the scores of the depressed group fell to 0.39, a significant improvement. This method of validation using groups of patients who are expected to be of different severity was also used by Carroll *et al.* (1973), with less satisfactory results. The SDS failed to discriminate between patients with depression in general practice (mean score 49.0), day patients (56.3) and in-patients (51.9). Indeed day patients scored higher than in-patients, against prediction and contrary to results obtained with the Hamilton Rating Scale in the same sample. The correlation of the SDS and the HDRS was only 0.41. Downing and Rickels (1972) found that the SDS failed to distinguish between depressed patients and non-depressed psychiatric patients.

This brings us to the second way of validating the SDS—against the observer-rated HDRS. Brown and Zung (1972) found a correlation with the HDRS of 0.79 in 65 patients. Davies *et al.* (1975) examined the concurrent validity of the SDS against the HDRS, the self-rated Beck Depression Inventory (BDI), and against a Visual Analogue Scale (VAS). The correlation with the HDRS was 0.62, with the BDI 0.73, and with the Visual Analogue Scale 0.62. Biggs *et al.* (1978) found an overall correlation with the HDRS of 0.80. However, as might be expected, the correlation was lowest at greatest severity, i.e. before treatment (0.45).

Validation against global clinical ratings of severity has also given variable results. Biggs *et al.* (1978) obtained a correlation of 0.69 in 26 depressed patients, with a significant differentiation between four severity levels. Downing and Rickels (in Hedlund and Vieweg, 1979b), on the other hand, obtained a correlation of only 0.22 in psychiatric patients and 0.49 in general practice.

Zung has developed an observer-rated scale, the Depression Status Inventory, to complement the SDS. This is composed of the same items as the SDS and appears to have no advantage over previously developed scales (Zung, 1972). Predictably, however, correlations with the SDS were high at 0.87. The SDS has also been examined for its value as a diagnostic instrument (Zung, 1965) but no satisfactory threshold value was found, and of course its prime purpose was for rating severity in already diagnosed populations. In addition Zung and Wonnacott (1970) looked at its ability to predict treatment response, which was also poor, unless it was factor analysed and factor scores were applied, a lengthy procedure for little gain. Zung (1967) found no effect of age, sex, marital status, education, income or literacy on the scores. There was, however, a correlation with the MMPI(D) scale of 0.59. In another study an even higher correlation of 0.70 with the MMPI was obtained (Zung *et al.*, 1965). The MMPI is a measure of personality, and such a high correlation may explain the insensitivity of the SDS to change in clinical state.

Beck Depression Inventory (BDI)

This was the first attempt to use self-ratings to assess the severity of the depressive condition. Beck (Beck *et al.*, 1961) was developing his ideas of cognitive theory and therapy for depression from psychoanalytic approaches, and derived the items of the inventory from this experience. It consists of 21 items, each with a 0–3 grading system. Each item consists of four or five self-evaluative statements of increasing severity, for example:

I do not feel sad	0
I feel blue or sad	1
I am blue or sad all the time and I can't snap out of it	2
I am so sad or unhappy that it is very painful	3
I am so sad or unhappy that I can't stand it	4

For some items two alternative statements are provided at the same weight. It is said that no underlying theoretical stance governed the choice of items, although they are biased towards a cognitive content (See Ch. 1, Table 1).

Although it is essentially a self-rating instrument the recommended method of use is by assisted self-rating. This means that the interviewer reads the statements aloud to the patient, who then chooses the statement which best describes his or her present condition. The merits of this system are that literacy is not essential (although an illiterate patient would require an excellent memory to retain all the statements long enough to reply) and clarification can be given if necessary. However, it forfeits the only real advantage of self-rating instruments, that of saving time. In practice many researchers use it as a true self-rating instrument after explaining the instructions to the subject.

Beck *et al.* (1961) initially standardized the instrument on two samples of mixed in-patients and out-patients, of whom 41% were diagnosed as psychotic, 43% neurotic and 16% personality disordered according to the DSM. There was a total of 409 patients in the samples. Four psychiatrists made four-point global ratings of severity based on appearance, thoughts, social performance and vegetative symptoms. The inter-rater reliability of the global ratings was high. The correlation between BDI score and global ratings in the two groups was 0.65 and 0.67. All items individually correlated significantly with the total score, showing reasonable homogeneity, although the mean item–total correlation was lower than the HDRS. The split half reliability of the scale was 0.86 or 0.93, depending on the statistic used to calculate it. The mean scores for each level of depression were:

No depression	10.9
Mild depression	18.7
Moderate depression	25.4
Severe depression	30.0

Other studies have found correlations with global severity scores of 0.77 (Bech *et al.*, 1975), 0.62 (Metcalfe and Goldman, 1965) and 0.76 (Crawford-Little and McPhail, 1973, using a visual analogue rating). Against the HDRS criterion, correlations have been found of 0.72 (Bech *et al.*, 1975a), 0.74 (Schwab *et al.*, 1967b), 0.58 (Miller *et al.*, 1985), 0.73 (Davies *et al.*, 1975) and 0.82 (Williams *et al.*, 1972). Kearns *et al.* (1982) found the BDI, in common with other self-rating scales, to be weak in differentiating moderate from severe depression. Correlations with other self-rating scales vary. Against a self-rated visual analogue scale Davies *et al.* (1975) obtained a correlation of 0.65 and Crawford-Little and McPhail 0.76. Against the Zung SDS, Davies *et al.* (1975) found a correlation of 0.73. The Lubin Adjective Check-lists correlate 0.40–0.66 (Lubin, 1965).

The validity of change in scores on the BDI (sensitivity) is shown in a number of ways. Beck *et al.* (1961) showed that 85% of change in BDI score in 33 patients was reflected in changes in global ratings. Metcalfe and Goldman (1965) found a reduction in BDI score in their sample of depressives from 26.2 on admission to 7.15 on discharge. Bech *et al.* (1975) found a correlation of 0.82 between change in BDI score and change in global rating, and 0.56 between change in BDI and change in HRS score. Bailey and Coppen (1976) found the percentage change in BDI scores to be lower than change in HDRS scores.

The individual items of the BDI correlate from 0.32 to 0.62 with the total score, indicating moderate internal consistency (Schwab *et al.*, 1967b). Five items of the scale correlate significantly with the suicide item of the HDRS, demonstrating the cognitive bias. Beck and Beamersderfer (1974) provided item–total correlations, which were significant for all items. Bech *et al.* (1975) subjected the items to the three criteria of calibration, ascending monotonicity and dispersion, and found that 12 of the 21 items were satisfactory on all these indicators. Nine of these twelve items also occurred in the list of the best 13 items in Beck's analysis, leading Bech to propose the use of this subscale under the title 'Depression Inventory Subscale'.

However, Kearns *et al.* (1982) found this subscale to be unsatisfactory in distinguishing between grades of depression on a five-point global scale and it has not been used in practice. Factor analysis has failed to yield consistent results (Beck and Beamersderfer, 1974).

Carroll Rating Scale (CRS)

In view of the poorer performance of self-rating scales compared with observer rating scales, and the lack of a self-rating scale with comparable items to the HDRS, Carroll *et al.* (1981) have attempted to construct a direct equivalent of the HDRS for self-rating use. They have taken the 17 items of the HDRS and supplied two or four self-evaluative statements for each item, depending on the maximum score for each item in the original. The statements are presented in random order rather than in item-related blocks, in contrast to the BDI, to reduce response bias. Each statement has to be answered 'yes' or 'no'. The effect of this is to transform the hierarchical scoring of the HDRS into a summed score. In other words, the score on each item of the CRS is a sum of answers to two or four questions. The maximum score is 52. Half the items require a 'yes' response and half a 'no' response to score as depressed.

In a general population sample the median score was 3, and a cut-off score of 10 would classify 9% of the general population as depressed. The reliability was examined in two ways using the split half method (Carroll *et al.*, 1981). The odd- and even-numbered questions correlated 0.87 and the 'yes' and 'no' answers correlated 0.74. All of the four categories in this analysis correlated well with the total score.

In a sample of 278 patients the correlation with the HDRS itself was 0.80. An item correlation showed that the CRS was not uniformly successful in matching the HDRS, and the median item correlation was only 0.60. However, within the CRS the internal consistency, as determined by item–total correlations, was similar to the HDRS. Four items correlated weakly in both scales: loss of libido, hypochondriasis, loss of weight and loss of insight. The factor analysis of the two scales yields similar results (Smouse *et al.*, 1981).

Comparison with the BDI, as the most prominent and successful of the self-rating scales, showed an overall correlation of 0.86 (N = 279). In this group the CRS–HDRS correlation was 0.71 and the BDI–HDRS correlation was 0.60. Thus it appears that the CRS is more successful in matching the HDRS than the other main self-rating scale (Carroll *et al.*, 1981).

Feinberg *et al.* (1981) compared the CRS, HDRS, Visual Analogue Scale and clinical global rating of depression (CGRD). The results are shown in Table 2.

Robbins *et al.* (1985) found that self-rating of depression in adolescents was poorer than the results in Table 2 suggest is the case for adults. They found a CRS–HDRS correlation of only 0.46.

Table 2

	CRS	CGRD	VAS
HRS	0.75	0.77	0.65
CRS		0.63	0.71
CGRD			0.56

Wakefield Self-Assessment Depression Inventory

This scale was constructed from the ten items of the Zung SDS which occurred most frequently in a depressed population (Snaith *et al.*, 1971; Zinkin and Birtchnell, 1968). Two extra items were added to cover anxiety, and the responses were reformulated from Zung's frequency-based ratings to 'definitely, sometimes, not much, not at all'. It will immediately be noticed that this system confounds certainty, frequency and intensity of symptoms in a way which could make ratings difficult or ambiguous.

Snaith *et al.* (1971) administered the scale to groups of depressed and normal subjects and found very little overlap in the scores. Three per cent of normals and 7.5% of depressives were misclassified. The mean normal score was 6.22 and the mean depressive score was 24–25. The correlation with HDRS scores was 0.89.

An ingenious attempt was made to judge the test–retest reliability. The problem with using test–retest reliability in depression self-rating scales is that if the tests are too close together the subject will remember their previous responses and respond the same way as before from memory. If they are too far apart in time the clinical state will very likely have changed. Treatment with ECT often causes a retrograde amnesia for the period immediately before each treatment. By giving one test just before ECT and the other shortly afterwards it was hoped that it would be possible to get round both problems and to calculate meaningful test–retest statistics. The problem with this argument is that between one test and the next a powerful antidepressant treatment has been given. Secondly, the retrograde amnesia of ECT is not so reliably produced that some recall might not have occurred. These opposing influences may have acted to produce a fairly low reliability of 0.68 between one occasion and the next—a figure which is hard to interpret.

In 47 patients who went on to complete a course of ECT with good clinical effect, Wakefield inventories were repeated after treatment. All items except sleep showed significant reductions in score. Apart from this, there is no information about sensitivity to change. Age represents a significant confounding variable when assessing differences between groups using the Wakefield, as the correlation with scale score is significant (Snaith *et al.*, 1971). Therefore the transferability of the scale is low.

Kearns *et al.* (1982), when comparing several rating scales against a clinical global rating, found that the Wakefield was the weakest of all in differentiating levels of severity, and recommended that it be dropped from use. It was especially poor at the upper end of the severity scale, where self-assessment inventories tend to perform badly, but in this study the Wakefield produced higher scores for the moderately depressed group than for the severely depressed group.

Levine–Pilowsky Depression Questionnaire

This questionnaire started life as an attempt to investigate the validity of the distinction between neurotic and endogenous depression (Pilowsky *et al.*, 1969). The reasoning went that previous attempts had used psychiatrists' ratings of symptoms as the basis for the statistical calculations, and that these would be contaminated by the theoretical orientation of the psychiatrists towards the two-state hypothesis. Subjects themselves, on the other hand, would have no such preordained orientation. A self-rating scale, completed before the psychiatric interview, would therefore help to clarify the distinction.

Fifty-seven items were drawn from textbook descriptions of depression (thus introducing some theoretical bias into the content). All of the common symptoms of depression were included. The response was in the form of a check-list, the subject answering 'yes' or 'no' to each item. The period of time referred to is not specified. All answers indicating depression are 'yes' answers, thus allowing a possibility of response bias. Nevertheless a clear distinction was found in the results of 200 depressed patients between endogenous depression and other depressions, including neurotic symptoms.

Further research using the questionnaire derived a decision rule for classifying patients on the basis of the results (Pilowsky and Boulton, 1970). This correctly predicted response to ECT. Pilowsky and McGrath (1970) showed that items in the questionnaire associated with the endogenous syndrome were the ones which improved during a course of ECT.

Finally, the use of the questionnaire as a measure of the severity of depression was explored (Pilowsky and Spalding, 1972). In the 1969 study of Pilowsky *et al.*, 25 of the items discriminated between the depressed and non-depressed groups. Nineteen of them also correlated significantly and negatively with the taxonomic classification of non-depression. These 19 were chosen. They include 5 mood, 3 social activity, 6 cognitive, 2 vegetative, 1 motor and 1 irritability question, plus the rather odd item 'Have you moved house in the past year?' The relationship of the scores to diagnosis, their sensitivity to change and their concurrent validity were examined.

Psychotic depressives obtained the highest scores and non-depressed patients the lowest. The two groups identified on the basis of full questionnaire results and classed as endogenous or non-endogenous using the decision rule had similar scores, showing a degree of independence from syndrome diagnosis. In 54 subjects tested at discharge, the degree of improvement noted on clinical global scales was similar to the improvements recorded with the questionnaire. However, this was only a brief analysis and is difficult to interpret. The concurrent measures against which it was validated were visual analogue scales, one of which was observer-rated and one self-rated. Against self-rating the correlation was 0.59, while against observer rating it was 0.62. These results are similar to concurrent validity statistics of other self-rating scales.

Visual Analogue Scales for Depression

Visual analogue scales could be constructed for each item of an inventory and then summed or averaged (see Ch. 1), but in practice the visual analogue scale for depression refers to a single line, usually 10 cm long, with the wording 'as depressed as I have ever been' to 'not at all depressed' (Aitken, 1969; Folstein and Luria, 1973).

It might be expected that reliability and validity would be poor, as the definition of depression is unspecified and, as far as the patient is concerned, might refer to sadness alone, anhedonia alone or any combination of the elements of the syndrome of depressive illness (Luria, 1975). Zealley and Aitken (1969) found that the correlation with a global severity score on admission to hospital was 0.78, and with the HDRS score was 0.79. However, after discharge, the validity was very low. The correlation with global severity was 0.13 and with HDRS was 0.06!

Nevertheless the technique has continued to attract researchers, perhaps because of the ease of administration and the spurious sense of accuracy which the results can give (they are usually given to the nearest millimetre from the left-hand or normal end of the line). Crawford-Little and McPhail (1973), using repeated measures on eight patients during treatment, obtained a correlation of 0.80 between the VAS completed by the patients and a similar scale completed by the psychiatrist. Against a self-rating inventory, the BDI, a correlation of 0.76 was found.

Davies *et al.* (1975) found the VAS to correlate 0.63 with the HDRS, 0.65 with the BDI, and 0.62 with the Zung SDS. Whatever figures can be produced for the reliability or concurrent validity of the VAS, the problem of interpretation of studies in which it is used as the sole measure of depression would remain, as there is no control over which part of the syndrome of depression is being tapped. Indeed it is a way of obtaining a self-rated global assessment, and therefore has the same status as asking the patient 'How ill are you?' without specifying how they are to judge what is meant by illness. However, as a rapid global assessment method at the end of a more complete rating scale it can be useful (Bech *et al.*, 1986; Aitken and Zealley, 1970).

von Zerssen Scales

Working in Munich, von Zerssen's group developed a check-list for measuring mood changes on repeated occasions (von Zerssen, 1973a and b; von Zerssen *et al.*, 1974). One scale can be used in normal subjects and medical patients (the well-being scale: *Befindlichkeits-Skala*, BS). There are two parallel forms of this (BS and BS′), so that it can be administered frequently without response bias. Each is a 28-item scale and they correlate together 0.9. They are useful to plot the course of change in depression, but they are not specific to depression. The authors therefore have developed a further scale containing specifically aspects of depressive symptomatology using items which appear to discriminate the depressed from the non-depressed state. Some of these are common to the Beck and the Zung scales. There are again two parallel forms, the DS and DS′, each consisting of 16 items. There was a good correlation between the BS and DS scales in both psychiatric and non-psychiatric populations. In an endogenously depressed group the correlation with global clinical ratings was 0.70–0.99, although this fell in a more heterogeneous group of patients. The scale was sensitive to change in depressive state with treatment and also to speed of change, being able to differentiate ECT from antidepressant-induced change.

MANIA RATING SCALES

Mania is not just the opposite of depression. It is one phase of the illness manic-depression, which was first described by Kraepelin. The opposite of sadness is euphoria or elation. While this is a common emotion in mania it is soon replaced or even eclipsed by irritability and anger if the illness goes unchecked. There is also sadness if the psychiatrist asks about it. Patients often weep as well as being hyperactive, over-talkative and energetic. Indeed this is sometimes such a confusing picture that forms have had to be recognized of 'mixed affective states' in which it is impossible to say which mood disorder predominates.

For the diagnosis of manic-depression the individual should have suffered a depressive or a manic illness or both at some time in their life. The ICD-9 sticks to this roughly Kraepelinian definition but most researchers now have agreed that it is important for many biological studies that patients are typed into Bipolar (having suffered mania and depression) or Unipolar Affective Disorder (having suffered one or the other, in practice almost exclusively depression, hardly ever mania).

As in depression, it is important to exclude schizophrenia before making the diagnosis. However, mixed forms occur and it is not always easy, and sometimes it is impossible, to distinguish them. In this case the diagnosis of schizoaffective disorder is sometimes made (schizomanic type).

Like depression the symptoms can be divided into a number of categories:

Affective: the abnormal mood
Motor: hyperactivity of movement and speech
Vegetative: poor sleep
Abnormal experiences: delusions (grandiose) and hallucinations (auditory, only if severe)

Hypomania is a term used to connote the illness before it is severe enough to be called mania. However, at what point does hypomania become mania? English psychiatrists have said that mania is hardly ever seen, so that hypomania is used as the descriptive term almost exclusively. This is not, however, very helpful. The Research Diagnostic Criteria returned to a two-level diagnostic system based on operational definitions of hypomania and mania, depending on severity and duration. In fact the symptoms are the same but of different severity, so that the same rating scales can be used for each.

The nature of mania militates against self-rating scales. Patients are often grandiose and lacking in insight. They feel very well and would scoff at the idea that they were ill, even after several episodes. In fact there are very few scales of mania available and specific scales only appeared in the early 1970s. There is much work which could still be done in refining this area of measurement in psychiatry.

Manic State (MS) Scale

This was first designed by Beigel and Murphy (1971) and Beigel *et al.* (1971) (see also Murphy *et al.*, 1974) for the rating of in-patient manics by nursing personnel. Before this time there were scales for observed behaviour which presented mania as one item and others which were for general psychopathology that were too big for regular use. This then was the first specifically manic scale.

Sixteen topics were first compiled based on the mania clinical literature. Five nurses then took part in discussion of these items to find the most appropriate wording and items for use in the scale. They developed 26 items to be tested. Each item was rated on frequency (how much of the time?) on a six-point scale; 0 = none. If there was a score on this scale the item was also rated on intensity (how intense is it?,) on a five-point scale; 1–5. The scores on these two scales were multiplied to give a score for each item from 0 to 25. Thirteen admissions with clinically diagnosed mania or depression were rated in the initial standardization.

Reliability between raters was carried out for the 12 nurses on the team. Items varied in reliability from 0.86 to 0.99. All ratings for the item 'patient dresses inappropriately' were 0, so there was no information on that item.

Next they looked at manic patients alone, of which there were six. Here reliabilities were from 0.68 to 0.99.

The ratings were made for the previous 8-hour nursing shift. As a validity study psychiatrists made independent global ratings for the same 8-hour shift on a 15-point scale. The reliability of this criterion scale was 0.98. A second criterion was a 14-item check-list of manic symptoms completed by nurses. The reliability of this criterion was 0.98.

Twenty-two of the 25 items were highly correlated with the psychiatrists' global scores. The same items were also correlated with the nurses' check-list scores. The total score on the Manic State Scale was highly significantly correlated with the global psychiatrists' scores (0.96) and with the nurses' scores (0.96).

When the six manics were compared with the total group of 13, six items were best at picking out the manics; these were 'Moves from one place to another', 'Has poor judgement', 'Is distractible', 'Is active', 'Is angry', and 'Jumps from one subject to another'. These may be the most reliable and sensitive of the items for detecting change in manic state.

The 26 items of the scale are:

1. Looks depressed
2. Is talking
3. Moves from one place to another
4. Makes threats
5. Has poor judgement
6. Dresses inappropriately
7. Looks happy and cheerful
8. Seeks out others
9. Is distractible
10. Has grandiose ideas
11. Is irritable
12. Is combative or destructive
13. Is delusional
14. Verbalizes depressive feelings
15. Is active
16. Is argumentative
17. Talks about sex
18. Is angry
19. Is careless about dress and grooming
20. Has diminished impulse control
21. Verbalizes feelings of well-being
22. Is suspicious
23. Makes unrealistic plans
24. Demands contact with others

25. Is sexually preoccupied
26. Jumps from one subject to another

In a further study (Murphy and Beigel, 1974) the group looked at 12 manic in-patients. In addition to the MS Scale a global scale was completed by psychiatrists. Eleven items individually correlated with the global scale. These were 2, 3, 5, 9, 11, 15, 16, 18, 20, 24 and 26. These items then best reflected common elements of mania. Other items reflected two apparent subtypes of mania: Elated–Grandiose (EG) and Paranoid–Destructive (PD).

EG items were 7, 10, 21, 23.
PD items were 4, 12, 13, 22.

Two items were included which related to depressive mood in mania, because of the observations, beginning with Kraepelin, that these symptoms were present. These two items correlated slightly positively with the total score, showing that depression is not the polar opposite of mania. The elation items were only correlated with the total score in the group of patients with the EG subtype and this group appeared to respond more readily to lithium carbonate than did the PD group.

Young *et al.* (1978) has criticized the scale for not being sufficiently explicit in the ratings of severity and for being unnecessarily long, with several paired items. The inter-rater reliability was poorer than the Mania Rating Scale they devised (0.60 versus 0.93; Young *et al.*, 1978) and it correlated less well with the global rating by psychiatrists (0.66 versus 0.88). It was also less sensitive in the middle range of severity, in contrast with the Petterson *et al.* (1973) scale and the Mania Rating Scale (Young *et al.*, 1978).

Blackburn *et al.* (1977) have modified the Manic State Scale for use by psychiatrists (see MMS, below).

Bech *et al.* (1975b) carried out a further analysis of the scale using the statistics of calibration, ascending monotonocity and dispersion (for definitions see Ch. 1).

In Bech's study the Manic State Scale was given by nurses and psychiatrists to 11 in-patients on admission and just before discharge. Validity of the whole scale was tested against a global rating scale (reliability 0.65). Reliability of the Beigel scale in the hands of the psychiatrists was 0.85. Validity was tested for the intensity × frequency score and the intensity score alone. For the 25-point rating the validity against global rating was 0.90 and for the intensity score alone it was 0.80–0.91.

When the three criteria were applied to each item six passed each test, i.e. they were correctly calibrated (frequently gave a score in this population) had ascending monotonicity (were sensitive to differences in severity) and had low dispersion (were reliably rated). These six items were:

3. Moves from one place to another
7. Looks happy and cheerful
8. Seeks out others
9. Is distractible
20. Has diminished impulse control
24. Demands contact with others

This item content is rather similar to the seven most valid items of Petterson's scale. The authors conclude that the Beigel scale is useful and valid to profile manic behaviour but that the shorter scale of six items may be sufficient and possibly more sensitive throughout the range of severity.

Modified Manic State (MMS) Rating Scale

The Manic State (MS) Scale was explicitly for use by nurses. Blackburn *et al.* (1977) wished to create a scale for use by psychiatrists, taking into account their greater experience of the psychopathology. Certain symptoms were found to be absent from the MS scale, for example sleep disturbance. Five items were added after consulting experienced psychiatrists. These were sleep, hallucinations, religiosity, disinhibition and lability of mood. Three pairs of items were condensed. These were anger/combativeness, sexual talk/sexual preoccupation and depressed look/depressed verbalization.

The resulting scale has 28 items, six for rating after consulting nurses. A glossary was compiled and the points on the rating scale defined. Sixteen manic patients were used for standardization. All fulfilled Feighner Criteria for mania. Inter-rater reliability was 0.79–0.85 after using a semi-structured interview based on the PSE. All items, with the exception of depression, were significantly correlated with total score, showing good internal consistency. The depression item was retained because the correlation was 0.24. The total scores correlated 0.65 with nurses' global ratings and 0.80 with doctors' ratings. Scores were observed to diminish over the course of the admission but for two patients this was not significant. Thus the scale is capable of measuring change, but no work has been carried out on its relative sensitivity against other scales.

Petterson Mania Rating Scale

In 1973 there was still only one published scale for mania. The increased interest in lithium as an antimanic drug led Petterson *et al.* (1973) to develop the Petterson mania scale from scratch. They were dissatisfied with the Beigel (MS) scale because it took a long time to complete, had too many non-specific items, and the items and scale steps were not explicitly defined. Starting with 22 items they eliminated several because they were not reliable or they relied on the report of the patient which, in mania, is often unreliable since insight is usually at a premium. There were eventually seven items plus a global rating and a global rating of change. The first seven items were:

Motor activity
Pressure of speech
Flight of ideas
Noisiness
Aggressiveness
Orientation
Elevated mood

All were rated 1–5 except orientation, which was rated 1–3. Each step was clearly defined. In the first study inter-rater reliability was judged for two psychiatrists rating the same interview. Before treatment, the items had reliabilities of 0.57 (pressure of speech) to 1.00 (motor activity). During treatment with lithium the reliability of the items was 0.48 (noisiness) to 1.00 (aggressiveness and orientation). These are satisfactory. At the second rating, during lithium treatment there was a significant fall in scores, patients scoring little above baseline, demonstrating adequate sensitivity to drug effects. However, no comparative trial of sensitivity in drug trials against other rating scales has been carried out.

Young *et al.* (1978) examined the Petterson scale, their own Mania Rating Scale, and the Manic State Scale (Beigel and Murphy, 1971) for inter-rater reliability, concurrent validation and sensitivity in various ranges of severity. This form of sensitivity is not quite the same as for change in drug trials, which looks at within-patient changes in score. Here they divided patients into four groups according to scores on global ratings of severity. They then examined the ability of the three scales significantly to distinguish between the adjacent levels of severity. The Petterson scale gave the grade 2 severity a lower score than the grade 1 severity (11.8 against 12.5) and thus cannot be said to be sensitive at the lower levels of severity. However, it distinguished grade 3 from grade 4 adequately. The Beigel scale had a similar problem distinguishing grades 2 and 3 so is not very good at moderate grades. Young's MRS, however, had a linear relation to the global severity ratings.

The relative inter-rater reliabilities of the scales showed the Petterson to be second to the MRS, with a correlation of 0.88 (MRS, 0.93; Manic State Scale, 0.60; global, 0.77).

Concurrent validity of the Petterson scale against the MRS was 0.89, against the Manic State Scale 0.65, and against a global rating 0.80.

This is therefore a valid, reliable and brief scale for use by psychiatrists, and has a high degree of item specificity for mania. Its main drawback is possibly a lack of sensitivity in the milder ranges.

Mania Rating Scale (MRS) (Young *et al.*, 1978)

The aim of this scale was to provide a scale with broader item content and greater sensitivity than the Petterson seven-item scale, but shorter and more explicit in item severity ratings than the Manic State (MS) Scale (Beigel and Murphy, 1971). This then is an 11-item scale, each with five explicitly defined grades of severity. Choice of items was determined by contemporary understanding of the illness and by the need for items to be rateable at all grades of severity. Depressive symptoms were omitted. The style of the scale follows the Hamilton Rating Scale for Depression in that each severity grade of each item is individually defined, and the information source is unrestricted. The scale validity was established by comparison with the Beigel and Murphy MS scale and the Petterson scale, as well as a global rating (see above).

Of the three scales the inter-rater reliability of the total scores was highest for the Mania Rating Scale (0.93 versus 0.77–0.88). Individual items had reliabilities of 0.66–0.95.

The correlations of the Mania Rating Scale with the other three ratings were from 0.71 to 0.89, showing good concurrent validity. The correlation of change in score with change in global score was 0.79, showing good validity and sensitivity.

The MRS also correlated best (but only just) with the number of days spent in hospital, giving it good predictive validity (0.66). Comparison with the Petterson and the Manic State scales in ability to distinguish severity grades showed it to be the most consistent over all grades of severity, the Petterson scale being poorer in the mild range and the Beigel in the middle range.

Bech–Rafaelson Mania Scale

Bech *et al.* (1978) have also constructed a scale to be shorter than the Manic State Scale but having a broader item content than Petterson's scale, which makes no distinctions between mood items and self-esteem. Neither does it have items for social contact, sleep or work activity. The Bech–Rafaelsen Mania Scale (Bech *et al.*, 1978) consists of 11 items, each defined on a 0–4 severity scale, with definitions for each point. When completed by psychiatrists (Bech *et al.*, 1979) the concordance between raters was 0.95 (W). The scale appears to be fairly homogeneous in that the item total correlations were between 0.72 and 0.94 except for sleep (0.48). This is a fairly popular scale which with the related melancholia scale forms a useful pair.

REFERENCES

Aitken, R. C. B. (1969). Measurement of feelings using visual analogue scales. *Proc. R. Soc. Med.* **62**, 989–993.

Aitken, R. C. B. and Zealley, A. K. (1970). Measurement of moods. *Br. J. Hosp. Med.* 215–224.

American Psychiatric Association (1980). *Diagnostic and Statistical Manual for Mental Disorders III*, APA, Washington, DC.

Asberg, M., Kragh-Sorensen, P., Mindham, R. H. S. and Tuck, J. R. (1973). International reliability and communicability of a rating scale for depression. *Psychol. Med.* **3**, 458–465.

Asberg, M., Montgomery, S. A., Perris, C., Schalling, D. and Sedvall, G. (1978). A comprehensive psychopathological rating scale. *Acta Psychiatr. Scand.* Suppl. 271, 5–69.

Bailey, J. and Coppen, A. (1976). A comparison between the Hamilton Rating Scale and the Beck inventory of depression. *Br. J. Psychiatry* **128**, 486–489.

Bech, P. and Rafaelsen, O. J. (1980). The use of rating scales exemplified by a comparison of the Hamilton and the Bech–Rafaelsen Melancholia scale. *Acta Psychiatr. Scand.* Suppl. 285, 128–131.

Bech, P. (1981). Rating scales for affective disorder: their validity and consistency. *Acta Psychiatr. Scand.* Suppl. 295, 1–101.

Bech, P. and Clemmesen, L. (1983). The diagnosis of depression: 20 years later, Acta *Psychiatr. Scand.* Suppl. 310, 9–30.

Bech, P., Gram, L. F., Dein, E., Jabobsen, O., Vitger, J. and Bolwig, T. G. (1975a). Quantitative rating of depressive states. *Acta Psychiatr. Scand.* **51**, 161–170.

Bech, P., Bolwig, T. G., Dein, E., Jacobsen, O. and Gram, L. F. (1975b). Quantitative rating of manic states. *Acta Psychiatr. Scand.* **52**, 1–6.

Bech, P., Rafaelsen, O. J., Kramp, P. and Bolwig, T. G. (1978). The Mania Rating Scale: Scale construction and interobserver agreement. *Neuropharmacology* **17**, 430–431.

Bech, P., Bolwig, T. G., Kramp, P. and Rafaelsen, O. J. (1979). The Bech–Rafaelsen Mania Scale and the Hamilton Depression Rating Scale. *Acta Psychiatr. Scand.* **59**, 420–430.

Bech, P., Gram, L. F., Reisby, N. and Rafaelsen, O. J. (1980). The WHO Depression Scale: relationship to the Newcastle scales. *Acta Psychiatr. Scand.* **62**, 140–153.

Bech, P., Allerup, P., Gram, L. F., Reisby, N., Rosenberg, R., Jacobsen, O. and Nagy, A. (1981). The Hamilton Depression Scale: evaluation of objectivity using logistic models. *Acta Psychiatr. Scand.* **63**, 290–299.

Bech, P., Kastrup, M. and Rafaelsen, O. J. (1986). Minicompendium of rating scales for states of anxiety, depression, mania, schizophrenia with corresponding DSM III syndromes. *Acta Psychiatr. Scand.* **73** (Suppl. 326), 1–35.

Beck, A. T. (1976). *Cognitive Theory and the Emotional Disorders*. International University Press, New York.

Beck, A. T. and Beamersderfer, A. (1974). Assessment of depression: The depression inventory. In *Psychological Measurement* (P. Pichot, ed.), Karger, Basel.

Beck, A. T., Ward, C. H., Mendelson, M., Mock, J. and Erbaugh, J. (1961). An inventory for measuring depression. *Arch. Gen. Psychiatry* **4**, 561–571.

Beigel, A. and Murphy, D. L. (1971). Assessing clinical characteristics of the manic state. *Am. J. Psychiatry* **128**, 44–50.

Beigel, A., Murphy, D. L. and Bunney, W. E. Jr (1971). The Manic State Rating Scale: scale construction, reliability and validity. *Arch. Gen. Psychiatry* **25**, 256–262.

Biggs, J. T., Wylie, L. T. and Ziegler, V. E. (1978). Validity of the Zung Self Rating Depression Scale. *Br. J. Psychiatry* **132**, 381–385.

Blackburn, I. M., Loudon, J. B. and Ashworth, C. M. (1977). A new scale for measuring mania. *Psychol. Med.* **7**, 453–458.

Boyle, G. J. (1985). Self report measures of depression: some psychometric considerations, *Br. J. Clin. Psychol.* **24**, 45–59.

Brown, G. L. and Zung, W. W. K. (1972). Depression scales; self or physician rating? A validation of certain clinically observable phenomena. *Compr. Psychiatry* **13**, 361–367.

Bunney, W. E. and Hamburg, D. A. (1963). Methods for reliable longitudinal observation of behaviour. *Arch. Gen. Psychiatry* **9**, 280–294.

Burdock, E. I., Hardesty, A. S., Hakerem, G. and Zubin, J. A. A. (1960). A ward behaviour rating scale for mental patients. *J. Clin. Psychol.* **16**, 246–247.

Carney, M. W. P. and Sheffield, P. B. (1972). Depression and the Newcastle scales: their relationship to Hamilton's scale. *Br. J. Psychiatry* **121**, 35–40.

Carney, M. W. P., Roth, M. and Garside, R. F. (1965). The diagnosis of depressive syndromes and the prediction of ECT response. *Br. J. Psychiatry* **111**, 659–674.

Carroll, B. J., Fielding, J. M. and Blashki, T. G. (1973). Depression rating scales: a critical review. *Arch. Gen. Psychiatry* **28**, 361–366.

Carroll, B. J., Feinberg, M., Smouse, P. E., Rawson, S. G. and Greden, J. F. (1981). The Carroll Rating Scale for Depression 1. Development, reliability and validation. *Br. J. Psychiatry* **138**, 194–200.

Checkley, S. A., Glass, I. B., Thompson, C., Corn, T. H. and Robinson, P. (1984). The growth hormone response to clonidone in endogenous as compared with reactive depression. *Psychol. Med.* **4**, 773–779.

Costello, C. G. and Comfrey, A. L. (1967). Scales for measuring depression and anxiety. *J. Psychol.* **66**, 303–313.

Crawford-Little J. and McPhail, N. I. (1973). Measures of depressive mood at monthly intervals. *Br. J. Psychiatry* **122**, 447.

Cronbach, L. J. (1946). Response set and test validity. *Ed. Psych. Measurement* **6**, 475–495.

Cronholme, B. D. and Ottosson, J.-O. (1960). Experimental studies of the mechanism of action of electroconvulsive therapy in endogenous depression. The role of the electrical stimulation and of the seizure studied by variation of stimulus intensity and modification by lidocaine of seizure discharge. *Acta Psychiatr. Scand.* **35** (Suppl. 145), 69–102.

Cronholme, B. D., Schalling, D. and Asberg, M. (1974). Development of a rating scale for depressive illness. In *Psychological Measurements in Psychopharmacology* (P. Pichot, ed.), Karger, Basel.

Davies, B., Burrows, G. and Poynton, C. A. (1975). Comparative study of four depression rating scales. *Aust. NZ J. Psychiatry* **9**, 21–24.

Downing, R. W. and Rickels, K. (1972). Some properties of the Popoff Index. *Clin. Med.* **79**, 11–18.

Dratcu, L., DaCosta Ribeiro, L. and Calil, H. M. (1987). Depression assessment in Brazil. The first use of the Montgomery Asberg Depression Rating Scale. *Br. J. Psychiatry* **150**, 797–800.

Feinberg, M., Carroll, B. J., Smouse, P. E. and Rawson, S. G. (1981). The Carroll Rating Scale for Depression 3, Comparison with other rating instruments, *Br. J. Psychiatry* **138**, 205–209.

Folstein, M. F. and Luria, R. E. (1973). Reliability, validity and clinical application of the visual analogue mood scale. *Psychol. Med.* **3**, 479–486.

Frank, J. F., Gliedman, L. H., Imber, S. D., Nash, E. H. and Stone, A. R. (1957). Why patients leave psychotherapy. *Arch. Neurol. Psych.* **77**, 283–299.

Gastpar, M. (1983). The ICD 9 and the SADD criteria for depression. *Acta Psychiatr. Scand.* Suppl. 310, 31–41.

Goodwin, F. K., Brodie, H. K. H., Murphy, D. L. and Bunney, W. E. Jr (1970). Administration of a peripheral decarboxylase inhibitor with l-dopa to depressed patients. *Lancet* **i**, 908, 7653.

Gurney, C. (1971). Diagnostic scales for affective disorders. *Proc 5th World Congress Psychiatry*, Mexico, p. 330.

Hamilton, M. (1960). Rating Scale for Depression. *J. Neurol. Neurosurg. Psychiatry* **23**, 56–62.

Hamilton, M. (1967). Development of a rating scale for primary depressive illness. *Br. J. Soc. Clin. Psychiatry* **6**, 278–96.

Hamilton, M. (1969). Standardised assessment and recording of depressive symptoms. *Psychiatr. Neurol. Neurosurg.* **72**, 201–205.

Hamilton, M. (1976). Comparative value of rating scales. *Br. J. Clin. Pharmacol.* **3** (Suppl. 1), 58–60.

Hedlund, J. L. and Vieweg, B. W. (1979a). The Hamilton Rating Scale for Depression: a comprehensive review. *J. Oper. Psychiatry* **10**, 149–165.

Hedlund, J. L. and Vieweg, B. W. (1979b). The Zung Self Rating Depression Scale, a comprehensive review. *J. Oper. Psychiatry* **10**, 51–64.

Holden, N. L. (1983). Depression and the Newcastle Scales: their relationship to the dexamethasone suppression test. *Br. J. Psychiatry* **142**, 505–507.

Katona, C. L. E. and Aldridge, C. R. (1983). Antidepressant effects of ECT. *Br. Med. J.* **286**, 1443.

Kearns, N. P., Cruickshank, C. A., McGuigan, K. J., Riley, S. A., Shaw, S. P. and Snaith, R. P. (1982). A comparison of depression rating scales. *Br. J. Psychiatry* **141**, 45–49.

Knesevich, J. W., Biggs, J. T., Clayton, P. J. and Ziegler, V. E. (1977). Validity of the Hamilton rating scale for depression. *Br. J. Psychiatry* **131**, 49–52.

Langevin, R. and Stancer, H. (1979). Evidence that depression rating scales primarily measure a social undesirability response set. *Acta Psychiatr. Scand.* **59**, 70–79.

Lubin, B. (1965). Adjective check lists for measuring depression, *Arch. Gen. Psychiatry* **12**, 57–62.

Luria, R. E. (1975). The validity and reliability of the visual analogue mood scale. *J. Psychiatr. Res.* **51–57**.

Maier, W. and Phillip, M. (1985). Comparative analysis of observer depression scales. *Acta Psychiatr. Scand.* **72**, 239–245.

Metcalfe, M. and Goldman, E. (1965). Validation of an inventory for measuring depression. *Br. J. Psychiatry* **111**, 240–242.

Miller, I. W., Bishop, S., Norman, W. H. and Maddever, H. (1985). The modified Hamilton Rating Scale for Depression; reliability and validity. *Psychiatr. Res.* **14**, 131–142.

Montgomery, S. A. and Asberg, M. (1979). A new depression rating scale designed to be sensitive to change. *Br. J. Psychiatry* **134**, 382–389.

Montgomery, S., Asberg, M., Traskman, L. and Montgomery, D. (1978). Cross cultural studies on the use of the CPRS in English and Swedish depressed patients. *Acta Psychiatr. Scand.* Suppl. 272.

Mowbray, R. M. (1972a). Rating scales for depression. In: *Depressive Illness. Some Research Studies* (B. M. Davies, B. J. Carroll and R. M. Mowbray, eds), Thomas, Springfield, Illinois.

Mowbray, R. M. (1972b). The Hamilton Rating Scale For Depression; A factor analysis. *Psychol. Med.* **2**, 272.

Murphy, D. L. and Beigel, A. (1974). Depression, elation and lithium carbonate responses in manic patient subgroups. *Arch. Gen. Psychiatry* **31**, 643–648.

Murphy, D. L., Beigel, A., Weingartner, H. and Bunney, W. E. (1974). The quantitation of manic behaviour. In *Psychological Measurements in Psychopharmacology*, Modern Problems in Pharmacopsychiatry Vol. 7 (P. Pichot, ed.), Karger, Basle, pp. 203–220.

Paykel, E. S. (1985). Clinical Interview for depression, development, reliability and validity. *J. Affect. Disord.* **9**, 85–96.

Petterson, U., Fyro, B. and Sedvall, G. (1973). A new scale for the longitudinal rating of manic states. *Acta Psychiatr. Scand.* **49**, 248–256.

Pietzecker, A. and Gebhart, R. (1983). Depressive syndromes and scales in the AMDP system. *Acta Psychiatr. Scand.* Suppl. 310, 65–84.

Pilowsky, I. and Boulton, D. M. (1970). Development of a questionnaire based decision rule for classifying depressed patients. *Br. J. Psychiatry* **116**, 647–650.

Pilowsky, I. and McGrath, M. D. (1970). Effect of ECT on response to a depression questionnaire. *Br. J. Psychiatry* **117**, 685–688.

Pilowsky, I. and Spalding, D. (1972). A method for measuring depression: validity studies on a depression questionnaire, *Br. J. Psychiatry* **121**, 411–416.

Pilowsky, I., Levine, S. and Boulton, D. M. (1969). The classification of depression by numerical taxonomy. *Br. J. Psychiatry* **115**, 937–945.

Prusoff, B. A., Klerman, G. L. and Paykel, E. S. (1972). Concordance between clinical assessments and patients self report of depression. *Arch. Gen. Psychiatry* **26**, 546–552.

Rafaelsen, O. J., Andersen, J., Bech, P., Clemmesen, L., Gjerris, A., Kastrup, M. and Kramp P. (1983). Multiaxial classification of depression—MULTICLAD-2 case record system. *Acta Psychiatr. Scand.* Suppl. 310, 85–100.

Rasch, G. (1960). *Probabilistic Model for Some Intelligence and Attainment Tests*, Danish Institute for Educational Research, Copenhagen.

Raskin, A. and Crook, T. H. (1976). The endogenous neurotic distinction as a predictor of response to antidepressant drugs. *Psychol. Med.* **6**, 59–70.

Raskin, A., Schulterbrandt, J., Reatig, N. and McKeon, J. T., (1969) Replication of factors of psychopathology in interview, ward behaviour and self report ratings of hospitalised depressives, *J. Nerv. Ment. Dis.* **148**, 87–98.

Raskin, A., Schulterbrandt, J. G., Reatig, N., Chase, C. and McKeon J. T. (1970). Differential reponse to chlorpromazine, imipramine and placebo. Arch. Gen. Psychiatry **23**, 164–73.

Robbins, D. R., Alessi, N. E., Colfer, M. V. and Yanchyshin, G. W. (1985). Use of the Hamilton Rating Scale for Depression and the Carroll self rating scale in adolescents. *Psychiatr. Res.* **14**, 123–129.

Rosenthal, N. E., Sack, D. A., Gillin, J. C., Lewy, A. J., Wehr, T. A. and Goodwin, F. G. (1984). Seasonal affective disorder; a description of the syndrome and preliminary findings with light therapy. *Arch. Gen. Psychiatry* **41**, 72–80.

Roth, M., Gurney, C. and Mountjoy, C. G. (1983). The Newcastle rating scales. *Acta Psychiatr. Scand.* Suppl. 310, 42–52.

Sartorius, N., Jablensky, A., Gulbinat, W. and Ernberg, G. (1980). WHO collaborative study: assessment of depressive disorders. *Psychol. Med.* **10**, 743–749.

Schwab, J. J., Bialow, M. R., Clemmons, R. S. and Holzer, C. E. (1967a). Hamilton rating scale for depression with medical in-patients. *Br. J. Psychiatry* **113**, 83–88.

Schwab, J. J., Bialow, M. R. and Holzer, C. E. (1967b). A comparison of two rating scales for depression. *J. Clin. Psychol.* **23**, 94–96.

Smouse, P. E., Feinberg, M., Carroll, B. J., Park, M. H. and Rawson, S. (1981).

The Carroll Rating Scale for Depression 2. Factor analyses of the feature profiles. *Br. J. Psychiatry* **138**, 201–204.

Snaith, R. P. (1977). Hamilton Rating Scale for Depression. *Br. J. Psychiatry* **131**, 431–432.

Snaith, R. P. (1981). Rating scales. *Br. J. Psychiatry* **138**, 512–514.

Snaith, R. P. and Taylor, C. M. (1985). Rating scales for depression and anxiety: a current perspective. *Br. J. Clin. Pharmacol.* **19**, 17S–20S.

Snaith, R. P. Ahmed, S. N., Mehta, S. and Hamilton, M. (1971). Assessment of the severity of primary depressive illness: the Wakefield self assessment depression inventory. *Psychol. Med.* **1**, 143–149.

von Zerssen, D. (1973a). Selbstbeurteilungsskalen zur Abschatzung des subjektiven befundes in psychopathologischen querschnitt- und langssehnittuntersuchungen. *Arch. Psych. Nerv.* **217**, 299–314.

von Zerssen, D. (1973b). Beschwerdenskalen bei depressionen. *Therapiewoche* **46**, 4426–4440.

von Zerssen, D., Strian, F. and Schwartz, D. (1974). Evaluation of depressive states, especially in longitudinal studies. In *Psychological Measurements in Psychopharmacology*, Modern Problems in Pharmacopsychiatry, Vol. 7, (P. Pichot, ed.), Karger, Basle, pp. 189–202.

Wechsler, H., Grosser, G. H. and Busfield, B. L. (1963). The depression rating scale. *Arch. Gen. Psychiatry* **9**, 334–343.

Welner, J. (1972). A multinational, multicentre double blind trial of a new antidepressant. In *Depressive Illness, Diagnosis, Assessment*, Treatment (P. Kielholz, ed.), Hans Huber, Bern.

Williams, J. G., Barlow, D. H. and Agras, W. S. (1972). Behavioural measurement of severe depression. *Arch. Gen. Psychiatry* **27**, 330–333.

Young, R. C., Biggs, V. T., Ziegler, V. E. and Meyer, D. A. (1978). A rating scale for mania: reliability, validity and sensitivity. *Br. J. Psychiatry* **133**, 429–435.

Zeally, A. K. and Aitken, R. C. B. (1969). Measurement of Mood. *Proc. R. Soc. Med.* **62**, 993.

Zinkin, S. and Birtchnell, J. (1968). Unilateral electroconvulsive therapy: its effects on memory and its therapeutic efficacy. *Br. J. Psychiatry* **114**, 973–988.

Zisook, S., Click, M., Jaffe, K. and Overall, J. E. (1980). Research criteria for the diagnosis of depression. *Psychiatr. Res.* **2**, 13–23.

Zung, W. W. K. (1965). A self rating depression scale. *Arch. Gen. Psychiatry* **12**, 63–70.

Zung, W. W. K. (1967). Factors influencing the self rating depression scale. *Arch. Gen. Psychiatry* **16**, 543–547.

Zung, W. W. K. (1972). The Depression Status Inventory: an adjunct to the self rating depression scale. *J. Clin. Psychol.* **28**, 539–543.

Zung, W. W. K. and Wonnacott, T. H. (1970). Treatment prediction in depression using a self rating scale. *Biol. Psychiatry 2*, 321–329.

Zung, W. W. K., Richards, C. B. and Short, M. I. (1965) Self rating depression scale in an outpatient clinic. *Arch. Gen. Psychiatry* **13**, 508–515.

The Instruments of Psychiatric Research
Edited by C. Thompson

CHAPTER 5

Anxiety

Chris Thompson
Southampton University,
Royal South Hants Hospital,
Southampton, UK

INTRODUCTION

Morbid anxiety is distinguishable from normal anxiety in terms of:

1. The severity of the psychological discomfort.
2. An inappropriate balance of psychological and physical components.
3. Attachment of anxiety to inappropriate stimuli, for example in the phobias.
4. Avoidance of the feared stimuli, also seen in phobias.
5. May be severe enough to cause performance decrements on psychometric tests.
6. Episodes of panic for no apparent reason.

From this list it can be seen that ratings of morbid anxiety, to be comprehensive, should take into account not only self-ratings of the psychological state but also ratings of physical discomfort, objective measures of autonomic symptoms (since patients' ratings of discomfort do not accurately reflect physiological changes), lists of feared stimuli, the degree to which they are avoided, and the frequency of panic attacks. Disruption of psychomotor performance will also in some cases provide important information, and in most cases the physician's ratings of the morbid anxiety state will be essential.

Most cases of anxiety fall into broad syndromes, and not all measures will have to be taken in all studies. It will depend on the diagnosis and on the measures which are expected to change with the intervention.

From the above it follows that it is essential to build into anxiety studies a standardized diagnostic instrument. This will firstly confirm that the patient suffers anxiety and not, say, depression or schizophrenia, in both of which anxiety can be a symptom. Secondly, some instruments will make subsidiary diagnoses, for example of panic disorder, anxiety state, phobic disorder or agoraphobia.

Ratings of severity depend crucially on the diagnosis. For example, there is little point in applying a rating scale for generalized anxiety to a panic disorder or a phobia since the anxiety is not present continuously. In phobias the frequency with which the feared stimulus is encountered, and therefore the severity of distress, depends on the degree of avoidance, which must therefore also be taken into account in the ratings.

In generalized anxiety states it may be of interest to have some of the following measures:

1. Patient self-rating of anxiety.
2. Psychiatrists' rating of observed anxiety.
3. Psychophysiological measures of autonomic function and central arousal.
4. Patients' ratings of physical symptoms.
5. Psychological performance tests.

Items (3) and (5) will not be dealt with in this chapter, which is about rating scales.

THE DIAGNOSIS OF ANXIETY STATES

The commonly used interview schedules, such as the Schedule for Affective Disorders and Schizophrenia (SADS) and the Present State Examination (PSE), contain items for establishing anxiety diagnoses. The DSM-III diagnoses can be made using the Structured Clinical Interview for DSM-III (SCID). These are covered in detail in Ch. 2.

An instrument which has been designed specifically with anxiety disorders in mind is the ADIS or Anxiety Disorders Interview Scale (DiNardo *et al.*, 1982). This is structured to make DSM-III anxiety disorder diagnoses and to screen out psychosis, substance abuse and major affective disorders. A judgement of whether anxiety or depression is primary also has to be made, partially based upon the results of the Hamilton Anxiety Scale and the Hamilton Depression Scale, both of which are included in the schedule.

OBSERVER-RATED ANXIETY AND PHOBIA SCALES

Hamilton Anxiety Scale (HAS)

Like the depression rating scale of the same author the anxiety rating scale was specifically developed to rate clinical anxiety in patients already diagnosed as suffering from an anxiety state. Hamilton (1959) states that it should not be used in conditions in which anxiety is associated with another clinical syndrome such as agitated depression, obsessions, hysteria, schizophrenia or organic psychoses. It is for use by trained raters after an ordinary clinical interview, no interview schedule being provided. The time period of enquiry is 1 week and more frequent ratings, which are often wanted in anxiety studies, are not strictly permissible.

Hamilton (1959) took 12 groups of symptoms which were regularly observed in anxiety states as his starting point. The addition of a rating of behaviour at interview made 13 items. Each was rated on a five-point scale from 0 to 4 in ascending order of severity. The symptom categories were:

Anxious mood
Tension
Fears
Insomnia
Cognitive symptoms
Depressed mood
Somatic symptoms (muscular and sensory)
Cardiovascular symptoms
Respiratory symptoms
Gastrointestinal symptoms
Genitourinary symptoms
Autonomic symptoms
Behaviour (general and physiological)

Definitions are given in the scale for all symptoms.

Hamilton (1959) found independent ratings of the same interview to correlate 0.89 with each other. Factor analysis gave two factors, the first one of general severity and the second a bipolar factor contrasting psychic with somatic manifestations. Robinson *et al.* (1965) found the two factors to correlate only −0.02, as would be expected for orthogonal factors. This is the same as the first two factors in the Taylor MAS (O'Connor *et al.*, 1956). Indeed, two anxiety factors appear to be a rather general finding in psychiatric patients (Buss, 1962).

In constructing this scale Hamilton's approach was to concentrate on the form of symptoms rather than the content, in distinction from the scales constructed previously by psychologists more interested in normal than abnormal mood. As a side effect of this, studies of phobic states and panic disorder may require to have added items. One example of this is the modification of Bech (1986) which takes account of panic attacks. This is accomplished by having two versions of the scale. The HAS-P assesses the attack itself, defined as a sudden onset of anxiety without obvious provocation. The rating involves recording the number of attacks in the last week and their average severity using the items of the HAS. The assessment is completed with the second version, the HAS-G used to rate the severity of anxiety between panic attacks.

Further studies generally have confirmed the characteristics of the HAS. Snaith *et al.* (1965) give an inter-rater correlation of 0.94. Kellner *et al.* (1968) found it to discriminate adequately between diazepam and placebo in a double-blind trial. Kellner *et al.* (1972) found it to correlate 0.58–0.83 with the Symptom Rating Test, a self-rating measure of neurotic distress.

In 1969 Hamilton reviewed its use in several drug trials and reported a modification by splitting the somatic item into two components—muscular and sensory—and rating each separately. It has successfully discriminated between active and inactive treatment in trials by Davison (1963), LeGassicke and McPherson (1965) and Robinson *et al.* (1965).

Lader and Marks (1971) and Tyrer (1976) have used a version of the HAS modified for visual analogue presentation of each item with success.

Clinical Anxiety Scale (CAS)

This is a modification of the HAS designed to select those items which are best able to correlate with global severity ratings of the patient and the doctor. For practical purposes it is limited to six items, although a number of other items were tested and shown to be valid.

The authors (Snaith *et al.*, 1982) identified 88 items from the Hamilton scale and used 63 of them in the analysis. A schedule was made up with scoring rules for each item from 0 to 4 and 0 to 2 for the behavioural rating items. The HAS score could be extracted from the ratings as well as individual item scores.

The test group were patients diagnosed as anxiety neurosis (ICD 300.0). The global rating was constructed from two ratings:

1. An independent researcher made a global assessment on a 0–6 point scale.
2. The patients rated themselves on two visual analogue scales of:

As anxious as it is possible to be ______________ very calm
As tensed up as it is possible to be ____________ very relaxed

The sum of these was divided by 5.

The final global rating then was the mean of the patient and doctor ratings, giving equal weight to each.

First 51 patients were given the schedule. Twenty-four items correlated with global severity better than $p<0.001$. After excluding items which might be contaminated by depression or drug effects, the ten best items were picked for further analysis. Scales varying in length from four to ten items were correlated against global severity. All were better than the HAS in both the first sample of 51 and in a subsequent sample of 27. The eventual six-item scale correlated with global severity 0.85 in the first and 0.67 in the second sample.

Taking a cut-off score of 4.0 on the global ratings as distinguishing moderate from severe anxiety the HAS failed to distinguish the two groups, while the six-item (and the four- and ten-item) CAS distinguished the two levels of severity at the $p<0.01$ level. The new scales are also more sensitive to change. The HAS correlates with change in global score 0.45, while the six-item scale correlates 0.74.

The six-item scale was chosen for convenience over ten items and for extra item coverage over four items. The items are:

Psychic tension
Ability to relax
Startle responses
Worrying
Apprehension
Restlessness

In addition, because of the inclusion in DSM-III of panic disorder an extra item is given for separate scoring and with no validation data for rating panic attacks in severity and frequency, these two aspects being confounded into a single scale 0–4.

The CAS items are largely confined to psychic tension as opposed to somatic symptoms, while the HAS has a wide coverage. Thus choice of scale will depend on the breadth of coverage required and this must be balanced against the greater sensitivity of the CAS. All items of the CAS are represented in the anxiety section of the PSE, suggesting that the two could well be used together: PSE to diagnose the syndrome and the CAS to record severity and change in severity.

Buss Anxiety Scale

This scale was set up to measure anxiety in all clinical situations (Buss *et al.*, 1955), and in this respect it is similar to the Zung scales and different from the Hamilton scales.

It is not really a scale at all, but a glossary of definitions like the PSE which is designed to remove some of the criterion variance involved when raters make judgements about the presence or absence and the severity of a symptom.

There are two categories: observed and reported symptoms of anxiety. The observed symptoms are restlessness, physiological concomitants and distractibility (assessed by raters during a serial sevens test, in which the subject is asked to subtract 7 from 100 then, without stopping, 7 from the result and so on to the end).

The reported symptoms are subjective feelings of tension, worry, somatic complaints, physiological concomitants, muscular tension and overall rating of anxiety (a clinical integration of the findings during the interview).

The intercorrelation between four psychologists who interviewed together but rated independently varied from item to item. It was highest for distractibility (0.93) and lowest for observed physiological concomitants (0.56).

In general the reported symptoms tended to be better than the observed. There was little relationship between observed and reported physiological concomitants (0.30) but a better one between restlessness (observed) and muscular tension (reported) of 0.61. The inter-rater reliability of the overall rating was 0.83, and the correlation between this integrated clinical rating and the sum of the individual items was 0.93. The scale was used to validate the A scale of the Taylor Manifest Anxiety Scale, and the correlation between that and the overall rating on the Buss inventory was 0.60.

The use of this inventory is likely to be problematic and cumbersome and it offers little advantage over the use of the more recently developed and better-validated instruments.

Covi Anxiety Scale

This scale quantifies the psychiatrist's clinical impression of a patient in three areas: first their verbal report (e.g. feels nervous, jittery, jumpy), then their behaviour (e.g. appears frightened, shaky, restless) and their somatic signs (e.g. sweating, trembling, heart pounding).

Each of these three areas is rated by the psychiatrist on a five-point scale. This has the virtue of simplicity and might be a psychometrically valid scale, but unfortunately no psychometric data have been found in the literature despite a careful search. Covi *et al.* (1979) and Covi and Lipman (1984) describe the scale and its use in two rather unorthodox studies, but give no references to psychometric studies. It might be sensitive to change since it consists of global ratings (see Symptom Rating Test section below).

Gelder–Marks Phobia Questionnaire

This assessment battery was first described during use in a trial of behaviour therapy for severe agoraphobia, the results of which although statistically significant were clinically unimpressive (Gelder and Marks, 1966). There are four sections and each item is rated on a five-point scale. Some items are directed at phobias themselves and are rated:

1. No uneasiness when meeting feared object
2. Uneasiness but no avoidance
3. Definite fear, tendency to avoid
4. Strong fear, avoidance if at all possible
5. Terrifying, panic attack when avoidance impossible

Technically this scale confounds the qualities of avoidance and fear, but practically there seems to be little difficulty with its use. The main phobia (i.e. agoraphobia in the study for which it was first described) is rated first, then 'other phobias' since agoraphobics tend to be multiply phobic.

The next section is for anxiety and depression. There are five questions about anxiety, covering physical, autonomic and psychic symptoms. There are then further questions about depression and obsessions rated on 1–5 scales.

Self-rating and observer-rating versions are available and reliability between the versions is high. For main phobia the assessor–patient correlation is 0.74–0.81, for other phobias 0.69–0.78, for anxiety 0.56–0.66 and for depression 0.45–0.61. For obsessions the reliability is a less satisfactory 0.47–0.60.

The inter-rater reliability of the assessor scale is 0.82 for main phobia, 0.80 for other phobia, 0.67 for anxiety, 0.59 for depression and 0.77 for obsessions.

These scales or alternative versions of them, some using an eight-point scale, have been extensively used in behaviour therapy research with considerable success in showing differential treatment effects between different types of treatment, including pharmacological treatment (e.g. clomipramine for agoraphobia).

BROAD-SPECTRUM OBSERVER-RATED SCALES CONTAINING ANXIETY ITEMS

Brief Psychiatric Rating Scale (BPRS)

The BPRS was initially developed from factor analyses of results of several larger sets of items, particularly Lorr's Multidimensional Scale for Rating

Psychiatric Patients (Lorr *et al.*, 1962). It is recommended for use where economy, efficiency and speed are important considerations. There is a rather rudimentary standard interview procedure, but for the most part ratings are designed to be made by expert psychiatrists using their clinical judgement to a degree most other scales try to avoid.

There are 16 items, each rated on a 0–6 scale of severity (Overall and Gorham, 1962; Overall, 1974). Because the scale covers all aspects of psychopathology, and unlike the Comprehensive Psychopathological Rating Scale selection of items is not encouraged, there is only one item for anxiety, which is labelled, reasonably enough, 'Anxiety'. It cannot for this reason be recommended for use in anxiety studies.

Comprehensive Psychopathological Rating Scale (CPRS)

The CPRS was devised in Scandinavia with the express aim of measuring change during treatment interventions (Asberg *et al.*, 1978). Thus items were selected after consultation with a number of departments of psychiatry and pharmaceutical companies, by a multidisciplinary group under the auspices of the Swedish Research Council (Montgomery *et al.*, 1978a). They avoided items reflecting long-term traits, those heavily influenced by socio-cultural values and those which were too closely associated with particular syndromes, the aim being to obtain scores of general psychopathology.

Each item has a brief definition and where necessary the instruction to differentiate from other similar items. All items are scored 0–3 on criteria of intensity, frequency and duration. All items are to be related to habitual level of functioning for the individual.

This is one of the very few scales which have been designed with cross-cultural studies in mind and hence is useful in multicentre studies of psychotropic drugs (Montgomery *et al.*, 1978b). As of 1978 it was available in Swedish, German, Danish, Finnish, Italian and English.

There are 40 items based on the report of the patient to the interviewer and a further 25 based on the interviewer's observations. A further item of global rating of severity and one of assumed reliability of information bring the total available items to 67. However, it is recommended that selections of items are made for the purposes of each investigation. There are seven items which tap anxiety, but this number varies depending on how specific the items are required to be. There appear to be a maximum of ten items: eight reported and two observed. These are:

3. Inner tension
9. Worrying over trifles (non-specific)
11. Phobias
19. Reduced sleep

23. Autonomic disturbances
25. Muscular tension
27. Derealization
28. Depersonalization
46. Autonomic disturbances (observed)
63. Muscular tension (observed)

The use of the scale by untrained raters has been tested against scores of psychiatrists trained in its use. Whether the untrained rater is a general practitioner, a psychologist or a nurse, the inter-rater reliabilities are all very high for the depression items—the only ones so tested (see also the Montgomery–Asberg Depression Rating Scale). The same has not been carried out with the anxiety items.

A similar problem *vis-à-vis* anxiety items arises with the cross-cultural comparison study. This was performed on 106 hospitalized depressed patients and the items selected for study were the 17 most commonly occurring ones, excluding most of the anxiety-related items.

It would clearly be a worthwhile study to check the reliability and validity of the anxiety items of the CPRS in further studies on the English version.

SELF-RATING SCALES FOR ANXIETY

Spielberger State–Trait Anxiety Inventory (STAI)

This scale was first developed in the 1960s when all available scales measured trait rather than state anxiety, and it was revised in 1983 (Spielberger *et al.*, 1983). A trait is a relatively enduring personality characteristic while a state is a psychological condition occurring at that moment in time. Thus all human beings will have high state anxiety at one time or another, especially under life-threatening conditions. At times of no or little threat some will have higher levels of anxiety than others. There was therefore a need for related scales which assessed both trait and state anxiety separately and as far as possible with the same items.

The STAI achieves this by using different instructions prefaced to two similar but not identical forms. The trait or T form (called Y2) asks subjects to rate how they *generally* feel and the state or S form (called Y1) asks them to rate how they feel at this moment. The state form can be modified for rating of any short period such as the last hour or the last day. About half of each scale is made up of 'anxiety present' items and half of 'anxiety absent' items (rated in opposite directions when scored). Subjects rate each on a four-point scale.

The scales have been through a large amount of development and testing, particularly for use in investigating psychological concepts and behaviour under various stress conditions of different groups. A bibliography and normal values for large populations are given in the manual (Spielberger *et al.*, 1983). It is only more recently that they have been used for psychiatric and psychopharmacological research. The anxiety items are not specified for clinical morbid anxiety and this is a drawback in clinical research.

Although the concurrent validity of the T scale against other personality scales of anxiety/neuroticism varies from 0.53 to 0.85, this does not guarantee that it really measures an unvarying trait. Indeed there is a consensus that trait anxiety tends to change as state anxiety changes. This may be because the instruction to rate 'how you are usually' is too difficult if high state anxiety has been present for some time.

To some extent the T scale does vary less than the S scale under conditions of varying threat. The correlation between S and T scales is around 0.65 under low stress conditions. The test–retest reliability of the S scale varies from 0.16 to 0.62. The T scale reliability is appreciably higher at 0.65–0.82. The S scores are of course supposed to change to a certain extent over time as threat levels change. In addition under levels of low threat the two scales correlate highly, as would be expected.

The T score has been shown to correlate satisfactorily with other personality measures of trait anxiety. There is no work on the correlation of the S score with observer or self-rated measures of anxiety states and this would make it a stronger scale for psychiatric use.

The problems with this scale appear to be particularly in the non-specific nature of the items of the S scale. It is so sensitive (theoretically a good thing for a scale to measure change) that it responds markedly to test anxiety and is really designed as a measure of perceived stress. This may not be appropriate for severely anxious patients. There are no items for accessory symptoms in anxiety states such as depression, as these have been studiously removed to purify the measure. The scale is contaminated by somatic items so its use in a general hospital or general practice population may be difficult to interpret. Nevertheless it is highly developed and is available in almost all languages.

The pre-1983 version has been replaced and the new version can be identified by the naming of the forms as X1 and 2 rather than Y1 and 2.

Taylor Manifest Anxiety Scale (TMAS)

Taylor (1953) developed this scale for recording the severity of manifest as opposed to latent anxiety. The items were drawn from the Minnesota Multiphasic Personality Inventory (MMPI), a widely used measure of individual differences in personality. Out of 200 items in the full scale, 65 were agreed by over 80% of clinicians to be indicative of manifest anxiety. Fifty of these items were found to have high correlations with the total score and the rest were dropped. A large number of buffer items were added to obscure the purpose of the inventory and reduce response bias, and this led to a 225-item inventory called the 'Biographical Inventory', again to obscure its purpose. In a normal population the median score is 13 and the mean is 14.6.

The following gives an idea of the items, with the anxiety response in parentheses:

I do not tire easily (false)
I frequently notice my hand shakes when I try to do something (true)

In normal subjects the test–retest reliability was 0.89 over 3 weeks, 0.82 over 5 weeks and 0.81 over 9–17 months, i.e. the scores are very stable, reflecting its origin as a personality questionnaire.

Scores depend on the buffer items. When the same items were scored after administration, either as part of the MMPI or of the Biographical Inventory, the correlation was only 0.68 with an 18-week gap.

Further revision aimed to simplify the language for a non-college population. The new version had a correlation of 0.85 with the old version (3-week gap) and the test–retest reliability of the new one was 0.88.

One hundred and three mixed psychiatric patients had a mean score of 34, which is the 98.8 percentile for normals. O'Connor and Stafford (1956) found by factor analysis five dimensions in the scale suggesting a lack of homogeneity.

De Bonis (1974) describes the TMAS as a personality instrument and this is to some extent confirmed by the findings of Kellner *et al.* (1968). These investigators gave seven different measures of anxiety concurrently to patients in a trial of diazepam against placebo and one other drug which was shown to be inactive. They used the 50-item version of the TMAS with no buffer items. All other instruments, including the Hamilton Anxiety Scale, global ratings, target symptom ratings, three main complaint ratings, the Symptom Rating Test and a check-list score, discriminated the active from inactive treatments. The TMAS did not, and neither did the neuroticism scale of the Eysenck Personality Inventory. This suggests that the TMAS is insensitive for use, at least in psychopharmacology, and that it has the characteristics of a personality measure.

Other studies have shown change during treatment using the TMAS but, unlike Kellner *et al.* (1968), have not compared its sensitivity to change with other instruments. Lorr *et al.* (1962) and Byrne. (1964) both used it successfully but in view of the Kellner *et al.* (1968) findings it cannot be recommended for the measurement of change.

Anxiety Status Inventory and Self-rating Anxiety Scale

These scales were reported by Zung (1974). The aims were to:

1. Include items of anxiety as a psychiatric disorder but not only in anxiety states (in contrast to the Hamilton Anxiety Scale).
2. It should quantify symptoms.
3. It should be short and simple.
4. There should be two formats: a self-rated (SAS) and an observer-rated (ASI) scale using the same item content. This allows subjective and 'objective' ratings of the same state.

The items were drawn from the clinical literature.

The ASI consists of 20 items, each with probe questions for use at interview. Five items are mood-directed and 15 are somatic directed.

All items are rated 1–4 (1 is 'no symptom') on the basis of intensity, duration and frequency of the symptom during the previous week. The scores were to be expressed as a percentage of the maximum (80) and this is called the 'z score' to distinguish it from the 'index' derived from the SAS.

The SAS consists of the same items with balanced positive and negative wording. Scoring is 1–4 based on the duration of the symptom in the past week. The index is the percentage of maximum score.

In comparison with the Taylor MAS both tests (SAS and ASI) were better at separating anxiety disorders from other psychiatric diagnoses but were still not completely specific for anxiety (Zung, 1974). The ASI and SAS correlated together 0.66 in all subjects and 0.74 in anxiety disorders (DSM-II diagnosis).

The different purposes of the scales compared with the Taylor MAS are reflected in low correlations of 0.30 and 0.33 with the SAS and the ASI, respectively.

Costello and Comrey Scales for Anxiety and Depression

These scales, first published in 1967, are inappropriate for use as ratings of clinical syndromes. The anxiety scale is said to 'measure the predisposition to develop anxious-depressive states', in fact something like the personality trait of neuroticism. It is very unlikely that the scales are at all sensitive to change.

The scales are the result of a study combining the best items of two previous sets of scales for measuring anxious moods and depressed moods developed by the authors independently. Twenty-nine items for mood states were combined with items from a truth scale and a social desirability scale to control for these sources of response bias, which are inherent in all self-rating scales but controlled for in few. This made a 42-item scale.

The results from a study of normal subjects showed four factors. The first was depression, the second anxiety, the third truth–social desirability and the fourth age–marital status. There was a correlation of 0.5 between the depression and the anxiety scales. The impure items were dropped to make the two scales for anxiety and depression.

In an undiagnosed psychiatric population the factor structure described above was upheld and the scales appeared to retain homogeneity. In these patients the correlation between the MMPI(D) scale and the Taylor MAS was 0.69, suggesting that these do not well separate anxiety and depression factors. The two new scales were better for this purpose, the depression scale correlating only 0.20 with the MAS and the anxiety scale correlating only 0.30 with the MMPI(D). The scale scores appeared not to be contaminated by the truth–social desirability factor to any great extent, and age and sex did not bias them.

The test–retest reliability for anxiety was 0.72 and for depression 0.79.

Social-evaluative Anxiety Scales

Social-evaluative anxiety is the experience of distress, discomfort, fear or anxiety in social situations, the avoidance of social situations and the fear of receiving a negative evaluation from others. The importance of the concept is that 8% of all phobic patients seen in out-patient psychiatric departments have social phobia, and the symptom of social phobia is commonly present in patients with other diagnoses such as depression.

Two scales were designed by Watson and Friend (1969); one for social avoidance and distress and the other for the fear of negative evaluation. Social Avoidance and Distress (SAD) consists of 28 items, such as:

I try to avoid situations which force me to be very sociable (avoidance)
I often find social occasions upsetting (distress)

Fear of Negative Evaluation (FNE) consists of 30 items, such as:

I rarely worry about seeming foolish to others (false)
I feel very upset when I commit some social error (true)

The two scales are quite homogeneous, i.e. the items all measure the same characteristic of the subjects. The item–total correlations of the SAD was 0.77 and of the FNE 0.72. The relationship of the scales to social desirability was also minimized, the correlation with a scale to measure social desirability set being only −0.25. Thus subjects are not responding with what they think are socially desirable responses.

The relationship between the scales and hence between the concepts vary from 0.32 to 0.51. Experimentally it was shown that people high on SAD avoided social situations and were anxious in social situations, thus validating that scale. Individuals high on FNE were more anxious in evaluative situations and tended to seek approval.

SELF-RATING SCALES FOR MIXED MOOD STATES

Anxiety is an integral component of depression and vice versa. For this reason many of the scales dealt with above, whether they are observer- or self-rated, have some items to grade the severity of the depression component.

The overlap between the two mood states is at its greatest in the milder disturbances, when they may be inextricably mixed. In this situation it makes sense to measure the two, giving them equal prominence. In mild disorders self-rating scales are generally adequate. A range of instruments have been developed for this task and they will be included here. They could just as well have been covered in the depression chapter (Ch. 4).

Hospital Anxiety and Depression Scale (HAD)

In this scale, Zigmond and Snaith (1983) attempted to overcome a problem in the use of symptom rating scales in hospital populations. Many patients, especially in general hospital practice, have physical as well as psychiatric conditions. Some of these, for example cardiac disease giving rise to palpitations, or gastrointestinal disease giving rise to constipation or nausea, could give misleadingly high scores on most of the depression or anxiety rating scales, which include ratings of somatic symptoms on the assumption that they are 'psychogenic'. A scale without this contamination would be valuable in self-assessment of mood disorders in a general hospital.

Depression items were included if they made no reference to physical functions. These items therefore referred almost exclusively to the anhedonic state, which is said to be the central feature of a depressive illness. Anxiety items were added from the Present State Examination. This is a little surprising as most of the anxiety items of the PSE rely on autonomic symptoms for their identification. The eventual items were modified by the failure of one of the depression items to show an adequate correlation with total scores and the removal of the worst anxiety item to retain the balance.

In a medical population the depression scale correlated 0.70 with an independent global rating, and the anxiety scale 0.74. Each subscale was independent in that they failed to correlate significantly with the global rating of the other mood (Zigmond and Snaith, 1983). The scale scores were independent of physical illness, as physically ill patients with low global severity scores of either depression or anxiety scored very low on the questionnaire.

The scale was assessed for its usefulness as a case-finding instrument in a general hospital population, a function for which it would be in competition with the General Health Questionnaire (see Ch. 6). However, the appropriate study to compare the two instruments in this population has not been carried out. Preliminary data show that as many as 20–25% of patients would be unclassifiable or borderline if the HAD was used as a screening instrument. Thus, if it was to be used, a low threshold score would have to be adopted to ensure that no cases were missed, and in this case there are likely to be as many false positive results as are found in general hospital populations with the GHQ.

Snaith (1985) has described how the scale can be used to follow improvements or exacerbations in a patient's progress during a stay in hospital. Fallowfield *et al.* (1987) showed it to be well accepted by general medical patients.

Aylard *et al.* (1987) confirmed some of the qualities of the HAD in four groups of patients, some medical, some psychiatric and some expected to be normal. They used the MADRS and the Clinical Anxiety Scale (CAS) as observer-rated criteria of the severity of depression and anxiety. After eliminating all those subjects with scores within the normal range the MADRS and CAS scores did not correlate significantly with each other. The HAD-D scale correlated with the MADRS but not the CAS and the HAD-A scale with the CAS but not the MADRS. However, this is to take the limiting case only, since the greater part of the screened groups were eliminated before the analysis. When these subjects were left in the analysis the HAD-A and D scales do correlate significantly. In oncology out-patients (Sensky *et al.*, 1989) A and D correlated 0.36, and in dialysands (Sensky, personal communication) 0.56. Thus the notion of independent dimensions at lower levels of severity appears to be unwarranted. Even in psychiatric patients the independence of the dimensions is not as good as at first seemed the case. Bromley *et al.* (in press) found the D–A correlation to be 0.49 in this group. In addition the HAD fared no better in this respect than older established scales (IDA, Zung or CCEI).

Aylard *et al.* (1987) also found low misclassification rates for severe depression or anxiety using cut-off scores on the appropriate observer-rated instruments as the criteria. However, in order to achieve this all the mild disorders had to be left out of the analysis, so the value of the HAD as a case-finding instrument must remain in doubt. However, none of this detracts from the value of the instrument to measure depression and anxiety in medically ill populations—its original purpose.

Symptom Rating Test (SRT)

This interesting and useful scale was devised and thoroughly developed by Kellner and colleagues. From the start it was designed as a scale of neurotic distress which would be sensitive to change. This differentiated it from case-finding instruments for use in epidemiological research and from personality questionnaires.

Several forms of the test are available, although the most commonly used is now the short form. At first the following versions were tested:

1. All versions started with a structured interview in which a check-list of symptoms was completed by the interviewer.
2. A self-rating scale was then completed by the patient. This was in several forms:
   (a) The answers were elicited on test cards or on pencil-and-paper tests. The test cards had printed on them the available responses to each item and were presented in random order for each item. This was an attempt to overcome response sets (Cronbach, 1946; Langevin and Stancer, 1979).
   (b) In the pencil-and-paper test the items were completed as in any other scale.
   (c) The time period to which the response referred could be set at the previous week or the previous day.
   (d) In some studies the short form only was used, in which the semi-structured interview to elicit the check-list was deleted.

The items were developed from the 100 commonest complaints of neurotic patients and 38 were chosen. Fifteen were somatic in nature and 23 were psychological complaints. Five different scales for rating the items were tried, two based on frequency, two on intensity and one on duration of the symptom when it occurred.

In development it was found that the pencil-and-paper and the test card versions correlated 0.90, suggesting that positional set is of little importance (Bedford *et al.*, 1979). In the pencil-and-paper test it was found that over 50% of patients preferred to record their responses on a box scale rather than on an unbroken line. This procedure was therefore adopted. Three subscales were identified on the basis of factor analysis: anxiety, depression and somatic complaints, and a fourth was added on an a priori basis—inadequacy. This analysis led to the construction of a shorter version of 30 items, on the basis that the remaining eight items conferred no greater advantage in terms of sensitivity or reliability.

The sensitivity to change of the five kinds of scale were tested in a study of 46 out-patients who were tested before and after treatment. It was found that the duration scale and one of the frequency scales discriminated poorly between the groups and were relatively insensitive to change (Sheffield and Kellner, 1970). On the basis of this analysis a single, best scale was constructed.

The reliability of the 1-week form was tested by giving it on consecutive days. Correlation between the two test times was 0.92–0.94 in two separate groups. This was better than the Manifest Anxiety Scale (Taylor, 1953) on the same groups. The reliability of change in scores was tested using a split half method in 40 in-patients during treatment. The reliability was 0.89.

All items of the scale discriminated significantly between 100 neurotic patients and 100 normal subjects. The change in scores was found to be as sensitive as psychiatrists' ratings using the Hamilton Anxiety Scale, a global rating or a rating of target symptoms (Kellner *et al.*, 1968). It performed better than the Eysenck Personality Inventory and equal to the Manifest Anxiety Scale in the task of discriminating normals and neurotics, misclassifying about 12–15% of subjects (Kellner and Sheffield, 1973). Depressed patients had higher scores than the remainder of the neurotic population. They were reduced after 3 weeks of treatment with an antidepressant but they remained higher than normals.

In addition to the 1-week and 1-day forms there is also a 1-hour form for use in studies of diurnal variation. The 1-day and 1-hour forms may also be useful in single-case cross-over designed studies (Kellner and Sheffield, 1968).

Evidence that the SRT is sensitive to change comes from a study in which it was given to 40 consecutive neurotic out-patients and 43 employees of a pharmaceutical company as a normal control. At the same time subjects were given the Eysenck Personality Inventory. In the normal population, i.e. those without a recent increase in neurotic symptoms, the two measures correlated significantly, but in the out-patient group they did not, suggesting that they measure different attributes (Kellner and Sheffield, 1967). When compared against other anxiety ratings in a study of the effects of diazepam, hydroxyzine pamoate or placebo, all ratings adopted gave significant results. These were the Manifest Anxiety Scale, global ratings, Hamilton Anxiety Scale, a check-list score and a score on three main complaints (N=24). As one scale was as good as another it was suggested that the SRT, being brief, was to be preferred.

Kellner (1971, 1972) conducted an exhaustive review of the literature on therapeutic trials with neurotic patients up to that time, looking for evidence that some forms of scoring of change were more sensitive than others. All the trials were double-blind, with random allocation of subjects. He classified them as follows:

Questionnaires
Check-lists of symptoms
Scales of individual symptoms, e.g. SRT
Scales of categories of symptoms, e.g. phobic anxiety, cognitive
Global scales
Ranking of treatment by preference

Medication guess
Compound scores of several methods
Rating of target complaints

He found that scales of both kinds and global ratings were commonly used. When attention was restricted to those trials in which one method discriminated between treatments while another failed, global scales succeeded 14 times when others did not; and if attention was further restricted to trials between a known successful drug and placebo, ten trials were found in which global scales were superior. This does not of course imply that global scales are all that is necessary, as they leave the profile of the improvement unknown. In a closer study of trials of known active drug against placebo Kellner (1972) found that the SRT was as sensitive as the other established techniques, such as the Hamilton Anxiety Scale. This he called a validation against the external chemical criterion, which is an essential part of the validation procedure for a scale to measure change.

Another validation exercise was to test the scales against the Personal Questionnaire (PQ; Shapiro, 1961). The PQ is tailored to each patient's symptoms and incorporates a defence against response bias (Sheffield and Kellner, 1970). The median correlation against the PQ for the 1-week SRT was 0.70 and for the 1-day SRT 0.89. The PQ takes much longer to construct and complete than the SRT.

Although the SRT is not designed as a case-finding instrument in the same way as the GHQ, Cochrane (1980) has compared it with the Langner 22-item index on this function. The attractions of the scale for this purpose are that it has been validated on criterion groups, it is brief, simple and very acceptable to patients, and it was designed with a subscale structure.

The author reduced the number of available responses per item from four to three. Patients scored a mean of 24.63 and a community sample scored 8.03. Females scored higher than males and unmarried higher than married subjects. Factor analysis showed a single dominant theme accounting for 77.9% of the variance, confirming previous studies which showed that its use as a unidimensional measure of severity of neurotic distress is valid (Kellner and Sheffield, 1973). A proportion of the subjects were retested at 1 week and a test–retest reliability of 0.91 was found in this stable sample.

There are two problems with the results of this study. First, it does not demonstrate the usefulness of the SRT as a screening instrument since there was no second stage consisting of a psychiatric interview, and therefore data on proportions of 'hits' and 'misses' are not available. Secondly, the factor analysis failed to support the subscale structure of the SRT. However, as the authors acknowledge, it was not designed for use in a non-clinical population. In general the SRT discriminated the normal and neurotic groups better than did the Langner 22-item index.

In a group of depressed patients in general practice all the SRT subscales correlated highly with each other. During the course of an antidepressant study the change in the SRT sum score correlated highly with the change in the Hamilton Depression Rating Scale (HDRS). The subscales showed varying correlations with the HDRS. Depression and somatic subscales had a correlation of a higher order of magnitude than anxiety and inadequacy subscales, suggesting that in some instances a two-factor solution may be appropriate (Thompson and Thompson, in press).

Leeds scales for Self-assessment of Anxiety and Depression

Snaith *et al.* (1976) developed a set of scales from the Wakefield Depression Inventory for screening and for measurement of severity of anxiety and depression. They started with 12 items from the Wakefield and added a further ten (two from the Symptom Rating Test; Kellner and Sheffield, 1973). These 22 symptoms were chosen to cover a wide range of the symptomatology, with the exception of obsessional symptoms, loss of libido, weight loss and restless sleep, as these items would have been impossible to construct in a self-rating format for use with all ages. Response was according to the ratings: definitely (3), sometimes (2), not much (1) and not at all (0). The wording of four items was reversed so that response set was to some extent overcome.

To validate items as measures of depression a new criterion was chosen. This consisted of the score on the Hamilton Depression Scale with the anxiety items removed, renamed the Symptoms of Depression Scale. The same operation was performed for anxiety by removing the depression items from the Hamilton Anxiety Scale, calling the result the Symptoms of Anxiety Scale. Both scales proved to have high inter-rater reliabilities. Global ratings of severity were also made.

Two scales were first constructed for use in already diagnosed groups of depressed and anxious patients. Those items of the original 20 were included if they achieved a correlation of more than 0.58 with the global severity scale (we are not told why this figure was chosen) and if they had a significantly higher mean score in the appropriate diagnostic group. Each scale comprised six items after this analysis:

Endogenous depression	*Anxiety neurosis*
Sadness of mood	Panic
Loss of enjoyment	Agoraphobia
Lack of energy	Palpitation
Apathy	Dizziness
Delayed insomnia	Fearful mood
Suicidal thoughts	Psychic tension

These scales were called the 'Leeds Self-assessment of Depression (SAD) Specific Scale and the Leeds Self-assessment of Anxiety (SAA) Specific Scale, respectively.

When assessing previously undiagnosed illness (for example in a screening study) an instrument is necessary which makes no diagnostic assumptions. Snaith *et al.* (1976) derived two such scales: one for the assessment of anxiety, the Leeds Self-assessment of Anxiety General Scale, and one for depression, the Leeds Self-assessment of Depression General Scale. Items for these scales were chosen if they fulfilled the criteria of (a) having a correlation with the appropriate observer rating of 0.52, and (b) having a significantly different contribution to the variance of the two observer ratings.

This procedure produced remarkably similar results to the previous exercise. In the depression scale, loss of appetite substituted for lack of energy. In the anxiety scale restlessness and irritability substituted for dizziness and psychic tension.

A further refinement was attempted by subtracting the Leeds SAA specific score from the Leeds SAD specific score for each patient. This was to give a diagnostic score for the distinction between anxiety and depression. With a theoretical maximum from −18 to +18 it was found that only one case of endogenous depression scored less than −4 and no case of anxiety neurosis more than +4 when the scores of the criterion groups were calculated. These scores were therefore proposed as the cut-off scores beyond which a diagnosis could be made of either anxiety or depression. Inside these limits a mixed state prevailed. However, in both the criterion and validation studies the majority of cases fell between these two limits, an uncomfortable finding which must cast a degree of doubt upon the validity of the original scales.

A similar problem occurred with the use of the general scales for case finding. About 33% of all cases fell at the mild or borderline illness level.

Irritability Depression Anxiety (IDA) Scale

Irritability is defined by Snaith *et al.* (1978) as a temporary psychiatric state characterized by impatience, intolerance and poorly controlled anger. It is a similar concept to hostility and, like hostility, may be inwardly or outwardly directed. It is often present in states of morbid anxiety or depression, hence the attempt in this scale to combine ratings of all three.

The starting point was to take items from the Buss–Durkee inventory of hostility and direction of hostility (HDHQ) and other items for anxiety and depression from this group's extensive past experience with such ratings. Ten items for each state were chosen to go into the analysis. Four irritability items were outwardly directed and four inwardly directed, with the remaining two items being unclear as to direction. The item wording was alternately healthy and unhealthy to control response bias, and the items were arranged in the order DIA DIA, etc.

The validating criteria were observer ratings of anxiety (the Symptoms of Anxiety Scale) and depression (the Symptoms of Depression Scale), which are both described under the Leeds scales. An observer rating for irritability separating outward and inward direction was constructed to validate the self-assessed irritability ratings. This gave results as a nine-point global rating. The validating scales all had high inter-rater reliability. Items were selected from the originals if they had a significant correlation with the relevant observer scale and a significantly higher correlation with that scale than with the others. Five of the anxiety and five depression items survived, and all eight directional irritability items. The subscales thus formed were found to have high correlations with the relevant observer scales (depression 0.75, anxiety 0.70, outward irritability 0.79 and inward irritability 0.84). Split half reliabilities of the scales varied from 0.72 to 0.93.

In a subsequent paper (Snaith and Taylor, 1985) the value of the irritability subscales has been questioned by further testing. Thus the *raison d'être* of the IDA scale is now in doubt.

Mood Adjective Check-lists (MACL)

Many investigators, especially psychologists, have attempted to develop mood rating scales using adjectives in either a check-list or a rating scale format. Strictly, these are not designed for use in psychiatric populations and may contain no information about aspects of the syndrome of depression other than intensity of mood. For psychotic depression they are of no use at all and for endogenous depression their use could be severely criticized.

The earliest version was developed by Nowlis and Nowlis for use in studies with students—the Mood Adjective Check-list (Nowlis and Nowlis, 1956). Clyde (1961) has also published a measure of several mood states. McNair and Lorr (1964) developed a version of this type of scale specifically for use with neurotic patients, called the Profile of Mood States (POMS). They took the MACL adjectives and eliminated those which were too hard to understand and added a four-point scale of intensity for each adjective. In studies of out-patient populations five mood states were identified: tension, anger, depression, vigour and fatigue. Factor scores were used to obtain scores for each patient on each scale, and adequate homogeneity within each was found. In several treatment trials the scores were found to change significantly with improvement in clinical state although the data given are unclear. Each scale was found to correlate significantly with a concurrently administered measure of that mood. Particularly the tension scale correlated 0.80 with the Manifest Anxiety Scale. Other correlations, although significant, were small in real terms and were related to scales whose clinical significance was uncertain. A further development of the POMS is a bipolar version with items worded 'much like this, slightly like this, slightly unlike this, much unlike this' (Lorr and McNair, 1984).

Lubin (1965) has also attempted to develop Depression Adjective Checklists (DACL), aiming at ease of administration. From a pool of 171 adjectives he developed seven lists consisting of between 32 and 34 adjectives. The split half reliabilities of these lists ranged from 0.82 to 0.93 and were all highly intercorrelated, so that they can be considered as equivalent. Correlations between all of the lists and the MMPI-D scale or the Beck Depression Inventory were all significant, although no correlation was above 0.66. Acceptability was high, with a mean completion time of only 2.5 minutes. The effects of response sets and other sources of bias are unknown but cannot be discounted. Their sensitivity to change is also unknown.

SCL-90 and Subscales, Especially the BSI

The Symptom Check-list-90 was designed at Johns Hopkins University for self-rating by patients and normal populations of a range of dimensions of psychopathology. Thus, it is suited to community studies of psychiatric illness but not particularly suited to studies of a single aspect of psychopathology or change in that aspect. There have been numerous versions of the Hopkins Symptom Check-lists (HSCL). The first was developed by J. Frank as an improvement measure for trials of psychotherapy, and items were culled from the Cornell Medical Index and a scale by Lorr (see Derogatis *et al.*, 1974 for review and Lorr *et al.*, 1953). Versions have been produced with 58 items (the basic version), 64 items, 35 items (ECDEU version), 53 items (Brief Symptom Inventory, see below) and 90 items (SCL-90).

The SCL-90 (and the Brief Symptom Inventory, BSI, retains these) has nine subscales constructed according to clinical expectations and factor analytically validated. They have the following titles:

Somatization
Obsessive-compulsive
Interpersonal sensitivity
Depression
Anxiety
Hostility
Phobic anxiety
Paranoid ideation
Psychoticism

Each of the 90 items is rated on a 0–4 scale by the respondent. The time for completion is about 10 minutes. In addition to the items relating to the subscales there are four more not subsumed under any but which load on several dimensions. Also there are three indices of global distress: the general severity index, combining the number of symptoms and the intensity of distress; the positive symptom distress index, which is a pure intensity measure, functioning as a measure of response style; and the positive symptom total, which is simply a count of the symptoms.

The anxiety dimension of the basic HSCL consists of the following items:

Nervousness or shakiness inside
Heart pounding or racing
Sweating
Suddenly scared for no reason
Trouble getting your breath
Trembling
Hot or cold spells
Feeling tense or keyed up
Faintness or dizziness
Feeling fearful
A lump in your throat

The test–retest reliability of this dimension is 0.80 and the internal consistency 0.84, with item–total correlations varying from 0.68 to 0.78.

The sensitivity of the HSCL has been established in drug trials with anxious neurotic patients, using meprobamate, chlordiazepoxide and other minor tranquillizers. However it is not just the anxiety dimension which shows responses to anxiolytic drugs. Four of the five dimensions of the basic HSCL and the total symptom score showed responses to treatment with diazepam in a trial against placebo and phenobarbital (Derogatis *et al.*, 1974). There appears to be a high degree of agreement between the various forms of the HSCL right down to the 35-item version; however, the 58-item version appears to be a little more sensitive to change than the smaller version, and although this has not been directly tested it is likely that the SCL-90 is more sensitive than the BSI (53 items).

The validity of the dimensions has been successfully tested against the diagnoses of psychiatrists, and the influence on the dimensional scores of factors such as sex, social class and other interferring variables has been shown to be small.

The Brief Symptom Inventory has been validated on large groups of in-patients, out-patients and normal subjects (Derogatis and Melisaratos, 1983). Scores for the patients are more than 2 standard deviations above the mean of normals on all subscales and on the three global ratings. The internal consistency of the scales is high, ranging from 0.71 to 0.85 (anxiety is 0.81 and phobic anxiety is 0.77). Test–retest reliability is also high, from 0.68 to

0.91 (anxiety is 0.79 and phobic anxiety is 0.91). High test–retest reliability is desirable in an instrument to detect psychopathology but may indicate an insensitivity to change. This impression is confirmed by high correlations with the relevant sections of the MMPI, a personality measure designed to tap enduring personality traits. This would confirm the impression of the comparison in sensitivity between the HSCL basic 58-item version and the very short 35-item version that the shorter scales are less sensitive to change, presumably because the baseline scores are necessarily numerically lower.

AUTONOMIC PERCEPTIONS OF ANXIETY

Autonomic Perceptions Questionnaire (APQ)

This was devised to investigate the relationships between anxiety, the physiological concomitants of anxiety, and the perception by the subject of that physiological perturbation (Mandler *et al.*, 1958). There had been no previous attempts to carry out this sort of research on humans.

The APQ consists of three sections. The first section deals with the meaning of the term anxiety for the subject, asking them to describe what anxiety was for them, and then asking them to refer to their own definition wherever the word anxiety occurred in the subsequent questions. The second section comprises 30 visual analogue scales covering areas of bodily reaction to feelings, heart rate, perspiration, temperature change, respiration, gastrointestinal disturbance, muscle tension and blood pressure. Twenty-one are for states of anxiety and nine for states of pleasure. The wording is, for example: 'When you feel anxious how often are you aware of any change in your heart action?' followed by a visual analogue scale labelled 'always' and 'never.'

The third section has 70 MMPI items relating to internal sensation: 50 are Taylor Manifest Anxiety Scale items and 20 are extras. A short version contains just the 20 MMPI and 14 of the TMAS items dealing specifically with body perceptions and is called the Body Perception Scale. It is heavily biased towards trait items as all items are drawn from a personality inventory.

The authors tested the scale in an experimental situation in which the top and bottom scorers on the APQ underwent stress while having physiological recordings. The scale score did relate to both the intensity of physiological change and the discrepancy between it and the perception, i.e. high scorers had more change than low scorers and also exaggerated that change, while low scorers had less change with stress and also underestimated the change.

The items were not very specific for anxiety since the correlation between scores on the APQ completed for states of anxiety and pleasure was 0.50.

There are two problems with this instrument. It is very bulky and time-consuming for the subject, and the items are probably not very amenable to short-term change since they are worded as personality items.

Tyrer (1976) constructed his own version for use in his study of the effects of propranolol on physiological anxiety, the perception of bodily symptoms and the mood of anxiety. The subject rates feelings at the present time on a VAS for eight different symptoms, labelled 'absent' to 'very severe'. In use this scale was also found not to be very sensitive, partly because the distribution of scores was very skewed, so it is necessary to carry out log transformation before analysis. Tyrer suggests that bodily symptoms show wide variations in severity during the day, so that a single rating each day may be inaccurate. However, the scores did show a relation to stress.

It has to be pointed out that it would be naive to use this scale as an estimate of what is happening physiologically. That can only be done by direct measurement. Correlation between the patient's impression of physiological change and the actual changes taking place is present but of a low order for most items.

Body Sensations Questionnaire (BSQ)

This scale was devised for use in studies of agoraphobic populations, particularly intervention by behaviour therapy (Chambless *et al.*, 1984). The driving hypothesis was that fear of feeling afraid, and of the internal cues signalling anxiety, is what distinguishes agoraphobic and generalized anxiety patients from others. The acceptance of this hypothesis is not necessary for acceptance of the scale's validity.

There are 17 items, derived initially from asking subjects about their autonomic sensations during exposure sessions in treatment. Each is rated on a five-point scale from 'not frightened or worried by this sensation' to 'extremely frightened by this sensation'. Hence this scale attempts not to give an accurate account of the intensity of the sensation but how frightening it was found by the subject. This then is slightly different from the APQ, which only attempts to quantify the sensations.

The scale was tested on a sample of agoraphobics and a sample of controls. All 17 items were homogeneous, with item total correlations higher than 0.35. The distribution was normal. Test–retest reliability was 0.67.

During behaviour therapy combined with cognitive therapy the BSQ showed a marked and significant reduction in score, suggesting that it can be a sensitive instrument to measure change in some types of therapy for one aspect of anxiety. Each item of the BSQ differentiated the agoraphobic from the normal group.

UNSCALED TECHNIQUES FOR ASSESSING ANXIETY

Patient Diary of Symptoms

Anxiety fluctuates greatly depending upon the situation in which patients find themselves, the syndrome from which they suffer (generalized anxiety, panic disorder or phobic disorder) and the efficacy of treatment. Thus ratings carried out at the time of interview or appointment will not always pick up accurately the correct picture of the clinical state. This is different from depression, where it is assumed with some justification that the state is more constant regardless of surroundings.

Thus asking the patient to keep a daily diary of anxiety symptoms can be a useful addition to the assessment of anxiety in the course of therapy. This is especially so in the case of syndromes which are predominantly episodic, such as panic disorder. In addition, ratings of the avoidance of anxiety-inducing situations may also provide added information about behavioural concomitants of anxiety, and may help to explain unexpected results, for example a reduction in anxiety may be due to increased avoidance behaviour even if the patient is having an inactive treatment. These kinds of data cannot be subjected to the same rigorous validation as the standard rating scales and has to be taken largely at face value.

Medication Guess or Drug preference

These are techniques used in early studies of anxiolytics such as those by Granville-Grossman and Turner (1966) and Bonn *et al.* (1972). They require the patient to guess which was the active medication in a cross-over trial of placebo versus test drug, or which medication they preferred in a cross-over trial of two active drugs.

The problem with this as anything more than a screening test is that the reasons for the choice are unknown. They may be absence of side effects as much as anxiolytic advantage. On the other hand, the side effects may alert the patient to the fact that the tablet is 'active', so that they may then report that tablet to be more anxiolytic in an effort not to appear silly to the doctor, or through a misguided attempt to help the doctor out.

Probably these problems are more theoretical than real but may account for the apparent sensitivity to drug effects of this method (Kellner, 1972). If used in conjunction with established rating scales they may still have a place but not as the main indicator of therapeutic effect.

REFERENCES

Asberg, M., Montgomery, S. A., Perris, C., Schalling, D. and Sedvall, G. (1978). A comprehensive psychopathological rating scale. *Acta Psychiatr. Scand.* Suppl. 271, 5–28.

Aylard, P. R., Gooding, J. H., McKenna, P. J. and Snaith, R. P. (1987). A validation study of three anxiety and depression self assessment scales. *Psychosom. Res.* **31**, 261–268.

Bech, P., Kastrup, M. and Rafaelson, O. J. (1986). Minicompendium of rating scales for states of anxiety, depression, mania, schizophrenia with corresponding DSM III syndromes. *Acta Psychiatr. Scand.* Suppl 326, 73.

Bedford, A., Edington, A. and Kellner, R. (1979). Changes in self rating of symptoms: A comparison of questionnaire graphic scales with test cards. *Br. J. Psychiatry* **134**, 108–110.

Bonn, J. A., Turner, P. and Hicks, D. C. (1972). Beta adrenergic receptor blockade with practolol in treatment of anxiety. *Lancet* **i**, 814–815.

Bromley, P. N., Easton, A. M. E. Morlay, S. and Snaith, R. P. (in press). The differentiation of anxiety and depression by rating scales. *Acta Psychiatr. Scand.*

Buss, A. H. (1962). Two anxiety factors in psychiatric patients. *J. Abnorm. Soc. Psychol.* **65**, 426–427.

Buss, A. H., Wiener, M., Durkee, A. and Baer, M. (1955). The measurement of anxiety in clinical situations. *J. Consult. Psychol.* **19**, 125–129.

Byrne, D. (1964). Assessing personality variables and their alteration. In *Personality Change* (P. Worchel and D. Byrne, eds), Wiley, New York.

Chambless, D. L., Caputo, C., Bright, P. and Gallagher, R. (1984). Assessment of fear of fear in agoraphobics: The body sensations questionnaire and the agoraphobic cognitions questionnaire. *J. Consult. Clin. Psychol.* **52**, 1090–1097.

Clyde, D. J. (1961). *Clyde Mood Scale*, GWU, Washington, DC.

Cochrane, R. (1980). A comparative study of the Symptom Rating Test and the Langner 22-item Index for use in epidemiological surveys. *Psychiatr. Med.* **10**, 115–124.

Costello C. G. and Comrey A. L. (1967). Scales for measuring depression and anxiety. *J. Psychol.* **66**, 303–313.

Covi, L. and Lipman, R. S. (1984). Primary depression or primary anxiety? A possible psychometric approach to a diagnostic dilemma. *Clin. Neuropharmacol.* **7**, Suppl 1.

Covi, L., Lipman, R. S., McNair, D. M. and Czerlinsky, T. (1979). Symptomatic volunteers in multicentre drug trials. *Prog. Neuropsychopharm.* **3**, 521.

Cronbach, L. J. (1946). Response set and test validity. *Ed. Psych. Measurement* **6**, 475–495.

Davison, K. (1963). Evaluation of a new tranquiliser, benzquinamide, by a sequential method. **109**, 539–543.

De Bonis, M. (1974). Content analysis of 27 anxiety inventories and rating scales. In *Psychological Measurements in Psychopharmacology*, Modern Problems in Pharmacopsychiatry, Vol. 7, (P. Pichot, ed.), Karger, Basle.

Derogatis, L. R. and Melisaratos, N. (1983). The Brief Symptom Inventory; an introductory report. *Psychol. Med.* **13**, 595–605.

Derogatis, L. R., Lipman, R., Rickels, K., Uhlenhuth, E. H. and Covi, L. (1974). The Hopkins Symptom Checklist (HSCL). In *Psychological Measurements in Psychopharmacology*, Modern Problems in Pharmacopsychiatry, Vol. 7 (P. Pichot, ed.), Karger, Basle.

DiNardo, P. A., O'Brien, G. T., Barlow, D. H., Waddell, M. T. and Blanchard, E. B. (1982). *The Anxiety Disorders Interview Schedule*, Centre for Stress and Anxiety Disorders, Albany, New York.

Fallowfield, L. J., Baum, M. and Maguire, G. P. (1987). Do psychological studies upset patients? *J. R. Soc. Med.* **80**, 59.

Gelder, M. G. and Marks, I. M. (1966). Severe agoraphobia; a controlled trial of behaviour therapy. *Br. J. Psychiatry* **112**, 309–319.

Granville-Grossman, K. and Turner, P. (1966). The effect of propranolol on anxiety. Lancet **i**, 788–790.

Hamilton, M. (1959). The assessment of anxiety states by rating. *Br. J. med. Psychol.* **32**, 50–55.

Hamilton, M. (1969). The diagnosis and rating of anxiety. In *Studies of Anxiety* (M. H. Lader, ed.), Headley Bros, Kent.

Kellner, R. (1971). Part 1. Improvement criteria in drug trials with neurotic patients. *Psychol. Med.* **1**, 416–425.

Kellner, R. (1972). Part 2. Improvement criteria in drug trials with neurotic patients. *Psychol. Med.* **2**, 73–80.

Kellner, R. and Sheffield, B. F. (1967). Symptom rating test scores in neurotics and normals. *Br. J. Psychiatry* **113**, 525–526.

Kellner, R. and Sheffield, B. F. (1968). The use of self rating scales in a single patient multiple cross over trial. *Br. J. Psychiatry* **114**, 193–196.

Kellner, R. and Sheffield, B. F. (1973). A self rating scale of distress. *Psychol. Med.* **3**, 88–100.

Kellner, R., Kelly, A. V. and Sheffield, B. F. (1968). The assessment of changes in anxiety in a drug trial: A comparison of methods. *Br. J. Psychiatry* **114**, 863–869.

Kellner, R., Gervais, R. H. and Pathak, D. (1972). A pilot study of the short term antianxiety effects of molindone HC1. *J. Clin. Pharmacol.* **12**, 472–476.

Lader, M. H. and Marks, I. M. (1971). *Clinical Anxiety*, Heineman Medical, London.

Langevin, R. and Stancer, H. (1979). Evidence that depression rating scales primarily measure a social undesirability response set. *Acta Psychiatr. Scand.* **59**, 70–79.

LeGassicke, J. and McPherson, F. M. (1965). A sequential trial of Wy 3498 (oxazepam). *Br. J. Psychiatry* **111**, 521–525.

Lorr, M. and McNair, D. M. (1984). *Manual of the Profile of Mood States, Bipolar Form (POMS-BI)*, Ed. and Ind. Testing Service, San Diego.

Lorr, M., Jenkins, R. L. and Holsopple, J. Q. (1953). Multidimensional scale for rating psychiatric patients. *VA Tech. Bull.* **10**, 507.

Lorr, M., McNair, D. M., Michaux, W. W. and Raskin, A. (1962). Frequency of treatment and change in psychotherapy. *J. Abnorm. Soc. Psychol.* **64**, 281–292.

Lubin, B. (1965). Adjective check lists for measuring depression. *Arch. Gen. Psychiatry* **12**, 57–62.

Mandler, G., Mandler, J. M. and Uviller, E. T. (1958). Autonomic feedback: the perception of autonomic activity. *J. Abnorm. Soc. Psychol.* **56**, 367–373.

McNair, D. M. and Lorr, M. (1964). An analysis of mood in neurotics. *J. Abnorm. Soc. Psychol.* **69**, 620–627.

Montgomery, S., Asberg, M., Jornstedt, L., Thoren, P., Traskman, L., McAuley, R., Montgomery, D. and Shaw, P. (1978a). Reliability of the CPRS between the disciplines of psychiatry, general practice, nursing and psychology in depressed patients, *Acta Psychiatr. Scand.* Suppl. 271, 29–32.

Montgomery, S., Asberg, M., Traskman, L. and Montgomery, D. (1978b). Cross cultural studies on the use of CPRS in English and Swedish depressed patients. *Acta Psychiatr. Scand.* Suppl. 271, 33–38.

Nowlis, V. and Nowlis, H. H. (1956). The description and analysis of mood. *Ann. NY Acad. Sci.* **65**, 345–355.

O'Connor, J. P., Lorr, M. and Stafford, J. W. (1956). Some patterns of manifest anxiety. *J. Clin. Psychol.* **12**, 160–163.

Overall, J. E. (1974). The Brief Psychiatric Rating Scale in psychopharmacology research. In *Psychological Measurements in Psychopharmacology*, Modern Problems in Pharmacopsychiatry, Vol. 7 (P. Pichot, ed.), Karger, Basel.

Overall, J. E. and Gorham, D. R. (1962). The Brief Psychiatric Rating Scale. *Psychol. Rep.* **10**, 799–812.

Robinson, J. T., Davies, L. S., Knowles, J. and Kreitman, N. (1965). A controlled trial of pericyazine in the treatment of anxiety states. In *Proceedings Leeds Symposium on Behaviour Disorders* (A. Jenner, ed.), May & Baker, Dagenham, pp. 221–227.

Sensky, I, Dennehy, M, Culbert, A., Begent, R., Newland, E., Rustin, G. and Thompson, C., (1989). Physicians' perceptions of anxiety and depression among their outpatients: relationships with patients and doctors' satisfaction with their interviews, *J. R. C. Phys*, 23, 33–38.

Shapiro, M. B. (1961). *The Personal Questionnaire: A Method of Measuring Change in the Symptoms of an Individual Psychiatric Patient*, IOP, London.

Sheffield, B. F. and Kellner, R. (1970). The temporal stability of self ratings of neurotic symptoms. *Br. J. Soc. Clin. Psychol.* **9**, 46–53.

Snaith, R. P. (1985). A mood chart for use in clinical practice, *B. J. Clin Soc. Psychiatry* **3**, 16–18.

Snaith, R. P. and Taylor, C. M. (1985). Rating scales for depression and anxiety: a current perspective. *Br. J. Clin. Pharmacol.* **19**, 17S–20S.

Snaith, R. P., Goodman, M. J. and Holman, R. M. (1965). The control of manifest anxiety in dermatological patients: a comparison between sodium amylobarbitone and pericyazine. In *Proceedings Leeds Symposium on Behaviour Disorders* (A. Jenner, ed.), May & Baker, Dagenham, pp. 221–227.

Snaith, R. P., Bridge, G. W. K. and Hamilton, M. (1976). The Leeds Scales for the self assessment of anxiety and depression. *Br. J. Psychiatry* **128**, 156–165.

Snaith, R. P., Constantopoulos, A. A., Jardine, M. Y. and McGuffin, P. A. (1978). Clinical scale for the self assessment of irritability. *Br. J. Psychiatry* **132**, 164–171.

Snaith, R. P., Baugh, S. J., Clayden, A. D., Hussain, A. and Sipple, M. A. (1982). The Clinical Anxiety Scale: an instrument derived from the Hamilton Anxiety Scale. *Br. J. Psychiatry* **141**, 518–523.

Spielberger, C. D., Gorsuch, R. L., Luchene, R., Vagg, P. R. and Jacobs, G. A. (1983). *Manual for the State–Trait Anxiety Inventory*, Consulting Psychologists Press. Palo Alto.

Taylor, J. A. (1953). A personality scale of manifest anxiety. *J. Abnorm. Soc. Psychol.* **48**, 285–290.

Thompson, C. and Thompson, C. H. (in press). The prescribing of antidepressants in general practice: a placebo controlled trial of low dose dothiep. In, *Human Psychopharmacology*.

Tyrer, (1976) *The Role of Bodily Feelings in Anxiety*, Oxford University Press, Oxford.

Watson, D. and Friend, R. (1969). Measurement of social evaluative anxiety. *J. Consult. Clin. Psychol.* **33**, 448–457.

Zigmond, A. S. and Snaith, R. P. (1983). The Hospital Anxiety and Depression Scale. *Acta Psychiatr. Scand.* **67**, 361–370.

Zung, W. W. K. (1974). The measurement of affects: depression and anxiety, In *Psychological Measurements in Psychopharmacology*, Modern Problems in Pharmacopsychiatry Vol. 7 (P. Pichot, ed.), Karger, Basle, pp. 170–188.

The Instruments of Psychiatric Research
Edited by C. Thompson

CHAPTER 6

Self-administered scales of neurotic symptoms

KEITH BRIDGES and DAVID GOLDBERG
*Department of Psychiatry,
University of Manchester,
Manchester, UK*

INTRODUCTION

This chapter is concerned with self-administered pencil-and-paper tests which aim to detect subjects who will turn out to have non-psychotic psychiatric illness when subsequently interviewed. These instruments are easy to administer and take only a brief period to complete. They depend on the subject being willing to perform the task as well as being able to read and understand the questions, although they can be administered by an assistant to people who are illiterate. They have been used in epidemiological surveys on patients receiving care from general practitioners, physicians and surgeons as well as on population samples in the community (Goldberg and Huxley, 1980; Mayou and Hawton, 1986). In addition to their use in research, they may be clinically useful in helping doctors detect 'hidden psychiatric morbidity' in patients consulting them (Johnstone and Goldberg, 1976).

Since the majority of non-psychotic illnesses are characterized by a disturbance of mood in which symptoms related to anxiety correlate with symptoms related to depression (Goldberg *et al.*, 1987), researchers may prefer a single scale that gives an indication of the overall mood disturbance. Such instruments include the General Health Questionnaire (Goldberg, 1972, 1978) and the Self-report Questionnaire (Harding *et al.*, 1980). However, several scaled instruments which detect specific groups of symptoms are also available and most can be used as general case detectors when the scaled scores are added together. These include the scaled version of the General Health Questionnaire (Goldberg and Hillier, 1979), the Symptom Check-list, of which there are several versions (Parloff *et al.*, 1954; Frank *et al.*, 1957) and the more recent Hospital Anxiety Depression Scale (Zigmond and Snaith, 1983).

None of these instruments make diagnoses but the total score for the responses of a patient is analogous to the erthrocyte sedimentation rate; those with positive or suspicious findings will require more intensive examination for definite identification and diagnosis (Goldberg, 1979). The total score, in fact, can be interpreted in three ways: as a measure of the severity of psychological disorder which presupposes a dimensional model of psychological disturbance; as a means of estimating the prevalence of psychiatric illness in a particular group of people; and as an indicator of morbidity by dichotomizing respondents into 'high scorers' and 'low scorers' using a threshold score distinguishing those which are probably ill from those which are probably normal.

These interpretations of the score of a self-administered questionnaire in epidemiological research depends on the validity of the instrument as assessed by comparing its performance against an external criterion of psychiatric disorder of known reliability and validity. This chapter we will therefore begin with an account of how the validity of an instrument can be determined. Following this will be a brief account of some being used in research; this will not be exhaustive but only concerned with those which appear to be of current interest.

VALIDITY

There is little point in carrying out validity studies if they have already been carried out with comparable patients; many studies may not, in fact, depend on knowing the validity coefficients if, for example, their purpose is to distinguish between different degrees of psychological disorder within a sample or to compare the amount of disturbance between two samples. The main purpose of carrying out additional studies would be to establish the best threshold for some new class of respondents or in some new cultural setting or because a new screening test is being studied.

Validity is concerned with the extent that the screening instrument actually measures what it is supposed to be measuring. The item content may look as though it is appropriate for what it purports to assess—its face validity—but it is not advisable to use any instrument in either clinical practice or research unless the following validity coefficients are known and acceptable. These are derived from a 2×2 contingency table of the screening instrument responses (low/high) versus psychiatric caseness (normals/cases) as shown in Table 1.

Table 1. Validity coefficients*

	Second-stage psychiatric assessment	
	Non-case	Case
Screening instrument	False positive	True positive
High scorers	*a*	*b*
	True negative	True negative
Low scorers	*c*	*d*

* When a sampling strategy is used this should be based on weighted data.

$$\text{Specificity} = \frac{c}{a + c} \times 100$$

$$\text{Sensitivity} = \frac{b}{b + d} \times 100$$

$$\text{Positive Predictive Value} = \frac{b}{a + b} \times 100$$

$$\text{Negative Predictive Value} = \frac{d}{c + d} \times 100$$

$$\text{Overall Misclassification Rate} = \frac{a + d}{N} \times 100$$

Validity Coefficients

Specificity

The specificity of a screening test is the proportion of correctly identified normals, or true negatives expressed as a percentage of non-cases.

Sensitivity

The sensitivity of a test is the proportion of correctly identified cases, or the true positives expressed as a percentage of the cases.

Both these coefficients are independent of prevalence. When they are known the prevalence of psychiatric morbidity, P_{est}, can be estimated using the following formula (Goldberg, 1978):

$$P_{est} = \frac{\%\text{ high scorers} - \%\text{ false positive rate}}{\text{sensitivity rate} - \text{false positive rate}}$$

$$\text{where false positive rate} = \frac{100 - \text{specificity}}{100}$$

and $$\text{sensitivity rate} = \frac{\text{sensitivity}}{100}$$

Positive Predictive Value

The positive predictive value (PPV) is the probability that an individual with a high score on the test will turn out to have a psychiatric illness at subsequent clinical examination.

Negative Predictive Value

The negative predictive valve is the probability that a person with a low score will turn out not to have a psychiatric illness when subsequently assessed.

Overall Misclassification Rate

The overall misclassification rate refers to the proportion of respondents who are wrongly classified by the instrument.

These last three validity coefficients are dependent on the prevalence of the psychiatric morbidity in the patient population being considered. For example, low values reported for the positive predictive value in community settings will reflect the low prevalence of minor mood disorders in random samples of the population. It is therefore meaningless to quote a PPV for a screening test without reference to a particular prevalence, and it will always be considerably worse in situations when the prevalence is low.

Concurrent Validity

This is also known as the criterion validity and refers to the extent the screening test responds to the severity of disorder rather than merely to the presence or absence of disorder. It is usually measured by a rank-order correlation coefficient between scores on the instrument and the severity score of some standardized clinical measure of psychiatric morbidity, such as the Present State Examination (Wing *et al.*, 1974) and the Clinical Interview Schedule (Goldberg *et al.*, 1970). As these standardized assessments are not themselves error-free, these correlations are likely to be underestimates depending on the reliability of the second-stage interview being used (Goldberg and Williams, 1988).

External Criterion of Psychiatric Caseness

Several authors have drawn attention to the methodological weakness of psychiatric caseness being determined by clinical judgement alone and the need for using standardized procedures linked to operational criteria of caseness (see, for example, Kendell, 1975; Goldberg, 1972; Cooper, 1979; Williams *et al.*, 1980; Goldberg and Bridges, 1987; Goldberg and Williams, 1988). Standardized psychiatric assessments include the PSE (Wing *et al.*, 1974), the CIS (Goldberg *et al.*, 1970) and the Psychiatrist Assessment Schedule (Dean *et al.*, 1983). Each uses somewhat different criteria for caseness, especially with regard to the length of time that symptoms must be present in order for the subject to be counted as a 'case'.

Wing and his colleagues developed the concept of an Index of Definition (ID) which is derived from PSE data using a computer program known as CATEGO. The ID ranges from 1 to 8, of which 5 and above are regarded as indicating a 'definite disorder' (Wing *et al.*, 1978). Some researchers, however, have made a 'clinical judgement' on the basis of information collected by the PSE (e.g. Rabins and Brooks, 1981; Stefannson and Kristjannson, 1985).

With regard to the CIS the criteria used for an operational definition of a 'case' are a weighted total item score of least 20 (where each reported symptom score, R_i, is left unweighted and each manifest abnormality score, M_i, is given a double weighting *so that the total score* $S = \Sigma R_i + 2\ \Sigma M_i$); an overall clinical severity rating of 2 or more using a five-point scale ranging from 0 = no psychiatric abnormality to 5 = severe psychiatric abnormality: and a psychiatric diagnosis according to the mental disorders section of the International Classification of Diseases, Injuries and Causes of Death (ICD-9; Goldberg *et al.*, 1970; Cooper, 1979, 1984). All respondents who fulfil at least two of these three criteria are classified as 'cases'.

The PAS consists of the short version of the PSE (first 40 items) together with 19 additional symptoms. In addition to the ID CATEGO and ICD, this allows psychiatric diagnoses to be made to DSM-III (American Psychiatric Association, 1980) and Bedford College (Finlay-Jones *et al.*, 1980) criteria (Dean *et al.*, 1983; Grayson *et al.*, 1987).

Some tests have been validated against other rating scales of reported reliability and validity administered during a psychiatric interview such as the Hamilton Depression Scale (Hamilton, 1960), the Montgomery–Asberg scale (MADRS) (Montgomery and Asberg, 1979; Kearns *et al.*, 1982) and the Clinical Anxiety Scale (CAS) (Snaith *et al.*, 1982).

In a two-stage study the criterion interview should take place as soon as possible after the questionnaire has been completed, as changes in the clinical state of respondents may result in lower validity coefficients than would otherwise be the case (Goldberg and Williams, 1988).

Survey Design

Detailed descriptions of different procedures used in epidemiological surveys are provided by Goldberg and Williams (1988). When the number of respondents is small then all the subjects could be interviewed using a standardized psychiatric assessment after they have completed the screening instrument. If the estimated prevalence of psychiatric disorder is between 25 and 35%, it is best to select a random sample of respondents for the second-stage interview. However, if the number of respondents is large and the estimated prevalence of disorder is low, then either a truncated random sample or a simple two-stage statified sampling procedure should be used, so that a greater proportion of time is spent on interviewing subjects who are likely to turn out to be cases. A truncated random sample is one in which all respondents with a score of zero are not selected for interview, but are assumed to be 'non-cases', and a random sample of those with a score of one or more are interviewed. The potential saving of second-stage interviewing is substantial, some, for example in random samples, between 35 and 47% score zero on the GHQ while in consulting samples about a quarter score zero. In all these procedures the psychiatrist carrying out the psychiatric assessment should be blind to the scores of the screening instrument.

Following the psychiatric assessment each subject is then categorized as either a 'case' or 'non-case' according to the operational criteria for 'caseness' that are being used. For every possible threshold score of the screening instrument a 2×2 contingency table of the screening instrument responses (low/high) versus psychiatric caseness (normals/cases) is then drawn up. When a truncated or stratified sampling procedure is used the number of 'cases' and 'non-cases' need to be proportionately increased, i.e. the data are weighted back so that these relate to the total number of respondents in each stratum (Table 2). The validity coefficients can then be calculated from these contingency tables (Table 1). The 'optimal' threshold score of the screening instrument which is chosen for the population being studied is the one which gives the most acceptable trade-off between sensitivity and specificity, i.e. the best compromise between high sensitivity and low false positive rate.

Receiver Operating Characteristics (ROC) Analysis

Recently there has been an interest in the use of a technique known as ROC analysis for determining this 'optimal' threshold score of the instrument. This technique can also be used to assess the ability of a screening instrument to discriminate between 'cases' and 'non-cases' using different threshold scores (i.e. the discriminating ability of an instrument across the total spectrum of morbidity, rather than describing the results of a validation study by present-

Table 2. Weighting procedure in two-stage sampling strategy

(a) Number of people in each stage of assessment

Response category of test	Assessment: Test$_{(1)}$	Assessment: Interviewed$_{(2)}$
High scorers$_{(h)}$	n_{h1}	n_{h2}
Low scorers$_{(l)}$	n_{l1}	n_{l2}

(b) Results of second-stage assessment: raw data$_{(r)}$

Response category of test	Psychiatric caseness: Non-cases	Psychiatric caseness: Cases
High Scorers	a_{hr}	b_{hr}
Low scorers	c_{lr}	d_{lr}

(c) Results of second-stage assessments: weighted data

Response category of test	Psychiatric casesness: Non-cases	Psychiatric casesness: Cases
High scorers	$\frac{a_{hr} \times n_{h1}}{n_{h2}}$	$\frac{b_{hr} \times n_{h1}}{n_{h2}}$
Low scorers	$\frac{c_{lr} \times n_{l1}}{n_{l2}}$	$\frac{d_{lr} \times n_{l1}}{n_{l2}}$

ing the sensitivity and specificity at the chosen threshold score), and it has the advantage of enabling clinicians to compare the relative performance, in terms of discriminating power, of two or more competing screening instruments.

It was originally developed for use with radar to separate observed variability from innate detectability of a signal (Swets, 1964). It produces a curve which has been described as 'a function which summarizes all possible performances of an observer faced with the task of detecting a signal in noise' (Egan, 1975). It has been used in various psychological studies (Swets, 1973) and in some branches of medicine, for example the assessment of diagnostic skills and techniques (Swets *et al.*, 1979; Berwick and Thibodeau, 1983; McNeil and Adelstein, 1976). It is thought to be particularly useful in epidemiological research (Erdreich and Lee, 1981), and several investigators have used this form of analysis in psychiatry (Mari and Williams, 1985, 1986; Bridges and Goldberg, 1986; Bellantuono *et al.*, 1987.

It is described in detail elsewhere (McNeill *et al.*, 1975; Metz, 1978; Hanley and McNeil, 1982; Erdreich and Lee, 1981; Goldberg and Williams, 1988) but is briefly outlined here. It is important to note that patients selected for the second-stage interview must be a random sample of those competing the first-stage questionnaire, and that for each threshold score the data should be weighted as described above before the validity coefficients are calculated.

The true positive rate (sensitivity) and the false positive rate (1−specificity) are then calculated from the contingency tables drawn up for each possible threshold score. By plotting these against each other for each threshold score, a graph is then constructed which summarizes the discriminating performance of the screening instrument across the total spectrum of morbidity (Fig. 1). If this discriminating power is no better than chance, i.e. the sensitivity is equal to the false positive rate for all threshold scores, then a straight line (a) on the principal diagonal is produced with an area underneath it of 0.5. A concave line (b) above this indicates discrimination, and the area under this curve can be used as an index of the discriminating ability of the instrument. An ideal screening instrument would produce a curve indicating 100% true positives before admitting to a single false positive, with an area underneath it of 1.0. In practice an ROC curve is always intermediate between this and the principal diagonal, and when two or more screening instruments are being compared the one with greatest discriminating ability will have a curve furthest away from the diagonal (c).

The researcher can select the threshold score that is most suitable for his

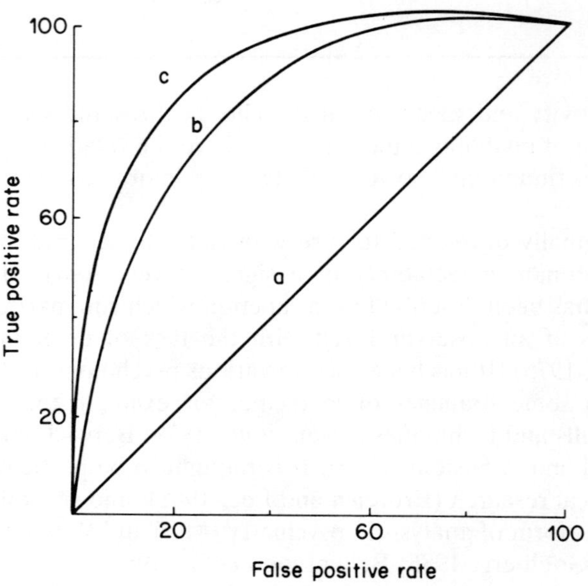

Fig. 1. Receiver Operating Characteristic (ROC) curves

purpose. This will depend on the relative costs and benefits associated with classifying a patient with an illness as normal and classifying a normal person as ill; the 'optimal' threshold score is at the point on the ROC curve which is the greatest perpendicular distance from the diagonal.

OTHER PRACTICAL ISSUES

Some investigators may wish to draw a sample in such a way that false positives are minimized but at the expense of losing some true positives, for example the selection of patients for teaching exercises involving medical students or trainee practitioners so that the teacher can focus teaching on respondents who have a high likelihood of being cases (Goldberg, 1986; Gask *et al.*, 1987) or in order to select patients who are to be considered for some intervention such as counselling (Johnstone and Shepley, 1986). The best strategy here is to raise the threshold, since this will increase the positive predictive value of the test. This would also have the effect of producing a sample whose average degree of disturbance is greater and thus less likely to remit spontaneously. An additional step would be to add a question about the duration of the disorder, since many of the disorders which are likely to remit spontaneously will be transient situational disturbances which are likely to have had a relatively short duration of episode. A question 'How long have you been feeling as you do at present?' could be added, and patients selected for the second-stage interview if they score above some raised threshold, and have been feeling this way for longer than 2 weeks.

Some investigators may wish to find as many cases of psychiatric disorder as possible. This is really the reverse of the last problem. Clearly, if the need is to be absolutely sure that no one is missed, then a screening instrument should not be used and everyone should be interviewed. However, a reasonable compromise is to lower the threshold of the screening test. The rational way of doing this is to first decide how much redundancy can be tolerated in the second-stage interviews by reference to the ROC curve, and then lower the threshold accordingly. For those using the GHQ, three further steps can be taken to avoid missing cases, particularly when a respondent with a long-standing disorder may have replied 'Same as usual' to all the questions and thus not been identified as a potential case. First, if medical records are available (for example in a general practice study) then long-standing cases are almost always known to medical staff; second, the questionnaire can be scored using the 'C-GHQ' method referred to earlier (Goodchild and Duncan-Jones, 1986); and third, two further questions can be added to the questionnaire: (1) 'Do you take any tablets or medicines for your nerves?' (2) 'Do you consider that you suffer from a nervous illness?' (Goldberg, 1983; Goldberg and Williams, 1988). Respondents answering 'yes' to either of these can then be regarded as 'high scorers' and proceed to the second-stage interview.

INSTRUMENTS IN COMMON USE

General Screening Tests

General Health Questionnaire (GHQ)

This is now the most widely used screening test and is available in versions as short as 12 items and as long as 60 (Goldberg, 1972; Goldberg and Williams, 1988). Since the questionnaire was designed for use in consulting settings, it focuses on breaks in normal functioning and is concerned with a person's inability to continue with normal 'healthy' functions and the experience of new phenomena of a distressing nature.

Each item consists of a question asking whether the respondent has experienced a particular symptom or item of behaviour within the previous few weeks on a four-point response scale ranging from less than usual to much more than usual. The GHQ-12 takes only 2 minutes to complete, while the GHQ-60 takes between 10 and 12 minutes. Each item is scored either as a 'Likert scale' ranging from 0 to 3 or as a bimodal response scale, so that only pathological deviations from normal signal possession of the item. This is known as the 'GHQ scoring' method, in which responses in either the third or fourth column (probably pathological) are scored as one while the others are scored as zero. This is not only a very simple method of scoring but has the advantage that it eliminates any errors due to 'end-users' and 'middle-users' since they will score the same irrespective of whether they prefer columns 1 and 4 or Columns 2 and 3 to indicate possession or non-possession of the item in question (Goldberg, 1972).

A modification of this scoring has recently been proposed for when this instrument is used on patients with chronic mood disorders and who are likely to respond 'No more than usual' to a number of the items (Goodchild and Duncan-Jones, 1985). This modification produces a more normal distribution of test scores and therefore has better statistical properties. However, further research is required to determine the applicability of this and it may be better in the meantime to use the two additional questions about use of psychotropic medication and history of nervous problems mentioned above.

The number of items with a morbid rating are counted to give a total GHQ score. This total score correlates highly with the total score derived from the Present State Examination (Banks, 1983; Newson-Smith and Hirsch, 1979; Henderson *et al.*, 1979; Duncan-Jones and Henderson, 1978; Rabins and Brooks, 1981; Robinson and Price, 1981) and the Clinical Interview Schedule (CIS; Goldberg, 1972; Goldberg, 1978). High correlations have also been reported with other psychiatric screening questionnaires, such as the Symptom Check-list (Goldberg *et al.*, 1976) and the Symptom Rating Questionnaire (Chan and Chan, 1983), as well as with scales specifically measuring depression, such as the Hamilton Depression Scale (Robinson and Price, 1981) and the Standardized Assessment of Depressive Disorders (Katschnig *et al.*, 1980).

A scaled version which consists of four subscales for somatic symptoms, anxiety and insomnia, social dysfunction and severe depression has been derived by factor analysis (Goldberg and Hillier, 1979; Goldberg, 1978). Each item is scored in the same way as the other versions of the GHQ. Like other versions of the GHQ, its total score correlates highly with the total score of the PSE (Banks, 1983; Rabins and Brooks, 1981) as well as the CIS (Bridges, 1983).

The GHQ has been translated into 16 languages and different versions have been validated in many countries, including England, Australia, the USA, Mexico, Austria, Hong Kong, Iceland, India, Jamaica, Japan, Nigeria, Spain and Yugoslavia (see Goldberg and Williams, 1988, for a comprehensive summary of these studies). When the performance of different versions of the GHQ are analysed using variance-weighted mean (VWM) validity coefficients obtained from these published studies—a procedure which takes into account the number of respondents in a study (see Goldberg and Williams, 1988, for details of how VWM is calculated)—it appears that the shorter versions have higher sensitivities, whereas the GHQ-60 has a better specificity (Table 3).

Table 3. Variance-weighted mean (VWM) validity coefficients from 43 validity studies of the GHQ

	Sensitivity (%)	Specificity (%)
GHQ-12	89 (85, 92)*	80 (77, 83)*
GHQ-28	84 (77, 89)	82 (78, 85)
GHQ-30	74 (70, 77)	82 (80, 83)
GHQ-60	78 (75, 82)	87 (86, 89)
All	76 (74, 78)	85 (84, 86)

* 95% confidence limits.
Reproduced with permission from Goldberg and Williams, 1988.

Patients with physical disorders may be over-represented among respondents classified as false positives because of their responses to items concerned with somatic symptoms and social dysfunction (Goldberg and Williams, 1988; Maguire *et al.*, 1974; Finlay-Jones and Murphy, 1979; Rabins and Brooks, 1981; Bridges and Goldberg, 1986). When this occurs the threshold score needs to be raised in order to obtain optimal discrimination between 'non-cases' and 'cases'.

Self-report Questionnaire (SRQ)

This is a 24-item screening questionnaire developed by the World Health Organization for use in developing countries in general medical settings. It can be found as an appendix in Harding *et al.* (1980) and Mari and Williams (1985), and has been translated into several languages, including Hindi, Arabic, Filipino and Portuguese. The first 20 items were designed to detect non-psychotic disorders. These were extracted from other screening instruments: the Patient Self-report Symptom Form developed and tested in Cali, Columbia (PASSR; Climent and Plutchick, 1980); the PGI Health Questionnaire developed by Wig and his colleagues in Chandigarh (Verma and Wig, 1977); the 'symptom' items on the shortened version of the Present State Examination (PSE; Wing *et al.*, 1974) and the General Health Questionnaire (Goldberg, 1972). The four additional items were taken from Foulds' Symptom Sign Inventory (Foulds and Hope, 1968) and selected to detect psychotic conditions. The SRQ response scale is simply 'yes' or 'no'.

Its validity has been assessed by Harding *et al.* (1980) using the PSE as second-stage assessment of psychiatric caseness. Subjects were normal and from four different countries. The threshold score which yielded optimal sensitivity and specificity was different in each study area: Union de Viviendo, Cali, Columbia—10/11; Raipur Rani, Haryana, India—5/6; Shagara Jebel Awalia, Khartoum Province, Sudan—3/4; and Sampaloc, Manila, Philippines—6/7. The sensitivity varied between 73% and 83%; and specificity varied between 72% and 85%, indicating tha the overall misclassification rate in a population with a psychiatric morbidity rate of 15% would vary between 18% and 24%. Dhadphale *et al.* (1983) report a sensitivity >93% and a specificity of 89% in a study in Kenya in which they matched psychiatric patients with controls for age, sex and education, and used the CIS as the external criterion. More recently Mari and Williams (1985, 1986) assessed its validity in patients attending three primary care clinics in the city of Sao Paulo, using the CIS (Goldberg *et al.*, 1970). According to their ROC analysis, the 'optimum' threshold score, i.e. the best compromise between high sensitivity and low false positive rate, was found to be 7/8. By using this threshold score, sensitivity was 83%, specificity 80%, overall misclassification rate 19% and the positive predictive value of the test 81%.

Cornell Medical Index Health Questionnaire

This is a large inventory which was originally designed to screen recruits in the Second World War. It consists of 195 questions which correspond closely to those asked in a comprehensive medical interview to which the respondent answers 'yes' or 'no'. The questions relate to bodily symptoms, past illnesses, family histories and behaviour and are organized into 18 sections each headed by a letter of the alphabet. The last six of these, sections M–R, contain 51 questions which are concerned with emotional disorder (Brodman *et al.*, 1949; 1956). In the two decades following its introduction it was used in several studies, including research on general hospital patients and in primary care (Culpan *et al.*, 1960; Brown and Fry, 1962; Shepherd *et al.*, 1966; Rawnsley, 1966;). Shepherd *et al.* (1966), however, found that this instrument misclassified a substantial proportion as probable normals: at least 30% of a series of 1484 Maudsley out-patients confirmed as cases at subsequent clinical interview had scores below a threshold score of 10. Another shortcoming reported by these workers was the stability of its scores over time, suggesting that the test gives more information about personality than about current illness. This is not unexpected since its questions often ask for broad generalizations and about how the subject usually feels.

From an analysis of the data obtained by Shepherd *et al.* (1966) a much shorter screening instrument was developed, consisting of the 20 items which best discriminated between 'non-cases' and 'cases' as determined by general practitioners (see Eastwood, 1975, appendix 1) and used in a study assessing the relationship between physical and mental illness in primary care. Although it was not possible to validate it in terms of sensitivity and specificity in this study, the correlation of its total score with the total severity score of the CIS was found to be +0.52 (Eastwood, 1971).

Murphy (1981) summarizes a number of the methodological weaknesses of studies assessing its validity as a screening instrument for psychiatric morbidity and now it is not thought to be a useful instrument for psychiatric research (Mann and Murray, 1979). However, there has recently been a renewed interest in its use in epidemiological studies in Iceland, in which the correlation of its total score with the total PSE score has been reported as +0.59 and +0.48 with the total score of the GHQ-30 (Stefansson and Kristjansson, 1985).

Instruments Detecting Specific Symptoms

In addition to the GHQ-28 other tests which detect specific symptoms are also available. Most of these have been derived by factor analysis and can be used as general case detectors as well, by adding the scaled scores together.

Symptom Check-list (SCL)

This was initially developed by Parloff *et al.* (1954) and further elaborated by Frank *et al.* (1957). It was originally known as the Johns Hopkins Symptom

Distress Check-list, when it consisted of only 59 items. It is now available in a variety of lengths, for example: the SCL-90 has nine subscales—depression, anxiety, somatization, obsessive-compulsive, interpersonal sensitivity, hostility, phobic anxiety, paranoid ideation and psychoticism (Derogatis *et al.*, 1974; Wilson *et al.*, 1985); the SCL-71 has five subscales—anxiety, depression, somatization, obsessive-compulsive and interpersonal sensitivity (Glass *et al.*, 1978); the SCL-64 has five subscales—depression, fear–anxiety, performance difficulty, somatization, general neurotic feeling (Rickels *et al.*, 1972); the SCL-58 has five subscales—depression, anxiety, somatization, obsessive-compulsive and irascibility (Derogatis *et al.*, 1971); and the SCL-25 has only two subscales—depression and anxiety (Hesbacher *et al.*, 1980). Each instrument is concerned with the current state of the respondent, and each item is rated using a frequency scale running from 'not at all' to 'extremely'. Typically the score for each response has been 1 to 4, and a common procedure for calculating the total score has been to divide the sum of the response scores by the number of questions answered (Murphy, 1981). Some workers, however, have preferred to use a total score without the division and an individual item rating of 0–3 (e.g. Goldberg *et al.*, 1976; Glass *et al.*, 1978).

At least three studies—two in the USA and one in the UK—have reported on its validity. Goldberg *et al.* (1976) assessed the validity of the SCL-35 version in primary care attenders using the CIS, and reported a sensitivity of 84% and a specificity of 72% when applying a threshold score of 15/16. The correlation of its total score was +0.70 with the total score of the psychiatric assessment and +0.78 with the total score of the GHQ-30. Glass *et al.* (1978) assessed the validity of the SCL-75 version in medical outpatients against a standardized psychiatric interview linked with diagnostic criteria developed by the Washington University School of Medicine at St Louis (Feighner *et al.*, 1972). Using a threshold score of 27/28 they report a sensitivity of 73% and a specificity of 71%. More recently, Wilson *et al.* (1985) assessed the concurrent validity of each of the subscales of the SCL-90 version in the UK using the PSE in a sample of men remanded to prison for psychiatric assessments. The reported correlations between these subscales and the syndromes derived from the PSE ranged from +0.34 to +0.51.

Hospital Anxiety Depression Scale (HAD)

Unlike the other scales this has scales derived from clinical experience rather than from factor analysis. It consists of two sets of seven questions—one representing an anxiety subscale, the other representing a depression subscale (Zigmond and Snaith, 1983). Each item is rated using a four-point frequency scale which is scored from 0 to 3. As the instrument was originally designed for use on patients with physical disorders, the items selected were based only on psychic symptoms of neurosis.

Several validity studies are at present under way (Snaith, 1986, personal communication) and recently Snaith and his colleagues reported concurrent validity for each scale using the MADRS (Montgomery and Asberg, 1979) and the CAS (Snaith *et al.*, 1982) as external criteria in hospital out-patients. In a subsample of patients with a definite mood disorder the correlation of the depression scale with the MADRS was +0.77, while the correlation between the anxiety scale and the CAS was +0.67. The correlations between the two scales was −0.04 (Aylard *et al.*, 1987). It is available in many languages, including European, Arabic, Chinese, Hebrew, Japanese and Urdu.

Other Instruments

Other tests exist which have either been superseded or require further research using standardized psychiatric research interviews to determine their validity and applicability. These include the Depression Adjective Check-list (Lubin, 1965, 1966); the Zung Self-rating Depression Scale (Zung, 1965; Zung *et al.*, 1965; Carroll *et al.*, 1973); the Profile of Mood States (McNair *et al.*, 1971); the short form of the Beck Depression Inventory (Beck *et al.*, 1974); the Rotterdam Scales designed for use with patients with cancer (De Haes, 1983; Trew and Maquire, 1982); the Middlesex Hospital Questionnaire (MHQ; Crown and Crisp, 1966; Crisp *et al.*, 1978); the Irritability–Depression–Anxiety (IDA) Scale, which as the name indicates has a subscale for irritability (Snaith *et al.*, 1978; Snaith and Taylor, 1985; Aylard *et al.*, 1987); and the Centre for Epidemiologic Studies Depression Scale (CES-D; Radloff, 1977), and more recently two scales detecting anxiety and depression in general medical settings (Goldberg *et al.*, 1988)

REFERENCES

American Psychiatric Association (1980). *Diagnostic and Statistical Manual of Mental Disorders*, 3rd edn, American Psychiatric Association, Washington.

Aylard, P. R., Gooding, J. H., McKenna, P. J. and Snaith, R. P. (1987). A validation study of three anxiety and depression self-assessment scales. *J. Psychosom. Res.* **31**, 261–268.

Ballantuono, C., Fiorio, R., Cortina, P., Zanotelli, R. and Tansella, M. (1987). Psychiatric screening in general practice in Italy: a validity study of the GHQ. *Soc. Psychiatry* (in press).

Banks, M. (1983). Validation of the GHQ in a young community. *Psychol. Med.* **3**, 349–354.

Beck, A. T., Rial, W. Y. and Rickels, K. (1974). Short form of depression inventory: cross validation. *Psychol. Rep.* **34**, 1184–1186.

Berwick, D. M. and Thibodeau, L. A. (1983). Receiver operating characteristic analysis of diagnostic skills. *Med. Care* **21**, 876–885.

Bridges, K. W. (1983). *A Study of Psychiatric Morbidity in Patients Admitted to an Adult Neurology Ward*, MSc thesis, University of Manchester.

Bridges, K. W. and Goldberg, D. P. (1986). The validation of the GHQ-28 and the use of the MMSE in neurological inpatients. *Br. J. Psychiatry* **148**, 548–553.

Brodman, K., Erdnan, A. J., Lorge, I., Wolff, G. and Broadbent, T. H. (1949). The Cornell Medical Index, *J. Am. Med. Assoc.* **140**, 530–540.

Brodman, K., Erdmann, A. J. and Wolf, H. G. (1956). *Cornell Medical Index Health Questionnaire Manual*, Cornell University Medical College, New York.

Brown, A. C. and Fry, J. (1962). The Cornell Medical Index Health Questionnaire in the identification of neurotic patients in general practice. *J. Psychosom. Res.* **6**, 185–190.

Carroll, B. J., Fielding, J. M. and Blashki, T. G. (1973). Depression rating scales: a critical review. *Arch. Gen. Psychiatry* **28**, 361–366.

Chan, D. W. and Chan, T. S. C. (1983). Reliability, validity and the structure of the General Health Questionnaire in a Chinese context. *Psychol. Med.* **13**, 365–371.

Climent, C. E. and Plutchick, R. (1980). Confiabilidad, validez y sensibilidad de los itemes de una escala de auto-repotaje de sintomas de enfermedad mental. *Rev. Colomb. Psiquiatria* **8**.

Cooper, B. (1979). Demographic and epidemiological methods in psychiatric research. In *Psychiatrie der Gegenwart*, Bd. I/1,2 Anfl. (K. P. Kisker, J. E. Meyer, C. Muller and E. Stromgren, eds), Springer-Verlag, Berlin.

Cooper, B. (1984). Home and away: the disposition of mentally ill old people in an urban population. *Soc. Psychiatry* **19**, 187–196.

Crisp, A. H., Jones, M. G. and Slater, P. (1978). The Middlesex Hospital questionnaire: a validity study. *Br. J. Psychiatry* **51**, 269–280.

Crown, S. and Crisp, A. H. (1966). A short clinical diagnostic self-rating scale for psychoneurotic patients. *Br. J. Psychiatry* **112**, 917–923.

Culpan, R. H., Davies, B. M. and Oppenheim, A. N. (1960). Incidence of psychiatric illness among hospital out-patients: an application of the Cornell Medical Index. *Br. Med. J.* **1**, 855–857.

Dean, C., Surtees, P. and Sashidharan, S. (1983). Comparison of research diagnostic systems in an Edinburgh community sample. *Br. J. Psychiatry* **142**, 247–256.

De Haes, J. C. (1983). Klachentenlijst voorkanker patienten: erste ervaringen. *Ned. Tijdschr. Psychol.* **38**, 403–422.

Derogatis, L. R., Lipman, R. S., Covi, L. and Rickels, K. (1971). Neurotic symptom dimensions. *Arch. Gen. Psychiatry* **24**, 454–464.

Derogatis, L. R., Lipman, R. S. and Covi, L. (1974). The SCL-90: an outpatient psychiatric rating scale. *Psychopharmacol. Bull.* **9**, 13–28.

Dhadphale, R., Ellison, R. H. and Griffin, L. (1983). The frequency of psychiatric disorders among patients attending semiurban and rural general out-patient clinics in Kenya. *Br. J. Psychiatry* **142**, 379–383.

Duncan-Jones, P. and Henderson, S. (1978). The use of a two stage design in a prevalence survey. *Soc. Psychiatry* **13**, 231–237.

Eastwood, M. R. (1971). Screening for psychiatric disorder. *Psychol. Med.* **1**, 197–208.

Eastwood, M. R. (1975). *The Relation between Physical and Mental Illness*, University of Toronto Press, Toronto and Buffalo.

Egan, J. A. (1975). *Signal Detection Theory and ROC Analysis*, Academic Press, New York.

Erdreich, L. S. and Lee, E. T. (1981). Use of relative operating characteristic analysis in epidemiology. *Am. J. Epidemiol.* **114**, 649–662.

Feighner, J. P., Robins, E., Guze, S. B. *et al.* (1972). Diagnostic criteria for use in psychiatric research. *Arch. Gen. Psychiatry* **26**, 57–63.

Finlay-Jones, R. A. and Murphy, E. (1979). Severity of psychiatric disorder and the 30-item GHQ. *Brit. J. Psychiat.* **134**, 609–616.

Finlay-Jones, R., Brown, G. W., Duncan-Jones, P., Harris, J., Murphy, E. and Prudo, R. (1980). Depression and anxiety in the community: replicating the diagnosis of a case. *Psychol. Med.* **10**, 445–454.

Foulds, G. A. and Hope, K. (1968). *Manual of the Symptom Sign Inventory (SSI)*, University of London Press, London.

Frank, J. D., Gliedman, L. H., Imber, S. D. *et al.* (1957). Why patients leave psychotherapy. *Arch. Neurol. Psychiat.* **77**, 283–299.

Gask, L., McGrath, G., Goldberg, D. and Millar, T. (1987). Improving the psychiatric skills of established general practitioners: evaluation of group teaching. *Med. Educ.* **21**, 362–368.

Glass, R. M., Allan, A. T. and Uhlenhuth, E. H. (1978). Psychiatric screening in a medical clinic. *Arch. Gen. Psychiatry* **35**, 1189–1195.

Goldberg, D. P. (1972). *The Detection of Psychiatric Illness by Questionnaire*, Maudsley Monograph 21, Oxford University Press, London.

Goldberg, D. P. (1978). *Manual of the General Health Questionnaire*, NFER/Nelson, Slough.

Goldberg, D. P. (1983). The use of screening questionnaires by family doctors. In *Report of VII World Congress of Psychiatry*, Plenum, Vienna.

Goldberg, D. (1986). Use of the General Health Questionnaire in clinical work. *Br. Med. J.* **293**, 1188–1189.

Goldberg, D. and Bridges, K. (1987). Screening for psychiatric illness in general practice: the general practitioner versus the screening questionnaire. *J. R. Coll. Gen. Pract.* **37**, 15–18.

Goldberg, D., Bridges, K., Duncan-Jones, P. and Grayson, D. (1988). Detecting anxiety and depression in general medical settings. *Br. Med. J.* **297**, 897–899.

Goldberg, D. P. and Hillier, V. F. (1979). A scaled version of the general health questionnaire. *Psychol. Med.* **9**, 139–145.

Goldberg, D. and Huxley, P. (1980). *Mental Illness in the Community: The Pathway to Psychiatric Care*, Tavistock, London.

Goldberg, D. P. and Williams, P. (1988). *The User's Guide to the General Health Questionnaire*, NFER/ Nelson, Slough.

Goldberg, D. P., Cooper, B., Eastwood, M. R., Kedward, H. B. and Shepherd, M. (1970). A standardised psychiatric interview for use in community surveys. *Br. J. Preventive Soc. Med.* **24**, 18–23.

Goldberg, D. P., Rickels, K., Downing, R. and Hesbacher, P. (1976). A comparison of two psychiatric screening tests. *Br. J. Psychiatry* **129**, 61–67.

Goldberg, D. P., Bridges, K., Duncan-Jones, P. and Grayson, D. (1987). Dimensions of neuroses seen in primary-care settings. *Psychol. Med.* **17**, 461–470.

Goodchild, M. E. and Duncan-Jones, P. (1985). Chronicity and the General Health Questionnaire. *Br. J. Psychiatry* **146**, 55–61.

Grayson, D. A., Bridges, K., Duncan-Jones, P. and Goldberg, D. P. (1987). The relationship between symptoms and diagnoses of minor psychiatrist disorder in general practice. *Psychol. Med.* **17**, 933–942.

Hamilton, M. (1960). A rating scale for depression. *J. Neurol. Neurosurg. Psychiatry* **23**, 56–62.

Hanley, J. A. and McNeil, B. J. (1982). The meaning and use of the area under a Receiver Operating Characteristic (ROC) curve. *Radiology* **143**, 29–36.

Harding, T. W., Arango, M. V. and Baltazar, J. (1980). Mental disorders in primary health care. *Psychol. Med.* **10**, 231–241.

Henderson, S., Duncan-Jones, P., Byrne, D., Scott, R. and Adcock, S. (1979). Psychiatric disorders in Camberra—A standardised study of prevalence. *Acta Psychiatr. Scand.* **60**, 355–374.

Hesbacher, P. T., Rickels, K., Morris, R. J. *et al.* (1980). Psychiatric illness in family practice. *J. Clin. Psychol.* **41**, 6–10.

Johnstone, A. and Goldberg, D. (1976). Psychiatric screening in general practice: A controlled trial. *Lancet* **i**, 605–608.

Johnstone, A. and Shepley, M. (1986). The outcome of hidden neurotic illness treated in general practice. *J. R. Coll. Gen. Pract.* **36**, 413–415.

Katschnig, H., Berner, W., Haushofer, M., Berfuss, M. and Seelig, P. (1980). Psychiatric case identification in general practice: self-rating versus interview. *Acta Psychiatr. Scand.* Suppl. 285, **62**, 164–175.

Kearns, N. P., Cruickshank, K. J., McGuigan, K. J., Riley, S. A., Shaw, S. P. and Snaith, R. P. (1982). A comparison of depression rating scales. *Br. J. Psychiatry* **141**, 45–49.

Kendell, R. E. (1975). *The Role of Diagnosis in Psychiatry*, Blackwell Scientific Publications, Oxford.

Lubin, B. (1965). Adjective checklists for the measurements of depression. *Arch. Gen. Psychiatry* **12**, 57–62.

Lubin, B. (1966). Fourteen brief depression adjective checklists. *Arch. Gen. Psychiatry* **15**, 205–208.

Maguire, G. P., Julier, D. L., Hawton, K. E. and Bancroft, J. H. J. (1974). Psychiatric morbidity and referral on two general medical wards. *Br. Med. J.* **1**, 268–270.

Mann, A. and Murray, R. (1979). Measurements in psychiatry. In *Essentials of Postgraduate Psychiatry* (P. Hill, R. Murray and A. Thorley, eds), Academic Press, London, pp. 77–98.

Mari, J. J. and Williams, P. (1985). A comparison of the validity of two psychiatric screening questionnaires (GHQ-12 and SRQ-20) in Brazil, using Relative Operating Characteristic (ROC) analysis. *Psychol. Med.* **15**, 651–659.

Mari, J. J. and Williams, P. (1986). Misclassification by psychiatric screening questionnaires. *J. Chronic Dis.* **39**, 371–378.

Mayou, R. and Hawton, K. (1986). Psychiatric disorder in the general hospital. *Br. J. Psychiatry* **149**, 172–190.

McNair, D. M., Lorr, M. and Droppleman, L. F. (1971). *EITS Manual for the Profile of Mood States*, Educational and Industrial Testing Service, San Diego.

McNeil, B. J. and Adelstein, S. J. (1976). Determining the value of diagnostic and screening tests. *J. Nuclear Med.* **17**, 439–448.

McNeil, B. J., Keeler, E. and Adelstein, S. J. (1975). Primer on certain elements of medical decision making. *New England J. Med.* **293**, 211–215.

Metz, C. E. (1978). Basic principles of ROC analysis. *Semin. Nuclear* Med. **8**, 283–298.

Montgomery, S. and Asberg, M. (1979). A new depression scale designed to be sensitive to change. *Br. J. Psychiatry* **134**, 382–389.

Murphy, J. (1981). *Psychiatric Instrument Development For Primary Care Research: Patient Self-Report Questionnaire*, Report to Division of Biometry and Epidemiology of the NIMH, Washington (unpublished).

Newman, S. C., Bland, R. and Orn, H. (1987). The General Health Questionnaire as a screening instrument in a community survey. *Psychol. Med.* (submitted).

Newson-Smith, J. and Hirsch, S. (1979). Psychiatric symptoms in self poisoning patients. *Psychol. Med.* **9**, 493–500.

Parloff, M. B., Kelman, H. C. and Frank, J. D. (1954). Comfort, effectiveness and self-awareness as criteria of improvement in psychotherapy. *Am. J. Psychiatry* **111**, 343–351.

Rabins, P. and Brooks, B. (1981). Emotional disturbance in multiple sclerosis patients: validity of the General Health Questionnaire. *Psychol. Med.* **11**, 425–427.

Radloff, L. S. (1977). The CES-D scale. A self-report depression scale for research in the general population. *Appl. Psychol. Measurements* **1**, 385–401.

Rawnsley, K. (1966). Congruence of independent measures of psychiatric morbidity. *J. Psychosom. Res.* **10**, 84.

Rickels, K., Lipman, R. S., Garcia, C. R. and Fisher, E. (1972). Evaluating clinical improvements in anxious outpatients: a comparison of normal and treated neurotic patients. *Am. J. Psychiatry* **128**, 1005–1009.

Robinson, R. and Price, T. (1981). Post-stroke depressive disorders: a follow-up study of 103 patients. *Stroke* **13**, 635–641.

Shepherd, M., Cooper, B., Brown, A. C. and Kalton, G. W. (1966). *Psychiatric Illness in General Practice*, Oxford University Press, London.

Snaith, R. P. and Taylor, C. M. (1985). Irritability: definition, assessment and associated factors. *Br. J. Psychiatry* **147**, 127–136.

Snaith, R. P., Constantopoulos, A. A., Jardine, M. Y. and McGuffin, P. (1978). A clinical scale for the self-assessment of irritability. *Br. J. Psychiatry* **132**, 164–171.

Snaith, R. P., Baugh, S. J., Clayden, A. D., Husain, A. and Sipple, M. A. (1982). The Clinical Anxiety Scale: an instrument derived from the Hamilton Anxiety Scale. *Br. J. Psychiatry* **141**, 518–523.

Stefansson, J. G. and Kristjansson, I. (1985). Comparison of the GHQ and the CMI. *Acta Psychiatr. Scand.* **72**, 482–487.

Swets, J. A. (1964). *Signal Detection and Recognition by Human Observers*, Wiley, New York.

Swets, J. A. (1973). The relative operating characteristic in psychology, *Science* **182**, 990–1000.

Swets, J. A., Pickett, R. M., Whitehead, S. F., Getty, D. J., Schmur, J. A., Swets, J. B. and Freeman, B. A. (1979). Assessment of diagnostic technologies. *Science* **205**, 753–759.

Trew, M. and Maquire, G. P. (1982). *A Further Comparison of Two Screening Instruments*, EORTC (Study group monograph), Amsterdam.

Verma, S. K. and Wig, N. N. (1977). Standardisation of a neuroticism questionnaire in Hindi. *Indian J. Psychiatry* **19**, 67–72.

Williams, P., Tarnopolsky, A. and Hand, D. (1980). Case definition and case identification in psychiatric epidemiology: review and assessment. *Psychol. Med.* **10**, 101–114.

Wilson, J. H., Taylor, P. J. and Robertson, G. (1985). The validity of the SCL-90 in a sample of British men remanded to prison for psychiatric reports. *Br. J. Psychiatry* **147**, 400–403.

Wing, J. K., Cooper, J. E. and Sartorius, N. (1974). *The Measurement and Classification of Psychiatric Symptoms*, Cambridge University Press, Cambridge.

Wing, J. K., Mann, S. A., Leff, J. P. and Nixon, J. M. (1978). The concept of a case in psychiatric population surveys. *Psychol. Med.* **8**, 203–217.

Zigmond, A. S. and Snaith, R. P. (1983). The hospital anxiety and depression scale. *Acta Psychiatr. Scand.* **67**, 361–370.

Zung, W. W. K. (1965). A self-rating depression scale. *Arch. Gen. Psychiatry* **12**, 63–70.

Zung, W. W. K., Richards, C. B. and Short, M. J. (1965). Self-rating depression scale in an outpatient clinic. *Arch. Gen. Psychiatry* **13**, 508–515.

The Instruments of Psychiatric Research
Edited by C. Thompson

CHAPTER 7

Anorexia nervosa and eating disorders

George I. Szmukler
Royal Melbourne Hospital,
Parkville, Victoria 3050, Australia

Department of Psychiatry,
University of Melbourne,
Melbourne, Australia

INTRODUCTION

A number of research instruments are presently available for use in the investigation of the eating disorders. Most have not been the subject of extensive development, nor carefully designed with a highly specific application in mind. As bulimia has been a more recent focus of study, instruments devised specifically for its assessment have been later in appearing. However, most instruments devised for anorexia nervosa have also been applied to these subjects. When bulimia is discussed note should be taken of which category of patient is being considered: Bulimia in association with co-existing anorexia nervosa ('bulimic anorexics'), bulimia in patients with a past history of anorexia nervosa who are now at a normal weight, and bulimia in subjects with no history of anorexia nervosa.

Some instruments have derived from particular theoretical standpoints, the constructs of Hilde Bruch (1973) having been particularly influential. The majority have been based on the results of clinical experience with an attempt to capture the phenomena deemed important at a clinical descriptive level.

Uses of Scales

Scales have been put to a number of uses in research. These include the following.

Detection of Cases in a Population

An important limitation of most of the scales used concerns their method of validation. This has usually involved an examination of their ability to discriminate cases presenting to clinics with a clear-cut diagnosis from control groups selected for having no evidence of an eating disorder. Cut-off scores have been arrived at which reveal little overlap between the groups. However, when applied in a community sample the ability of such scales to discriminate cases from non-cases is restricted by two major factors. The first is a limitation imposed by the prevalence of the disorder in a community sample. It is a mathematical fact that even a screening instrument with an impressively high 'specificity' and 'sensitivity' will have a limited 'positive predictive value' when cases are uncommon in the population studied. Secondly, there are subjects in the community who are not clearly cases or non-cases; they fall somewhere in between, being termed for example, 'borderline' or 'partial' syndromes. Both issues have been of importance in studies of anorexia nervosa. A more detailed discussion is available in Williams *et al*. (1982) and Szmukler (1985). The Eating Attitudes Test (EAT) (Garner and Garfinkel, 1979) has been most used in case detection studies.

Definition of the Nature of the Psychopathology

Some scales have attempted to embrace a wide range of psychopathological features in the eating disorders and then have been used to study their nature further, for example, by applying factor analytical methods to scores obtained in a population of subjects.

A quite specific application in anorexia nervosa research has been the endeavour to elucidate the clinical observation of the denial of emaciation which is so striking in many cases. A variety of measures have been designed to examine the patient's accuracy of body size estimation or 'body image disturbance'.

Measuring Change

Scales designed to rate psychopathology and abnormal behaviour have been used to assess severity or to measure change over time or with a course of treatment. It is important to bear in mind that changes measured by most of the scales have not been thoroughly correlated with changes that clinicians would regard as significant.

Measuring Fundamental Traits Relevant to the Disorders

As knowledge about the eating disorders has accrued, theories about fundamental disturbances have developed and these have formed the bases of more ambitious rating scales which seek to go beyond the 'surface phenomena' to underlying variables or traits. The Eating Disorders Inventory [5 (Garner and Olmstead, 1984)] and the SCANS [6 (Slade and Dewey, 1986)] are examples of these.

As an Aid to Diagnosis

In some instances researchers have substituted self-report inventories for interview-based clinical diagnoses, particularly in studies on larger population samples. This is an indefensible practice. No questionnaire at present available approaches even remotely the reliability of a clinical assessment. Some more recently developed semi-structured interviews may, however, find a useful application in sharpening diagnostic assessments.

An important caveat applies with most instruments when used with patients with anorexia nervosa. This is an illness in which disturbance is usually denied by the subject who usually strives, initially at least, to avoid treatment. She will therefore often respond to rating instruments in a manner which minimizes the psychopathology which she knows is being sought. In the author's experience with the EAT administered to in-patients with anorexia nervosa, for example, about 10–15% of subjects produced clearly unreliable scores. This phenomenon has been further investigated by Vandereycken and Vanderlinden (1983).

INSTRUMENTS SELECTED FOR REVIEW

Instruments have been selected for more detailed discussion in this chapter if they have fulfilled satisfactory formal psychometric criteria for reliability and validity or if a reasonable amount of experience has been accumulated in their usage, permitting an evaluation of their usefulness. For each measure a brief general description will be given, psychometric properties described where available and a brief account given of its main applications so far.

Instruments will be grouped as follows:

1. Self-report inventories:
   (a) Anorexia nervosa
   (b) Bulimia
2. Observer-rated measures
3. Structured interview measures
4. Body-size estimation techniques

Self-report Inventories

Anorexia Nervosa

Eating Attitudes Test. This questionnaire was developed by Garner and Garfinkel (1979) and comprises 40 items representing a broad range of symptoms and behaviours common in anorexia nervosa. Items were selected which covered the range of phenomena clinically evident in patients with anorexia nervosa and the questionnaire is relatively atheoretical. Each item is presented in a six-point forced-choice format based on frequency ('always', 'very often', 'often', 'sometimes', 'rarely' and 'never'). The EAT takes about 10 minutes to complete and is easily scored.

The alpha reliability coefficient for internal consistency has been reported as 0.79–0.94. Test–retest reliabilities have not been reported but the general impression of those who have used it extensively suggests that this is satisfactory.

The initial validation and cross-validation of the EAT was based on comparisons of scores in populations of anorexics, normal controls and obese subjects. A best cut-off score of ≥30 was arrived at which identified all cases of anorexia nervosa but also 13% of the normal controls. EAT scores in the normal controls were only modestly correlated with measures of dieting, weight fluctuations and 'neuroticism' and 'extroversion' on the Eysenck Personality Inventory. Administration of the EAT to a small group of recovered patients showed scores in the normal range, suggesting that the measure was sensitive to clinical change.

Further assessments of the properties of the EAT were reported by Garner *et al.* (1982) on a larger sample of 160 female patients with anorexia nervosa and a normal control group of 140. A factor analysis was performed of the 40 scale items. Three factors were extracted accounting for 40.2% of the variance. Items loading on the first factor, labelled 'dieting', related to an avoidance of fattening foods and a preoccupation with slimness. The second factor, termed 'bulimia and food preoccupation', consisted of items reflecting thoughts about food and those suggesting bulimia. The third factor, termed rather oddly 'oral control', loaded for items related to self-control of eating and perceived pressure from others to gain weight. With regard to the second factor it should be noted that 52% of the patients with anorexia nervosa studied had bulimic episodes as well. These patients had significantly higher factor scores on the second factor and significantly lower scores on the third factor than the pure 'restrictor' group of anorexics. There were no significant differences in total EAT scores between the bulimic and restrictor anorexics.

The authors went on to propose an alternative 26-item version of the EAT (EAT-26) (Garner *et al.*, 1982) in which 14 items not loading on the three factors extracted were eliminated. A cut-off score of ≥20 permitted a correct classification of 84% of cases using a discriminant function analysis on the combined groups of cases and controls, a figure comparable to that using a cut-off of ⩾30 on the EAT-40. Both EAT scores showed significant correlations with a number of other psychometric measures: body size estimates, body dissatisfaction (using an adapted version of the Berscheid *et al.* (1973) Body Dissatisfaction Scale), and the Hopkins Symptom Check-list (Derogatis *et al.*, 1974). Some of the factors correlated more highly than others with these measures. It should, however, be noted that the factor analysis performed in this study is suspect since the number of subjects was not really sufficient for the number of items included.

The EAT has been applied in numerous studies and these have helped to define its strengths and limitations.

As a screening test for eating disorders in general population samples its use is severely compromised by the problems mentioned earlier, particularly the low population prevalence of clinically diagnosable disorder (see Szmukler, 1985, for a detailed discussion of relevant studies). At the same time, however, it must be admitted that there is currently no more satisfactory instrument. The user must expect a positive predictive value (PPV) for cases of anorexia nervosa of 0–10% in a population where the prevalence is 1% or less, even with a specificity and a sensitivity each greater than 0.9. Furthermore, experience suggests that the EAT should be separately validated for different population groups even when they may appear quite similar. For example, the PPV for anorexia nervosa or for a 'partial syndrome' of anorexia nervosa differed substantially when the EAT was employed as a screening instrument in same-aged populations of schoolgirls from private schools and state schools in the same part of London (Eisler and Szmukler, 1985). The loading of scores on the major factors extracted was also systematically and significantly different in the two populations.

The factor structure of the EAT has been re-examined in other studies, this time when administered to normal populations. Wells *et al.* (1985) and Eisler and Szmukler (1985) reported similar results when the EAT was applied to large populations of schoolgirls. Four major factors were extracted: (a) 'dieting'; (b) 'food preoccupation'; (c) 'vomiting' and (d) 'social pressure to eat'. From these studies it appears that the dieting factor dominates the EAT score and is difficult to interpret for those who are overweight or who have been overweight. It would appear to be an indicator of serious psychopathology only when the subject is thin or where the preoccupation is extreme or where binge-eating is present, particularly if it is associated with vomiting. The second and third factors in both of these studies did not resemble closely those of Garner *et al.* (1982) derived from a patient group.

The EAT has been shown to change over the course of treatment (Channon and DeSilva, 1985; Steinhausen, 1985). The predictive capabilities of the EAT for eventual outcome has not been much evaluated. It has been suggested that the factor scores mentioned above might prove useful here but this has not been demonstrated.

Little attention has been focused on self-report inventories as measures of outcome for anorexia nervosa, probably because weight and menstruation provide good objective markers of clinical improvement. It appears that changes in EAT scores may lag behind those of body weight and in one study they appeared to be a reasonable predictor of weight one year later (Channon and DeSilva, 1985).

Eating Disorder Inventory (Garner and Olmstead, 1984). Whereas the EAT examines symptoms and behaviours observed in anorexia nervosa, the Eating Disorder Inventory (EDI) was constructed to assess a number of psychological and behavioural disturbances believed to be in some manner more fundamental. The EDI is a 64-item self-report measure with eight subscales:

1. Drive for thinness
2. Bulimia
3. Body dissatisfaction
4. Ineffectiveness
5. Perfectionism
6. Interpersonal distrust
7. Interoceptive awareness
8. Maturity fears.

The format is similar to the EAT, with forced-choice items based on frequency. The EDI usually takes less than 20 minutes to complete.

A number of these scales are attempts to measure features described, in particular by Bruch, as underlying the disorder. These are more of the nature of predisposing factors or relatively specific psychological deficits. 'Ineffectiveness', assessing feelings of general inadequacy and of not feeling in control of one's life, and 'Interoceptive awareness', measuring the subject's difficulties in recognizing and accurately identifying emotions or some visceral sensations, particularly hunger and satiety, are examples. 'Perfectionism' is commonly regarded as an important predisposing trait and 'Maturity fears' attempts to measure the wish to retreat from the challenges of becoming an adult, a common psychodynamic formulation for patients with anorexia nervosa.

The EDI was constructed and validated on three separate samples of patients with anorexia nervosa and three of normal controls. Reliability and validity data are reported in detail by Garner and Olmstead (1984). Reliability coefficients and item–total correlations were good. Criterion-related validity was assessed by comparing EDI scores with the clinical judgements of experienced clinicians familiar with the patient's psychological presentation. The clinicians were asked to rate the patient on each of the subscales of the EDI. Correlations between the patients' scores on each scale and those of the consultants ranged between 0.43 and 0.68, all being highly significant. The 'Bulimia' subscale was demonstrated to discriminate well between 'restrictor' and 'bulimic' anorexics; other subscales also revealed significant differences between these two groups. It is not clear to what extent these differences might have been weight-related since the bulimic subgroup weighed significantly more.

Evidence was also presented that the EDI might have changed significantly with clinical improvement since a group of recovered patients scored within the normal range. Numerous correlations between EDI scales and other measures were found, including the EAT, body size estimation and the HSCL. Details may be found in Garner and Olmstead (1984). (This reference supersedes the earlier report on the EDI by Garner *et al.*, (1983).

The authors emphasize that the EDI was not designed to replace the EAT. The latter was empirically derived from a pool of items reflecting symptoms of anorexia nervosa, while the former was theoretically or deductively constructed. However, the factor 'dieting' on the EAT correlates very highly (about 0.8) with 'Drive for thinness' and the factor 'bulimia and food preoccupation' on the EAT just as highly with 'Bulimia' on the EDI.

To date the EDI has not had sufficient time to establish clearly its real value, but the fact that it has been so carefully constructed will ensure its popularity. Included among the possible applications proposed by the authors are the identification of subtypes of anorexia nervosa in clinical populations and a clearer definition of psychological traits which distinguish them, the assessment of change as a result of treatment, and as a screening instrument to detect subjects with significant eating disturbances in non-clinical populations. As far as the last is concerned there seems little reason to believe that the EDI will be superior to the EAT.

A good example of the use of the EDI is provided by Garner *et al.* (1984). Patients with anorexia nervosa were compared with 'weight-preoccupied' (WP) and 'non-weight-preoccupied' (NWP) women drawn from college and ballet school samples. 'Weight preoccupation' was defined on the basis of an extreme score on the 'drive for thinness' subscale of the EDI. The results indicated that the WP subjects could be differentiated from the AN patients on some EDI subscales (Ineffectiveness, Interpersonal distrust, Lack of interoceptive awareness) but not on others. Further analysis based on EDI data suggested that two groups of subjects could be discerned in the WP group: one which resembled the AN patients closely on all of the EDI scales, and the other only superficially. Further studies might demonstrate whether this differentiation may have value, for example, in predicting the development of a clinical eating disorder.

Cooper *et al.* (1985) have questioned whether the EDI does in fact measure psychological dimensions fundamentally related to anorexia nervosa or whether some of the disturbances are similar to those in non-eating disordered psychiatric patients. In a small study they found that psychiatric outpatients who were 'cases' on the GHQ (Goldberg and Hillier, 1979) scored similarly to anorexics on 'Ineffectiveness' and 'Interpersonal distrust', 'Ineffectiveness', 'Interpersonal distrust' and 'Interoceptive awareness' scores were significantly correlated with GHQ scores, suggesting that they might be expressions of increasing levels of psychological disturbance and not specific to eating disorder patients.

Anorexic Attitudes Questionnaire (AAQ). This questionnaire, devised by Goldberg *et al.* (1980), has been used in a few studies. It is a self-report inventory specifically designed for administration to in-patients. Its 63 items have been subjected to a factor analysis, dubious in validity, since it was applied to only 105 patients. Fifteen 'interpretable' factors were extracted, including some related to 'fear of becoming fat', 'denial of illness', 'loss of appetite', 'achievement', 'hypothermia', 'food is sickening', 'attitudes to staff' and 'hobby cooking'. Four factors were shown to have some prognostic validity, being significantly correlated with weight gain in hospital, whilst some of the others were noted to change over the period of hospitalization. This questionnaire has been further studied in a short form covering seven of the original scales given to a small group of adolescent anorexic in-patients (Steinhausen, 1986). The scales showed low intercorrelations, suggesting that they were tapping separate attitudinal dimensions. Three of them correlated significantly with the EAT, while three changed significantly over the patients' hospitalizations. The 'denial of illness' scale did not correlate significantly with a separate clinical judgement of the extent to which patients denied their illness. So far, therefore, there is little to suggest that the AAQ has more to offer than the EAT or EDI unless one is particularly interested in attitudes to staff and parents, but here its validity is unproven.

SCANS (Setting Conditions for Anorexia Nervosa Scale) (Slade and Dewey, 1986). This is an ambitious scale specifically designed to detect people at risk for the development of an eating disorder. It is theoretically derived, being based on a 'functional–analytic model' of anorexia nervosa (Slade, 1982). This model holds that eating disorders will develop in subjects predisposed by certain 'setting conditions' to a need for bodily control, the latter then being reinforced by a variety of contingencies if dieting proves successful. The 'setting conditions' involve two major constructs: 'general dissatisfaction with life and with oneself' and 'perfectionistic tendencies'. The former construct is related to 'adolescent conflicts', 'interpersonal problems' and 'stress and failure experiences'. It is hypothesized that a combination of the above will result in the need for the subject to control some aspect of her life completely and that this will be the control of the body, especially its shape.

The SCANS comprises 40 items aimed at measuring the 'setting conditions', with only two items directly referring to body weight and shape. A validation on two large normal population samples (drawn from sixth form schoolgirls, female technical college students and student nurses) has been reported as well as on patient groups. Two independent principal component analyses suggested that the two major theoretical setting conditions were reasonably well approximated by the scale, with scores being quite readily derived for subscales called 'general dissatisfaction and loss of control' and 'perfectionism'. Cut-off points were arrived at, post hoc, which best discriminated the control subjects (n=722) from eating disorder patients (n= 40). The best discrimination involved a combination of both major constructs, each above a certain level, with only about 15% of each group being thus misclassified. Concurrent validity was assessed by comparing EAT scores in the control groups for those subjects scoring above the cut-off points on both scales with those scoring below. The differences were highly significant but not particularly large in absolute terms. It was surmised that the 14% of controls who scored highly might contain those most at risk for developing an eating disorder.

A second report (Kiemle *et al.*, 1987) aimed to provide further data on the concurrent validity of the SCANS. This study included interviews with samples of high and low scorers. In this instance 8.5% of subjects scored above the cut-offs on the SCANS. Four out of five girls with a 'partial syndrome' of anorexia nervosa were high scorers, and high scorers were significantly more preoccupied with weight and shape. An analysis in terms of sensitivity, specificity and so on was not performed, but the positive predictive value for the partial syndrome appeared to have been about 20%.

However, it must be remembered that the SCANS was not designed to detect cases but potential cases and therefore its success can only be determined by follow-up of high scorers. The fact that there is a significant relationship between this measure and problematic eating behaviours is of interest and tends to provide some support for Slade's (1982) model. However, it is also possible on the cross-sectional data presented to hypothesize that the causal relationship runs in the opposite direction. The construction of a screening instrument which will accurately predict the future development of a relatively uncommon disorder seems a tall order.

Bulimia

The EAT and EDI have been used in the study of bulimic subjects, but neither was designed specifically for this group. A number of such scales have been reported but most have been used in one-off studies, without any investigation of their psychometric properties.

The Binge Scale (Hawkins and Clement, 1980) has been used in a number of studies but its properties have never been adequately determined. The same may be said of the Binge Eating Scale (Gormally *et al.*, 1982). The Restrained Eating Inventory (Herman and Polivy, 1975) and a later related scale, the Eating Inventory (EI, Stunkard and Messick, 1985) have been used in research on bulimic subjects but these are primarily concerned with attempts at dietary restraint in order to control body weight, particularly in the obese, rather than with bulimic phenomenology. The notion of 'counter-regulation', i.e. of overeating rather than undereating following a food pre-load, derives from work using the former scale and this may have some relevance for mechanisms in bulimia, but there has been recent evidence casting doubt on the validity of the Restrained Eating Inventory in this regard (Stunkard and Messick, 1985). Correlations between the EAT, EDI and the EI have been investigated and they reveal some overlap between various factors on each scale (Berland *et al.*, 1985).

Two scales, recently developed, deserve consideration since attempts have been made to investigate their psychometric properties; these are considered next.

The Bulimia Test (BULIT) (Smith and Thelen, 1984). This is a 32-item, multiple-choice, self-report measure which attempts to cover the features of bulimia as articulated in DSM-III (American Psychiatric Association, 1980). The scale has undergone a series of validation stages on patient groups as well as large control groups and is one of the few measures in which validation through interviews of samples of high and low scorers has been essayed. Inter-item correlation coefficients were satisfactory and differences between controls and patients highly significant. A cut-off score was determined post hoc which resulted in an excellent discrimination between a group of normal control subjects (n=94) and a group of bulimic patients (n=20). The next stage involved the administration of the BULIT to a non-clinical population of 652 female college students followed by validating interviews of high scorers and stratified samples of low scorers. The sensitivity was reported as 0.64, the specificity as 0.89, the positive predictive value as 74% and the negative predictive value as 84%. There is some question in this author's mind as to the correctness of the calculations in the report but the errors made would, if anything, probably underestimate the sensitivity and specificity. The BULIT was also shown to be significantly correlated with the EAT (r=0.68) and the Binge Scale (Hawkins and Clement, 1980) (r=0.93) and had a high test–retest reliability (0.87) over 2 months.

The 'BITE' (Henderson and Freeman, 1987). This self-report measure has been validated on two groups of binge eaters and controls. The second version contains 30 items relating to symptoms, behaviour and dieting (Symptom subscale) with a second subscale of six items measuring the severity of behaviour. The maximum score on the Symptom subscale is 30, with 20 as the criterion score. The severity subscale has a maximum of 39 but 5 is regarded as a severe disorder. In the second validation study there was no overlap between controls and patients. A high inter-item reliability coefficient of 0.96 was reported for the symptom subscale. There were also high correlations with most scales of the EDI and the EAT. The BITE showed sensitivity to change in a group of 27 treated patients. The test–retest reliability at least 1 week apart in controls was 0.86 and 15 weeks apart in patients was 0.68. The BITE takes less than 10 minutes to complete. The authors suggest that the scale might prove useful in studying bulimia in a 'systematic way' and as a measure of change. Its value in epidemiological studies cannot be predicted until it is tested against a validating interview in normal population groups.

Observer-rated Measures

Only one scale has been used with any degree of frequency and this is one of the earliest devised—the Anorexic Behaviour Scale (ABS) (Slade, 1973). Two observers, usually nurses on the ward, rate the presence or absence of 22 typical anorexic behaviours. It is simply scored and Slade demonstrated that high inter-rater reliability could be achieved. The scale can also be filled out by parents, thereby rating the patient's behaviour at home, but this application has not been adequately investigated. Some of the behaviours rated are not easily engaged in by patients in a restrictive hospital programme and this may give a false impression of improvement.

Structured Interview Measures

Nearly all of the rating instruments used in research on the eating disorders so far have been of the self-report type. However, there are a variety of phenomena which cannot be satisfactorily covered in such a format. These concern primarily the reliability of the patient's self-rating given a propensity for denial and the fact that many of the features of the eating disorders are difficult to define accurately. A good example of the latter is the word 'binge', which for some subjects might mean a totally inadequate meal while for others an intake of over 2000 kcal. Other features which are central to most conceptualizations of anorexia nervosa and which are difficult to assess by questionnaire alone concern the patient's attitudes to her weight and the extent of her fear of 'fatness'. The opportunity for the patient to enlarge on these experiences should make their assessment more accurate and reliable.

It seems likely that the next phase of clinical research in the eating disorders will rely increasingly on interview schedules. Unfortunately, so far no standardized interview has achieved substantial recognition in research, although a few have recently appeared.

'Morgan and Russell Scales'. These scales were devised to measure a broad range of clinically relevant dimensions in a long-term outcome study (Morgan and Russell, 1975). They have subsequently been used in a number of similar studies to permit comparisons between different cohorts (Hsu *et al.*, 1979; Morgan *et al.*, 1983; Russell *et al.* 1987). The scales rated are nutritional status, menstruation, mental state, psychosexual functioning and social functioning. No information is available concerning inter-rater reliability, nor is there a published glossary to assist with a more precise definition of ratings than the sketchy points given for each scale. The scales have obvious clinical face validity, and the pattern of scores in the studies cited when set against other outcome variables suggest good concurrent validity. However, the coverage of specific features of the eating disorders is brief and bulimia is not separately considered.

Eating Disorders Interview. This was devised by the author for use in epidemiological studies of the eating disorders (Mann *et al.*, 1983). The interview aims at the detection of behaviours and attitudes common in patients with anorexia nervosa and bulimia but has been designed to elicit these in 'normal' population samples. Data are collected which permit a diagnosis of an eating disorder to be made and also allow for the definition of a category of subject described as having a 'partial syndrome' of anorexia nervosa. The items may also be scored on two major scales: 'food avoidance' and 'preoccupation with weight'. The interview has been used in a number of studies (Mann *et al.*, 1983; Szmukler, 1983; Hooper and Garner, 1986). The ratings have been shown to have adequate inter-rater reliability following some training. The interview schedule has not been published but copies are available from the eating disorders unit at the Institute of Psychiatry.

Two other semi-structured interview schedules have recently been developed.

The Eating Disorder Examination (EDE; Cooper and Fairburn, 1987) has been devised to examine only the specific psychopathology of the eating disorders and covers both anorexia nervosa and bulimia. There are 62 items and the previous 4 weeks is the time interval rated. The items cover the whole range of behaviours and attitudes found in these disorders. For each item there is at least one mandatory probe question as well as a number of optional subsidiary questions. These questions help the interviewer elicit sufficient information to make an adequate rating, but further questions of the interviewer's own choosing are permitted to further clarify any points.

Clear instructions are provided as to how to make ratings. The majority of ratings are made on seven-point scales with at least four clearly defined anchor points. Items are rated in terms of their severity, or their frequency at a certain level of severity. The interview takes between 30 and 60 minutes to administer and a brief training in its use is recommended by the authors. Inter-rater reliability has been examined and is reported as very satisfactory. So far no studies have been reported in which it has been applied.

The other recently developed scale is the Clinical Eating Disorder Rating Instrument (CEDRI) (Palmer *et al.*, 1987). This is also a semi-structured clinical interview comprising 31 items, each of which is rated on a four-point scale. Definitions are provided for each point. There are three groups of items: behavioural patterns, attitudes towards eating and weight, and symptoms not directly related to eating or weight but commonly present in patients with eating disorders (e.g. depressed mood, suicidal feelings, obsessional symptoms). The previous 4 weeks is again the period covered. Inter-rater reliability is again high.

As neither of the last two scales has been used in a reported investigation it is difficult to make any judgements about their value. The EDE appears comprehensive in its coverage of the specific features of anorexia nervosa and bulimia.

Body-size Estimation Measures

A specific aspect of the psychopathology of anorexia nervosa which permits fairly ready quantitative measurement and which is believed to represent a fundamental disturbance of the disorder is the patient's apparent overestimation of her body size, so that even when she is emaciated she claims to be fat. There is now an extensive body of literature in this field and it is beyond the scope of this chapter to deal with this complex area in detail. However, a brief description of the types of measures used and some of the methodological problems encountered will be given.

Four techniques have been applied:

(i) *Image-marking Method* (Askevold, 1975). This requires that the subject stand before a large blank sheet of paper and mark with a pen points corresponding to the outline of certain body parts, for example, shoulders, chest, hips.

(ii) *Movable Caliper Technique* (Slade and Russell, 1973). The basic apparatus consists of two indicators, usually illuminated, which move simultaneously in the horizontal plane. The patient is required to indicate when the indicators represent the outer edges of a particular body part.

(iii) *Distorting Photograph Technique* (Garner *et al.*, 1976). The subject views her body using a projected photograph which can be distorted along the horizontal axis, enabling the image to be made from 20% 'thinner' to 20% 'fatter' than the actual size. The subject is asked to indicate when the image corresponds to the way her body looks.

(iv) *Video Distortion Techniques.* (Touyz *et al.*, 1984; Freeman *et al.*, 1984). Video cameras may be modified electronically to produce controlled distortion of objects in a horizontal plane. Variations from 20% 'thinner' to 40% 'fatter' are possible. The video image of the patient is varied continuously by the experimenter and the patient is asked to indicate when she believes the image to be an accurate representation of her body.

Techniques (i) and (ii) above measure width estimation at particular sites (e.g. face, bust, hips) while (iii) and (iv) provide a single, whole-body estimate. Overestimation is usually expressed as an index (Body Perception Index, BPI) which is calculated by dividing the patient's estimate by the true width and multiplying by 100.

A seminal study by Slade and Russell (1973) showed that patients with anorexia nervosa significantly overestimated their body dimensions when compared with normal controls although they accurately estimated the size of a neutral object. Further, this overestimation decreased as the patients gained weight and the extent of overestimation prior to discharge from hospital significantly predicted the degree of weight loss following discharge.

However, later studies have demonstrated many methodological pitfalls with these techniques. Most important is their sensitivity to subtle aspects of the experimental conditions. The results may be greatly influenced by, among other factors, the precise nature of the instructions given to the patient and the expectancy aroused in her, the provision of visual or tactile cues, the instruction to try again, whether a meal has been eaten shortly beforehand, the degree of illumination in the testing room, the age of the subject and her absolute body size (Slade, 1985; Norris, 1984; Button *et al.*, 1977; Crisp and Kalucy, 1974; Garner and Garfinkel, 1981; Proctor and Morley, 1986; Halmi *et al.*, 1977). It is also possible that the different techniques employed may be measuring different facets of the patient's experience of her body (perceptual, cognitive and affective), and that they may not be comparable (Slade, 1985). These influences obviously make the assessment of the reliability of the measures difficult.

In general, patients with anorexia nervosa and bulimia have been found to overestimate more than controls but this is far from universal, there being a great deal of variance and overlap. The predictive validity of overestimation has been supported by a number of reports, but it has been suggested (Ben-Tovim and Crisp, 1984) that this may be an artefact since overestimation is greater when the patient's true dimensions are narrower, and they are narrower when the patient is most underweight. The degree of weight loss may thus be the key factor (Ben-Tovim and Crisp, 1984).

Great care must therefore be taken if it is planned to use body-size estimation techniques in an investigation.

CONCLUSIONS

The number of measures for use in the eating disorders is increasing rapidly; each issue of the *International Journal of Eating Disorders*, for example, seems to present a new scale. Scales are generally being evaluated in a more sophisticated manner and psychometric principles are more likely to have been observed in their design. Still, there seems to have been insufficient attention to designs for specific purposes, for example for epidemiological studies or to measure change. Semi-structured interviews are likely to become more important in the next phase of research in these disorders, allowing finer-grained assessments to be made. In the history of research in the eating disorders rating scales have reflected the major directions of investigation but perhaps even more often they have determined those directions. They are thus important tools which must be treated with care. When applied in a study, attention should always be paid to how well the measure has performed its job and, wherever possible, data given which extend our knowledge of its psychometric properties. It is hoped that this overview will help the reader to choose an appropriate scale for a particular project and perhaps to develop a useful new scale to fill some of the many current gaps.

REFERENCES

American Psychiatric Association (1980). *Diagnostic and Statistical Manual* (3rd edn), American Psychiatric Association, Washington, DC.

Askevold, F. (1975). Measuring body image. *Psychother. Psychosom.* **26**, 71–77.

Ben-Tovim, D. and Crisp, A. H. (1984). The reliability of estimates of body width and their relationship to current measured body size among anorexic and normal subjects. *Psychol. Med.* **14**, 843–846.

Berland, N. W., Thompson, J. K. and Linton, P. H. (1985). Correlation between the EAT-26 and the EAT-40, the Eating Disorder Inventory, and the Restrained Eating Inventory. *Int. J. Eating Disord.* **5**, 569–574.

Berscheid, E., Walster, E. and Hohrnstedt, G. (1973). The happy American body: A survey report. *Psychol. Today* Nov., 119–131.

Bruch, H. (1973). *Eating Disorders*, Basic Books, New York.

Button, E., Fransella, F. and Slade, P. D. (1977). Reappraisal of body perception disturbance in anorexia nervosa. *Psychol. Med.* **7**, 235–243.

Channon, S. and DeSilva, W. P. (1985). Psychological correlates of weight gain in patients with anorexia nervosa. *J. Psychiatr. Res.* **19**, 267–271.

Cooper, Z. and Fairburn, C. The Eating Disorder Examination: a semi-structured interview for the assessment of the specific psychopathology of eating disorders. *Int. J. Eating Disord.* **6**, 1–8.

Cooper, Z., Cooper, P. J. and Fairburn, C. G. (1985). The specificity of the Eating Disorder Inventory. *Br. J. Clin. Psychol.* **24**, 129–130.

Crisp, A. H. and Kalucy, R. S. (1974). Aspects of perceptual disorder in anorexia nervosa. *Br. J. Med. Psychol.* **47**, 349–361.

Derogatis, L., Lipman, R., Rickels, K., Uhlenhuth, E. H. and Covi, L. (1974). The Hopkins Symptom Checklist (HSCL): A self-report symptom inventory. *Behav. Sci.* **19**, 1–15.

Eisler, I. and Szmukler, G. I. (1985). Social class as a confounding variable in the Eating Attitudes Test. *J. Psychiatr. Res.* **19**, 171–176.

Freeman, R. J., Thomas, C. D., Solyom, L. and Hunter, M. A. (1984). A modified video camera for measuring body image distortion: technical description and reliability. *Psychol. Med.* **14**, 411–416.

Garner, D. M. and Garfinkel, P. E. (1979). The eating attitudes test: an index of the symptoms of anorexia nervosa. *Psychol. Med.* **9**, 273–279.

Garner, D. M. and Garfinkel, P. E. (1981). Body image in anorexia nervosa: Measurement, theory and clinical implications. *Int. J. Psychiatr. Med.* **11**, 263–284.

Garner, D. M. and Olmstead, M. P. (1984). *Eating Disorder Inventory Manual.* Psychological Assessment Resources Inc.

Garner, D. M., Garfinkel, P. E., Stancer, H. C. and Moldofsky, M. D. (1976). Body image disturbance in anorexia nervosa and obesity. *Psychosom. Med.* **28**, 327–337.

Garner, D. M., Olmstead, M. P., Bohr, Y. and Garfinkel, P. E. (1982). The eating attitudes test: Psychometric features and clinical correlates. *Psychol. Med.* **12**, 871–878.

Garner, D. M., Olmstead, M. P. and Polivy, J. (1983). Development and validation of a multidimensional eating disorder inventory for anorexia nervosa and bulimia. *Int. J. Eating Disord.* **2**, 15–34.

Garner, D. M., Olmstead, M. P., Polivy, J. and Garfinkel, P. E. (1984). Comparison between weight-preoccupied women and anorexia nervosa. *Psychosom. Med.* **46**, 255–266.

Goldberg, D. P. and Hillier, V. F. (1979). A scaled version of the General Health Questionnaire. *Psychol. Med.* **9**, 139–145.

Goldberg, S. C., Halmi, K. A., Eckert, E. D., Casper, R. C., Davis, J. M. and Roper, M. (1980). Attitudinal dimensions in anorexia nervosa. *J. Psychiatr. Res.* **15**, 239–251.

Gormally, J., Black, S. Daston, S. and Rardin, D. (1982). The assessment of binge eating severity among obese persons. *Addict. Behav.* **7**, 47–55.

Halmi, K. A., Goldberg, S. C. and Cunningham, S. (1977). Perceptual distortion of body-image in adolescent girls: distortion of body image in adolescence. *Psychol. Med.* **7**, 253–257.

Hawkins, R. C. and Clement, P. F. (1980). Development and construct validation of a self-report measure of binge eating tendencies. *Addict. Behav.* **5**, 219–226.

Henderson, M. and Freeman, C. P. L. (1987). A self-rating scale for bulimia: the 'BITE'. *Br. J. Psychiatry* **150**, 18–24.

Herman, C. P. and Polivy, J. (1975). Anxiety, restraint and eating behaviour. *J. Personality* **84**, 666–672.

Hooper, M. S. and Garner, D. M. (1986). Application of the Eating Disorder Inventory to a sample of black, white and mixed race schoolgirls in Zimbabwe. *Int. J. Eating Disord.* **5**, 161–168.

Hsu, L. K., Crisp, A. H. and Harding, B. (1979). Outcome of anorexia nervosa. *Lancet* **i**, 61–65.

Kiemle, G., Slade, P. D. and Dewey, M. E. (1987). Factors associated with abnormal eating attitudes and behaviours: Screening individuals at risk of developing an eating disorder. *Int. J. Eating Disord,* **6**, 713–724.

Mann, A. H., Wakeling, A., Wood, K., Monck, E., Dobbs, R. and Szmukler, G. I. (1983). Screening for abnormal eating attitudes and psychiatric morbidity in an unselected population of 15-year-old schoolgirls. *Psychol. Med.* **13**, 573–580.

Morgan, H. G. and Russell, G. F. M. (1975). Value of family background and clinical features as predictors of long-term outcome in anorexia nervosa: Four-year follow-up study of 41 patients. *Psychol. Med.* **5**, 355–371.

Morgan, H. G., Purgold, J. and Wellbourne, J. (1983). Management and outcome in anorexia nervosa: A standardized prognostic study. *Br. J. Psychiatry* **143**, 282–287.

Norris, D. L. (1984). The effects of mirror confrontation on self-estimation of body dimension in anorexia nervosa, bulimia and two control groups. *Psychol. Med.* **14**, 835–842.

Palmer, R., Christie, M., Cordle, C., Davies, D. and Kenrick, J. (1987). The Clinical Eating Disorder Rating Instrument (CEDRI): a preliminary description. *Int. J. Eating Disord.* **6**, 9–16.

Proctor, L. and Morley, S. (1986). 'Demand characteristics' in body-size estimation in anorexia nervosa. *Br. J. Psychiatry* **149**, 113–118.

Russell, G. F. M., Szmukler, G. I., Dare, C. and Eisler, I. (1987). An evaluation of family therapy in anorexia nervosa and bulimia nervosa. *Arch. Gen. Psychiatry.* **44**, 1047–1056.

Slade, P. D. (1973). A short anorexic behaviour scale. *Br. J. Psychiatry* **122**, 83–85.

Slade, P. D. (1982). Towards a functional analysis of anorexia nervosa. *Br. J. Clin. Psychol.* **21**, 167–179.

Slade, P. (1985). A review of body-image studies in anorexia nervosa and bulimia nervosa. *J. Psychiatr. Res.* **19**, 255–265.

Slade, P. D. and Dewey, M. E. (1986). Development and preliminary validation of SCANS: a screening instrument for identifying individuals at risk of developing anorexia and bulimia nervosa. *Int. J. Eating Disord.* **5**, 517–538.

Slade, P. D. and Russell, G. F. M. (1973). Awareness of body dimensions in anorexia nervosa—cross-sectional and longitudinal studies. *Psychol. Med.* **3**, 188–199.

Smith, M. C. and Thelen, M. H. (1984). Development and validation of a test for bulimia. *J. Consult. Clin. Psychol.* **52**, 863–872.

Steinhausen, H-C. (1985). Evaluation of inpatient treatment of adolescent anorexic patients. *J. Psychiatr. Res.* **19**, 371–375.

Steinhausen, H. C. (1986). Attitudinal dimensions in adolescent anorexic patients: An analysis of the Goldberg anorectic attitude scale. *J. Psychiatr. Res.* **20**, 83–87.

Stunkard, A. J. and Messick, S. (1985). The Three-Factor Eating Questionnaire to measure dietary restraint, disinhibition and hunger. *J. Psychosom. Res.* **29**, 71–83.

Szmukler, G. I. (1983). Weight and food preoccupation in a population of English schoolgirls. In *Understanding Anorexia Nervosa and Bulimia* (G. J. Bargman, ed.), Fourth Ross Conference on Medical Research, Ross Laboratories, Ohio, pp. 21–27.

Szmukler, G. I. (1985). The epidemiology of anorexia nervosa and bulimia. *J. Psychiatr. Res.* **19**, 143–153.

Touyz, S. W., Beumont, P. J. V., Collins, J. K., McCabe, M. and Jupp, J. (1984). Body shape perception and its disturbance in anorexia nervosa. *Br. J. Psychiatry* **144**, 167–171.

Vandereycken, W. and Vanderlinden, J. (1983). Denial of illness and the use of self-reporting measures in anorexia nervosa patients. *Int. J. Eating Disord.* **2**, 101–107.

Wells, J. E., Coope, P. A., Gabb, D. C. and Pears, R. K. (1985). The factor structure of the Eating Attitudes Test with adolescent schoolgirls. *Psychol. Med.* **15**, 141–146.

Williams, P., Hand, D. and Tarnopolsky, A. (1982). The problem of screening for uncommon disorders—a comment on the Eating Attitudes Test. *Psychol. Med.* **12**, 431–434.

The Instruments of Psychiatric Research
Edited by C. Thompson

CHAPTER 8

Suicide and attempted suicide

KEITH HAWTON
University Department of Psychiatry and Warneford Hospital, Oxford, UK

INTRODUCTION

Much research concerning suicidal behaviour, both fatal and non-fatal, has focused on the prediction of suicidal acts. It is not surprising therefore that several scales have been developed in an effort to refine such prediction. Thus there are scales for assessing risk of completed suicide in psychiatric populations, and other scales for assessing risk of suicide following attempted suicide. Some attention has also been paid to the somewhat easier problem of identifying among suicide attempters those who are at greatest risk of making repeat attempts. Other scales have been developed to provide a quantitative description of suicidal behaviour, often for the purpose of investigating relationships between degrees of severity of suicidal acts and clinical and social variables.

This chapter reviews rating scales in each of these areas, concentrating largely on those which in the author's opinion are most useful for research. The rationale behind the scales is explained and details provided of their use, scoring and, where available, their qualities, such as their reliability and validity. Comment is included on their usefulness and limitations in both research work and clinical practice, together with a brief review of research investigations in which they have been used.

SUICIDE RISK

Several efforts have been made to develop scales to identify individuals who are at risk of killing themselves. Research has concentrated on populations already known to have higher than the general population risk of suicide, namely psychiatric patients (especially those suffering from depression) and suicide attempters (these are discussed later). Most attention has been paid to the development of general scales which include a range of demographic and psychosocial variables. The Risk Estimator for Suicide provides one example. Recently attention has also focused on cognitive variables associated with suicide risk, including pessimism (the Hopelessness Scale) and suicidal ideation (the Suicidal Ideation Scale).

The usefulness of measures intended to predict suicide is severely limited, largely by the nature of suicide itself. Several factors contribute to this limitation (Hawton, 1987). First, suicide is rare, even in relatively high-rate groups. Second, the variables that can be identified as predictors are crude, each by itself having low predictive power. Even when these variables are combined in a scale the highest efficiency which can be obtained is of the order of 80%. This means that if a population of psychiatric patients has an annual suicide rate of 1%, then in order to identify eight out of ten individuals who might be expected to kill themselves in a year out of a total population of 1000, a further 192 individuals who will not kill themselves will also be identified as possible suicides. Third, while some risk factors are permanent (e.g. sex) or change predictably (e.g. age), others can change unpredictably. Thus, for example, an employed person may become unemployed, with consequently considerably increased risk of suicide, or a social drinker may begin to abuse alcohol, again thereby becoming at increased risk. Fourth, since it is unethical and indeed impractical to set up a treatment study which includes a no-treatment group in order to study the efficacy of a predictive scale for suicide, such a scale can only tell us who is at risk *in spite of* available treatment.

Risk Estimator for Suicide

This interviewer-rated scale will only be mentioned briefly in order to illustrate the type of scale that has been developed in this area. It contains 15 items which were identified from a prospective study of a large sample of depressed and/or suicidal psychiatric inpatients, 4.9% of whom committed suicide during a 2-year follow-up period (Motto *et al.*, 1985). The items include demographic (e.g. age, occupation), psychosocial (e.g. financial circumstances, stress) and clinical characteristics (e.g. sleep duration, suicidal ideas), plus a single item concerning the interviewer's reaction to the patient. Each item is given a weighted score, and the total score is used to assess relative risk of suicide during the following 2 years. In a preliminary field test volunteer crisis workers took on average 4.5 minutes to complete the scale (Motto, 1985).

An independent field test failed to demonstrate significant predictive value for this scale (Clark *et al.*, 1987). While the authors of the study accepted that their results did not definitely invalidate the scale, their study demonstrated the necessity for repeated testing and refinement in order to develop an adequate scale of this kind. An abortive study by Pokorny (1983), which included several scales thought to be predictive of suicide, demonstrated just how far we are from finding an efficient predictive measure of suicide.

The usefulness of scales of this kind in research is probably limited, except in themselves serving to increase our knowledge of predictors which can then be used clinically. However, because of the limitations already noted, clinical assessment of suicide risk should not lean heavily on rating scales; they should only be used as an adjunct to other aspects of clinical assessment and in order to remind clinicians of some of the factors which should be assessed.

Hopelessness Scale

Recent work has demonstrated the importance of pessimism or negative attitudes towards the future in suicidal risk and behaviour. The Hopelessness Scale (Beck *et al.*, 1974b), which is the most well known and tested scale to measure such attitudes, is self-rated and contains 20 statements, each of which is rated true or false. Each response is scored 0 or 1, the possible total range of scores therefore being from 0 to 20.

The author has not been able to find any reports of the test–retest reliability of the Hopelessness Scale. However, the correlations between individual items and the total score have been shown to be satisfactory (Beck *et al.*, 1974b).

Validity

Reasonable validity was demonstrated by Beck *et al.* (1974), who compared patients' ratings on the scale with ratings of hopelessness made by clinicians and with scores on a self-rated semantic differential test of hopelessness. They also demonstrated that the Hopelessness Scale score correlated more highly (0.63) with the pessimism item on the Beck Depression Inventory (p. 109) than with any other item on the depression scale.

Utility

The Hopelessness Scale has been used quite widely in research into suicidal behaviour. It has also been used to study depression, including the effects of psychological and physical treatments of depressed patients (e.g. Rush *et al.*, 1982).

The two main uses of the Hopelessness Scale in suicide research have been in the evaluation of factors contributing to suicidal intent and in the prediction of suicide. Several studies have demonstrated that while suicidal intent (see below) associated with attempted suicide correlates with both depression (Beck Depression Inventory score) and hopelessness, the latter is the key factor and accounts for the statistical association between depression and suicidal intent (Minkoff *et al.*, 1973; Beck *et al.*, 1975b; Wetzel *et al.*, 1980; Dyer and Kreitman, 1984). This led to the prediction that risk of eventual suicide would be increased among patients with high scores on the Hopelessness Scale, and that the risk would bear more relation to hopelessness scores than to depression scores. Both predictions have recently received support in a long-term prospective study of psychiatric in-patients admitted to hospital because of depression and suicidal ideas (Beck *et al.*, 1985). Patients with scores of 17 or more on the Hopelessness Scale appear to be at particular risk. However, the false positive rate is extremely high, even in this subgroup of very high scorers, thus demonstrating the limitation of this measure as with other predictors of suicide.

It has been shown that scores on the Hopelessness Scale are sensitive to changes in depression, and that a psychological treatment (cognitive therapy) of depression has more impact than an antidepressant on hopelessness scores (Rush *et al.*, 1982).

The Hopelessness Scale is clearly a useful research instrument for studying both suicidal behaviour and depression. Furthermore, it can readily be used in clinical practice. Most patients find it easy to complete, and it can form part of the clinician's general assessment of suicide risk, including during treatment of depression.

Scale for Suicide Ideation

Suicidal phenomena can be divided broadly into suicide attempts, completed suicide, and suicidal thoughts or ideation. The Scale for Suicide Ideation (included in full in Beck *et al.*, 1979) was developed to measure this third category. Specifically it assesses the intensity of current suicidal intent. It is an interviewer-rated 19-item scale, each item being scored 0, 1 or 2 and the range of total scores therefore being 0–38. The items cover the extent of suicidal thoughts, and their characteristics, as well as the patients' attitude towards them, the extent of any wish to die, possible desire to make an actual suicide attempt, details of any plans for an attempt, internal deterrents against an attempt, and subjective feelings of control and/or 'courage' regarding a proposed attempt. Questions necessary to complete the scale can be incorporated into a clinical interview.

Reliability

An inter-rater reliability coefficient of 0.83 was obtained for two assessors rating the same interviews with 25 patients (Beck *et al.*, 1979). Internal consistency of the scale has also been shown to be satisfactory.

Validity

Beck *et al.* (1979) stated that concurrent validity of the scale was tested by comparing scores against clinical evaluations and psychological inventory scores, but no results were given. However, the scale differentiated reasonably well between depressed patients hospitalized because of suicidal ideas and other, non-hospitalized, depressed patients with equivalent depression scores.

Utility

The Scale of Suicidal Ideation has not been used extensively in research, except as a dependent variable in order to allow the influence of other factors (e.g. depression and hopelessness) over suicidal thoughts to be evaluated (e.g. Wetzel, 1976; Beck *et al.*, 1979). It should be useful in further studies of this kind, and also in the evaluation of treatment outcome in suicidal depressed patients or suicide attempters. In clinical work the scale may prove a helpful adjunct when investigating suicide risk.

SEVERITY OF SUICIDE ATTEMPTS

Broadly speaking there are two types of scale for assessing the severity of suicide attempts: those which examine the extent to which death appears to have been the intended outcome ('suicidal intent') and those more concerned with the physical danger or consequences of an attempt. It is important to distinguish between these two aspects of attempts because, contrary to popular opinion, there is a very low correlation between suicidal intent and medical seriousness of attempts, especially for self-poisoning (Fox and Weissman, 1975). The danger of an attempt only shows a higher correlation with suicidal intent in individuals who are aware of the likely medical consequences of their attempts (Beck *et al.*, 1975a).

Suicidal Intent Scale

This interviewer-rated scale consists of two parts (Table 1). The first concerns factual aspects of the attempt and the circumstances in which it occurred. The information necessary to complete this section can be obtained from the

Table 1. Suicidal Intent Scale

I *Objective circumstances related to suicide attempt*

1. Isolation:
   0 = somebody present
   1 = somebody nearby, or in visual or vocal contact
   2 = no one nearby or in visual or vocal contact

2. Timing:
   0 = intervention probable
   1 = intervention unlikely
   2 = intervention highly unlikely

3. Precautions against discovery/intervention:
   0 = no precautions
   1 = passive precautions, e.g. avoiding others but doing nothing to prevent their intervention, alone in room with unlocked door
   2 = active precautions, e.g. locked door

4. Acting to get help during/after attempt:
   0 = notified potential helper regarding attempt
   1 = contacted but did not specifically notify potential helper regarding attempt
   2 = did not contact or notify potential helper

5. Final acts in anticipation of death (e.g. will, gifts, insurance):
   0 = none
   1 = thought about or made some arrangements
   2 = made definite plans or completed arrangements

6. Active preparation for attempt:
   0 = none
   1 = minimal to moderate
   2 = extensive

7. Suicide note:
   0 = absence of note
   1 = note written but torn up, or thought about
   2 = presence of note

8. Overt communication of intent before the attempt:
   0 = none
   1 = equivocal communication
   2 = unequivocal communication

II *Self-report*

9. Alleged purpose of attempt:
   0 = to manipulate environment, get attention, revenge
   1 = components of '0' and '2'
   2 = to escape, solve problems

10. Expections of fatality:
    0 = thought that death was unlikely
    1 = thought that death was possible but not probable
    2 = thought that death was probable or certain.

11. Conception of method's lethality:
    0 = did less to self than thought would be lethal
    1 = was unsure if action would be lethal
    2 = equalled or exceeded what he thought would be lethal

12. Seriousness of attempt:
    0 = did not seriously attempt to end life
    1 = uncertain about seriousness to end life
    2 = seriously attempted to end life

13. Attitude toward living/dying:
    0 = did not want to die
    1 = components of '0' and '2'
    2 = wanted to die

14. Conception of medical rescuability:
    0 = thought that death would be unlikely with medical attention
    1 = was uncertain whether death could be averted by medical attention
    2 = was certain of death even with medical attention

15. Degree of premeditation:
    0 = none, impulsive
    1 = contemplated for 3 hours or less before attempt
    2 = contemplated for more than 3 hours before attempt

Reproduced by permission of Dr A. T. Beck.

patient and/or from other informants. The second section records the patient's reported thoughts and feelings preceding and following the attempt. The first section contains more reliable items than the second, especially if information is obtained from other informants as well as the patient. However, the second part is necessary because introspective information is very valuable in assessing suicidal intent.

The Suicidal Intent Scale takes about 10 minutes to complete and the necessary questions can readily be incorporated into a routine clinical interview. Each item in the scale is scored 0–2 (as shown in Table 1) and the total score (range 0–30) across all the items obtained. The scores for the two sections can be used separately if wished. Higher scores correspond to greater suicidal intent. A manual which provides further guidance on scoring is available.

Reliability

The inter-rater reliability of the Suicidal Intent Scale appears to be good ($r = 0.95$ for 45 cases) (Beck *et al.*, 1974a). When the first part of the scale was scored by two experienced raters from case-notes for 25 completed suicides the inter-rater reliability was 0.91 (Beck *et al.* 1974c).

Validity

One type of assessment of the validity of the Suicidal Intent Scale has been based on comparison of the scores of 194 completed suicides and 231 attempted suicides on the first section of the scale (Beck *et al.*, 1974c). The former had a mean score of 7.68 and the latter 5.73 ($t = 9.04$, $p<0.001$). Another type of assessment (Pierce, 1984) has been to compare the full scale scores of attempters who repeated attempts (mean = 15.58) with those who did not (mean = 12.45; $t = 2.18$, $p<0.02$). However, this is not a true measure of validity since the scale was not designed to assess risk of repetition. One would expect suicidal intent to correlate with risk of eventual suicide. This expectation received some support in a study of a slightly modified version of the scale (Pierce, 1981), although this study included only a small number of actual suicides.

Utility

The Suicidal Intent Scale has proved extremely valuable in research investigations. It can be used to describe groups of attempters, to provide a means of subdividing attempters, and to examine the possible associations of suicidal intent with other characteristics of attempters (e.g. sex, age, psychiatric history and psychiatric disorder) or their attempts (e.g. medical danger, methods used, repeats versus first attempts). The first section of the scale can be completed from well-documented case-notes, although this is not generally recommended because of the variations between clinicians in both the questions they ask and the extent of information they record in case-notes. Rarely, for example, do even carefully trained assessors ask attempted suicide patients whether or not a suicide note has been left (Catalan *et al.*, 1980).

As already noted, suicidal intent has been shown to be more closely related to hopelessness than to depression (Minkoff *et al.*, 1973; Beck *et al.*, 1975b; Wetzel *et al.*, 1980; Dyer and Kreitman, 1984), and to be correlated with the medical danger of an attempt in those aware of the possible medical consequences of their acts (Beck *et al.*, 1975a). Using a modified version of the scale, Pierce (1977) demonstrated that higher scores (on at least one of the two sections of this scale) are found for suicide attempters who are socially isolated, use methods other than self-poisoning for their attempts, have physical illnesses and drink heavily. James and Hawton (1985) found that suicidal intent did not appear to influence whether attempters' relatives felt sympathetic or guilty about their attempts, but that the higher the intent score the more anger they felt towards the attempters.

Anyone planning to incorporate the scale in research investigations should ensure that raters get experience in using it with pilot cases beforehand. The main tendency is to over-rate and therefore score patients too highly. Raters should consult the manual frequently while becoming acquainted with the scale and, if possible, carry out their own inter-rater reliability check before beginning a study.

The Suicidal Intent Scale is also valuable in clinical practice. It can easily be incorporated in the assessment of suicide attempters (Hawton and Catalan, 1987) and, apart from the score providing useful additional information, its use can help ensure that important questions are included in the enquiry. However, undue reliance should not be placed on the score when, for example, deciding on after-care. Information concerning other factors (e.g. psychiatric history, mental state, current problems) is also necessary when making such decisions.

Assessment of Physical Danger of Attempts

Several workers have developed measures to assess the physical aspects of suicide attempts, although none appears to be particularly good. A simple scale such as that described by Kessel (1966) for deliberate self-poisoning is probably as useful as any. He classified overdoses according to the estimated consequences of what the patient took, should medical treatment not have been received, into: *certain survival, unlikely to die, critical* and *fatal*. An even simpler scale was derived from Kessel's by Pierce (1977), who used only three categories, again based on whether death would have occurred without medical treatment: *no* (0), *uncertain* (1) and *yes* (2). Kessel combined his scale with another simple scale concerning 'action by the patient at the time of the act to avoid or ensure discovery' (*ensure discovery, neutral, avoid discovery*) to develop an Index of Endangering Life, in which the predictable outcome of the act was classified as: *death, death probable, death unlikely* and *certain to survive* (see Kessel, 1966, for further details).

Pierce (1977) demonstrated that medical risk scores correlate with scores on the Suicidal Intent Scale, and are higher in older and male attempters.

Scales such as these are not very useful in clinical practice, but can be utilized in research studies such as when comparing clinical or motivational characteristics of attempters with the physical danger of their attempts. Ideally, the ratings should be made by independent clinicians presented with full descriptions of the nature of attempts, such as method used, number and type of tablets, and extent of any alcohol consumed with the attempt.

REPETITION OF ATTEMPTED SUICIDE

Attempted suicide is often repeated. Thus between 12% and 25% of hospital-referred attempters are re-referred to hospital for further attempts within a year (Hawton and Catalan, 1987). Identification of those patients likely to make repeat attempts is therefore important, both in clinical and research work.

Risk of Repetition Scale

This scale was developed by Buglass and Horton (1974) using a careful and elaborate research procedure. In summary, items which distinguished repeaters (those who made repeat attempts during the year following an index attempt) from non-repeaters among a large cohort of suicide attempters were first identified. These items were then tested and validated on two further large cohorts of attempters.

The Risk of Repetition Scale is simple, consisting of only six items (Table 2). These are rated by an interviewer. One point is allocated for each item, total scores thus ranging from 0 to 6, the higher the score the higher the risk of repetition during the year after an attempt.

Table 2. Risk of Repetition Scale

1. Sociopathy[a]
2. Problems in the use of alcohol[b]
3. Previous in-patient psychiatric treatment
4. Previous out-patient psychiatric treatment
5. Previous parasuicide (suicide attempt) resulting in general hospital admission
6. Not living with a relative

Reproduced by permission of the Royal College of Psychiatrists.
Definitions provided by Buglass and Horton (1974):
[a] Sociopathy: predominant distress of the patient's situation falls on society.
[b] Problems in the use of alcohol: includes 'excessive drinking' as well as alcohol addiction.

Reliability

The author is unaware of any published reports of the reliability of the Risk of Repetition Scale. There is little room for disagreement between raters for items 3–6 (Table 2). However, items 1 and 2, and especially item 1, pose more uncertainty. It would be wise therefore for anyone proposing to use this scale for research to carry out their own inter-rater reliability check beforehand.

Validity

There was good support for the scale's validity in the original report by Buglass and Horton (1974). Thus the percentages of attempters making repeat attempts within a year of a first attempt were, for example, for one of the years studied: score = 0 (5% repeaters); 1 (9%); 2 (16%); 3 (27%); 4 (37%); 5 or 6 (48%). Such findings have been replicated by other workers, including the author (Hawton, 1979).

Utility

The Risk of Repetition Scale has proved useful in research, especially in describing groups of attempters. It also has a potential research use for identifying target groups of attempted suicide patients (e.g. high-risk groups) when evaluating special treatment procedures, especially if it is hoped that the treatment will have an impact on repetition rates. However, while the predictive power of this scale is quite impressive, it should be noted that at least 50% of repeaters will not score highly on it.

Although the Risk of Repetition Scales is highly relevant in clinical work, assessment of risk of repetition in the individual patient should not rely solely on scores on the scale. Attention must also be paid to other factors, including, for example, whether the patient's problems appear likely to change, available supports, and psychiatric disorder. The scale has not been evaluated specifically in adolescent or elderly attempters.

SUICIDE FOLLOWING ATTEMPTED SUICIDE

The association between attempted suicide and completed suicide is extremely important. Thus approximately half of those individuals who kill themselves have made a previous attempt (Ovenstone and Kreitman, 1974). Furthermore, the risk of eventual suicide among attempted suicides is many times that of the general population. Approximately 1% of attempters die by suicide within a year of their attempts (Buglass and Horton, 1974; Hawton and Fagg, 1988) and approximately 3% have died by suicide within 3–8 years of an attempt (Buglass and McCulloch, 1970; Hawton and Fagg, 1988). Not surprisingly, considerable effort has gone into trying to develop scales which can help identify those attempters most at risk of suicide.

Scale for Assessing Suicide Risk of Attempted Suicides (Tuckman and Youngman Scale)

This scale (Table 3) was developed on the basis of a follow-up study of 3800 suicide attempters known to the police department in Philadelphia. The study extended over several years from the time of the initial attempts (Tuckman and Youngman, 1968). There were in all 48 deaths from suicide during the follow-up. In Table 3, three items from the original scale ('attempt between 6.00 a.m. and 5.59 p.m.', 'immediate discovery/attempt reported by person making attempt' and 'no self-reported intent to die') have been omitted because findings for these were in the opposite direction to the original hypotheses and may well have been chance findings.

Table 3. Tuckman and Youngman Scale for Assessing Suicide Risk of Attempted Suicides

1. Age 45 years or more
2. Male
3. White
4. Separated, divorced or widowed
5. Living alone
6. Unemployed or retired
7. Poor physical health (acute or chronic condition in the 6-month period preceding the attempt)
8. Nervous or mental disorder, including alcoholism
9. Medical care within 6 months
10. Attempt by hanging, firearm, jumping or attempted drowning
11. Attempt during April to September ('warm months')
12. Attempt in own or someone else's home
13. Suicide note
14. Previous attempt or threat

Each item is scored 0 (absent) or 1 by the clinician. The risk of suicide increases in proportion to the total number of items with a positive score. In Tuckman and Youngman's (1968) original study attempters scoring positively on two to five factors had a suicide rate of 6.98 per 1000, those who scored 6–9 a rate of 19.61 per 1000, and those with a score of 10–12 a rate of 60.61 per 1000.

Reliability and Validity

The author is unaware of any reliability studies on this scale. The validity of the scale was demonstrated in the original study, as noted above. However, this level of prediction is not impressive when one considers the number of false positive cases. Furthermore, Resnick and Kendra (1973) did not find that it was very effective in a study of patients admitted to psychiatric hospitals, although the methodology in their study was unusual. However, some of the items have been confirmed by other workers as distinguishing eventual suicides from survivors (e.g. Pallis *et al.*, 1982; Hawton and Fagg, 1988).

Post-attempt Risk-assessment (parasuicide) Scales

These interviewer-rated scales have been developed in an attempt to refine the prediction of suicide following attempted suicide. They are two basic scales: a 'short' six-item version (Table 4) and a 'long' 18-item version. These were the result of a study in which suicides were compared with attempted suicides on a large number of variables (Pallis *et al.*, 1982). Each of the items is weighted on the basis of discriminant· function coefficients to which a constant value has been added in order to eliminate negative values. The weighted scores can be used to assign attempted suicide patients to categories of 'low', 'medium', 'high' and 'extremely high' risk of suicide.

Table 4. Post-attempt Risk Assessment Scale: short version

	Item	Item category	Weights	Assigned Weight
1.	Age	Up to 44	0.12	
		45 and over	5.00	
2.	Sex	Male	6.41	
		Female	5.00	
3.	Social class	Upper (I and II)	6.64	
		Lower (III–V)	5.00	
4.	Work status	Employed	2.65	
		Retired	2.40	
		Other	5.00	
5.	Living Arrangements	Alone	5.84	
		Not alone	5.00	
6.	Suicidal communication in the last year	Yes	7.50	
		No	5.00	
			Total of assigned weights	

Reproduced by permission of the Royal College of Psychiatrists.

Reliability

Reasonable inter-rater reliability was reported by Pallis *et al.* (1982) on the basis of the assessment of a small number of patients.

Validity

The predictive value of the two versions of the scales was investigated in a 2-year follow-up study of attempted suicides (Pallis *et al.*, 1984). Each scale was tested alone and in combination with a modified version of the Suicidal

Intent Scale (items 1–7 in Table 1). Both scales proved useful in identifying the eventual suicides, the long scale somewhat more than the short scale (although the latter was especially effective in predicting risk during the first year after attempts), and their value was improved by combining them with the modified version of the Suicidal Intent Scale. However, the problems already discussed concerning assessment of suicide risk are all encountered with the use of these scales. In particular, they have a high false positive rate, mis-identifying a large proportion of eventual survivors as potential suicides.

Utility

Pallis suggests that the short-version scale might be utilized (together with the Suicide Intent Scale) in clinical work as part of the routine assessment of suicide attempters. However, the use of weighted scores might put off clinicians. The long-version scale is only likely to be useful in research investigations, but it requires further study before it can be generally recommended as a research instrument.

RECOMMENDED READING

Beck, A. T., Resnik, H. L. P. and Lettieri, D. J. (1974). *The Prediction of Suicide*. Charles Press, Philadelphia (republished in 1986).

Hawton, K. and Catalan, J. (1987). *Attempted Suicide: A Practical Guide to its Nature and Management*. Oxford University Press, Oxford.

Kreitman, N. (ed.) (1977). *Parasuicide*. Wiley, Chichester.

REFERENCES

Beck, A. T., Schuyler, D. and Herman, J. (1974a). Development of suicidal intent scales. In: *The Prediction of Suicide* (A. T. Beck, H. L. P. Resnik and D. J. Lettieri, eds), Charles Press, Maryland.

Beck, A. T., Weissman, A., Lester, D. and Trexler, L. (1974b). The measurement of pessimism: The Hopelessness Scale. *J. Consult. Clin. Psychol.* **41**, 861–865.

Beck, R. W., Morris, J. B. and Beck, A. T. (1974c). Cross-validation of the Suicidal Intent Scale. *Psychol. Rep.* **34**, 445–446.

Beck, A. T., Beck, R. and Kovacs, M. (1975a). Classification of suicidal behaviors: I. Quantifying content and medical lethality. *Am. J. of Psychiatry* **132**, 285–287.

Beck, A. T., Kovacs, M. and Weissman, A. (1975b). Hopelessness and suicidal behavior: An overview. *J. Am. Med. Assoc.* **234**, 1146–1149.

Beck, A. T., Kovacs, M. and Weissman, A. (1979). Assessment of suicidal intention: The Scale for Suicide Ideation. *J. Consult. Clin. Psychol.* **47**, 343–352.

Beck, A. T., Steer, R. A., Kovacs, M. and Garrison, B. (1985). Hopelessness and eventual suicide: A 10 year prospective study of patients hospitalized with suicidal ideation. *Am. J. Psychiatry* **145**, 559–563.

Buglass, D. and Horton, J. (1974). A scale for predicting subsequent suicidal behaviour. *Br. J. Psychiatry* **124**, 573–578.

Buglass, D. and McCulloch, J. W. (1970). Further suicidal behaviour: The development and validation of predictive scales. *Br. J. Psychiatry* **116**, 483–491.

Catalan, J., Marsack, P., Hawton, K. E., Whitwell, D., Fagg, J. and Bancroft, J. H. J. (1980). Comparison of doctors and nurses in the assessment of deliberate self-poisoning patients. *Psychol. Med.* **10**, 483–491.

Clark, D. C., Young, M. A., Scheftner, W. A., Fawcett, J. and Fogg, L. (1987). A field test of Motto's Risk Estimator for Suicide. *Am. J. Psychiatry* **144**, 923–926.

Dyer, J. A. T. and Kreitman, N. (1984). Hopelessness, depression and suicidal intent in parasuicide. *Br. J. Psychiatry* **144**, 127–133.

Fox, K. and Weissman, M. (1975). Suicide attempts and drugs: Contradiction between method and intent. *Soc. Psychiatry* **10**, 31–38.

Hawton, K. (1979). *Evaluation of Short-term Psychiatric Intervention following Acts of Self-poisoning*, Unpublished DM thesis, University of Oxford.

Hawton, K. (1987). Assessment of suicide risk. *Br. J. Psychiatry* **150**, 145–153.

Hawton, K. and Catalan, J. (1987). *Attempted Suicide: A Practical Guide to its Nature and Management*, 2nd edn, Oxford University Press, Oxford.

Hawton, K. and Fagg, J. (1988). Suicide and other causes of death following attempted suicide. *Br. J. Psychiatry* **152**, 359–366.

James, D. and Hawton, K. (1985). Overdoses: Explanations and attitudes in self-poisoners and significant others. *Br. J. Psychiatry* **146**, 481–485.

Kessel, N. (1966). The respectability of self-poisoning and the fashion of survival. *J. Psychosom. Res.* **10**, 29–36.

Minkoff, K., Bergman, E., Beck, A. T. and Beck, R. (1973). Hopelessness, depression and attempted suicide. *Am. J. Psychiatry* **130**, 455–459.

Motto, J. A. (1985). Preliminary field-testing of a Risk Estimator for Suicide. *Suicide Life Threat. Behav.* **15**, 139–150.

Motto, J. A., Heilbron, D. C. and Juster, J. P. (1985). Development of a clinical instrument to estimate suicide risk. *Am. J. Psychiatry* **142**, 680–686.

Overstone, I, and Kreitman, N. (1974) Two syndromes of suicide, *Br. J. Psychiatry* **124**, 336–45.

Pallis, D. J., Barraclough, B. M., Levey, A. B., Jenkins, J. S. and Sainsbury, P. (1982). Estimating suicide risk among attempted suicides: I. The development of new clinical scales. *Br. J. Psychiatry* **141**, 37–44.

Pallis, D. J., Gibbons, J. S. and Pierce, D. W. (1984). Estimating suicide risk among attempted suicides. II. Efficiency of predictive scales after the attempt. *Br. J. Psychiatry* **144**, 139–148.

Pierce, D. W. (1977). Suicidal intent in self-injury. *Br. J. Psychiatry* **130**, 377–385.

Pierce, D. W. (1981). Predictive validation of a suicide intent scale. *Br. J. Psychiatry* **139**, 391–396.

Pierce, D. (1984). Suicidal intent and repeated self-harm. *Psychol. Med.* **14**, 655–659.

Pokorny, A. D. (1983). Prediction of suicide in psychiatric patients: Report of a prospective study. *Arch. Gen. Psychiatry* **40**, 249–257.

Resnick, J. H. and Kendra, J. M. (1973). Predictive value of the 'Scale for Assessing Suicide Risk' (SASR) with hospitalized psychiatric patients. *J. Clin. Psychol.* **29**, 187–190.

Rush, J., Beck, A. T., Kovacs, M., Weissenburger, J. and Hollon, S. T. (1982). Comparison of the effects of cognitive therapy and pharmacotherapy on hopelessness and self-concept. *Am. J. Psychiatry* **139**, 862–866.

Tuckman, J. and Youngman, W. F. (1968). A scale for assessing suicide risk of attempted suicides. *J. Clin. Psychol.* **24**, 17–19.

Wetzel, R. D. (1976). Hopelessness, depression and suicide intent. *Arch. Gen. Psychiatry* **33**, 1069–1073.

Wetzel, R. D., Margulies, T., Davis, R. and Karam, E. (1980). Hopelessness, depression and suicidal intent. *J. Clin. Psychiatry* **41**, 159–160.

The Instruments of Psychiatric Research
Edited by C. Thompson

CHAPTER 9

Assessment of drug and alcohol use

John Strang,[1] Brendan Bradley[2] and Tim Stockwell[3]
[1]*Drug Dependence Clinical Research and Treatment Unit, Maudsley Hospital, London UK*

[2]*Department of Experimental Psychology, University of Cambridge, Cambridge, UK*

[3]*National Centre for Research into the Prevention of Drug Abuse, South Perth Australia*

INTRODUCTION

Drug use is not a unitary phenomenon. Any study of drug use or of its effects must identify what exactly is the subject of study. Drugs may be grouped according to their legal status, their extent of use, the route of use and many other groupings in addition to their pharmacological category. Grouping must be done after identifying the characteristic which is relevant to the particular enquiry.

In this chapter we will discuss the assessment of 'drug use' in its widest sense with reference to mood-altering substances in general—whether sold in supermarkets and pubs, prescribed by doctors or obtained from illicit suppliers. Changing patterns of alcohol and other drug use—and changing theoretical models—demand that no one substance can be studied in isolation from any other: too many people are users of many substances, too many of which satisfy similar functions (e.g. Busto *et al.*, 1983).

Studies of drug use and drug problems are perhaps more dogged by assumptions of causal relationships than any other field. Despite warnings of the dangers of confusing causes, correlates and consequences, the warnings are insufficiently heeded. Drug use does not occur in isolation from other behaviours and can only be understood within the social context in which it occurs. Consequently its study may involve consideration of socio-cultural and economic setting, family history, personal history, pre-morbid personality, psychological and psychiatric disturbance, biochemical milieu, etc. In each case, instruments for study should be used from the general field with adaptation/addition so as to increase the relevance to the drug and alcohol field. The study of depression in heroin addicts or problem drinkers does not need entirely new instruments for the identification and quantification of depression—but there must be a recognition that the scoring of results needs to take note of contamination from drug effects themselves, and the interpretation of the findings must allow due consideration of the context in which the data were collected. With these caveats, the drug researcher may benefit greatly from work outside this specialist field.

ASSESSING THE EXTENT OF ALCOHOL AND OTHER DRUG USE IN A COMMUNITY

There are numerous difficulties with gaining accurate information about people's use of mood-altering substances. Even with such legally available drugs as tobacco and alcohol people have a variety of reasons for over- or underestimating their use, ranging from poor memory through embarrassment to self-deception.

The most straightforward method of gaining such information is simply to go out and ask a representative sample of a community what they use, i.e. perform a community survey. Even with regard to alcohol use the resulting estimates of the total amount consumed in a community from such methods fall well short of the known volume of alcohol sales provided by the drinks industry (Plant, 1987).

The would-be researcher should not, however, be deterred from collecting such data. Firstly, comparisons can be made between, for example, different social classes, ages, sexes and regions. Such differences are not entirely due to differences in reporting bias, as can be borne out by cross-validation with more objective measures. Thus the fact that men consistently use more illicit drugs and alcohol than women is confirmed both from self-report data as well as data concerning drug-related accidents and deaths. The general principle then emerges that no research should rely on any one measure of drug use: ideally a wide range should be included in order to validate findings.

In the alcohol field, several methods have been developed which appear to enable subjects to be more open about their drinking habits. Some studies have found that respondents in 'door-to-door' community surveys provide higher estimates of their drinking when given a general lifestyle interview, including alcohol as only one variable, as compared with interviews which only focused on alcohol use. An excellent and very simple 'Health Questionnaire' has been developed for use in health settings which enquired about smoking, drinking, dieting and exercise (Anderson, 1987). Wallace and Haines (1985) successfully employed this questionnaire in a postal survey of patients registered with a London general practice and obtained a 75% completion rate.

Lucas *et al.* (1977) found a high level of agreement between information elicited by a computer and by a psychiatrist, although patients reported higher levels of alcohol consumption to the computer. Duffy and Waterton (1984) have confirmed that people consistently give higher estimates of their drinking to a computer than to an interviewer. Clearly we urgently need to develop self-assessment questionnaires and computer programs which tackle the whole range of substance use and other health behaviours. Skinner and colleagues at the Addiction Research Foundation in Toronto are currently evaluating such a computerized self-administered health check—also in the health centre context (Skinner and Horn, 1984).

The Drug Abuse Screening Test (DAST) has been developed by Skinner and Goldberg (1986) and adapts items from the MAST so as to be appropriate to substance abuse in general. The authors report the emergence of a dependence factor which is characterized by an inability to stop drug use, problems in getting through the week without drugs, and withdrawal signs and symptoms when use of the drug is stopped.

The marked increase in illicit drug use (especially heroin) in the last decade drew departmental and ministerial attention to the need for local estimates of prevalence of drug use (DHSS Health Circular 84/14). The subsequent dismal attempts at local estimates (DHSS, 1985) highlighted the need for more effective monitoring systems. A large bank of data on opiate addiction exists in the Home Office Addicts Index (for description see Edwards, 1981) derived from doctor–patient consultations. However, despite a statutory requirement to provide such data (Misuse of Drug Act 1971), compliance by doctors is poor (Strang and Shah, 1985). Deficiencies in the items of data recorded have recently been highlighted (Stimson, 1987). The advent of HIV/AIDS and the absence of data on route of drug use in this data bank have prompted the introduction of a modified national notification form for doctors (HS 2A/1 (REV), Home Office, 1987) including the request for information on injecting practice. In a special version of the notification form for the north-west, a simple matrix has been used for recording recent drug use so that details of substance, source, route(s), quantity, frequency and duration of use are systematically obtained (see Fig. 1). This matrix format can successfully be extended to use by a range of non-medical statutory and non-statutory workers (Strang, 1989) so that a more accurate picture can be built up of local patterns of drug use, and the different client profiles of different agencies. In a comparison of the information gathered both nationally and on a local database from a variety of agencies and practitioners, it was found that, over a 4-month period, community drug team workers

PROBLEM DRUG USE: For each drug recently used (prescribed or not), complete the following information:

	Drug name	Prescribed or not	How often (times per day/wk/month)	How much (quantity or cost)	Route	Duration (of this drug use)**	Age of 1st use
Drug 1 (main)							
Drug 2							
Drug 3							
Drug 4	Alcohol	—			—		

**or drug from same pharmacological group

Fig. 1. Drug-taking matrix record

reported 3.74 as many episodes of notifiable drug misuse to the local database as had been notified by doctors to the Home Office Addicts Index, although there was evidence of high levels of lost data to both systems (Donmall *et al.*, in preparation).

Hartnoll and his colleagues have demonstrated how it is possible to draw on data already being collected and to estimate approximate prevalence (Hartnoll *et al.*, 1985) using an approach that could be (and has been) used elsewhere (Levy, 1985; Haw, 1985; Parker *et al.*, 1988).

ASSESSMENT OF INTOXICATION

Assessment of degree of intoxication should not be confused with assessing the level of a drug in an individual's bloodstream due to variations in individual tolerance. As shown in Fig. 2 the risk of having a driving accident arises far more dramatically above the legal limit in a young, inexperienced drinker than in their maturer counterparts.

One objective measure of alcohol intoxication has improved upon the traditional test of having someone to try and walk in a straight line. An instrument has been developed for measuring 'body sway' which has already found research applications (Topham, 1983).

In many research contexts it is possible to rely on subjects' self-reported levels of intoxication. Simple rating scales having been used and validated

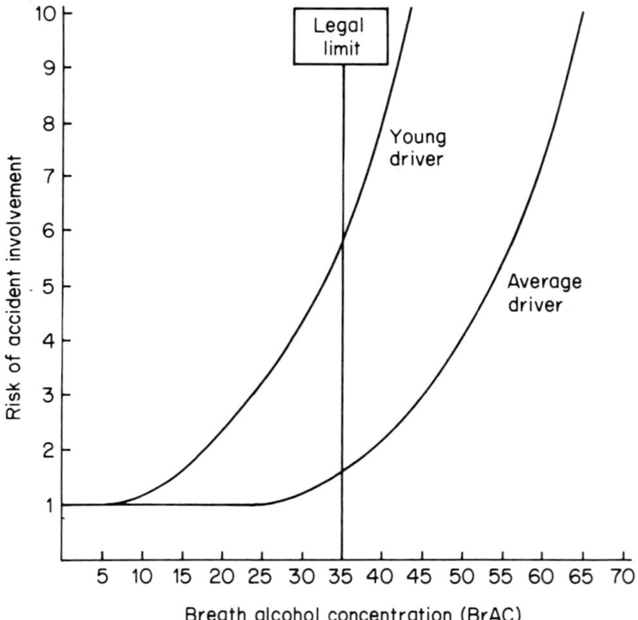

Fig. 2. Accident risk and breath alcohol concentration. The graph has been adapted from TRRL Leaflet No. LF762 (Jan. 1979)

such as 'I have a pleasant glow from alcohol' rated on 5 points from 'not at all' to 'a great deal' (Stockwell *et al.*, 1982). Clearly self-report scales of intoxication are not appropriate for studies of higher levels of intoxication—observer ratings will be needed here. Stockwell *et al.* (1984) found that observer's ratings of facial flushing following alcohol consumption were very reliable.

Over the last decade there has been a large body of work looking at the relationship between benzodiazepines and impairment of psychomotor function (e.g. Hindmarch, 1980; Lader, 1983; Aranko *et al.*, 1985; Lader, 1987). Workers such as Hindmarch have used a large number of tests of psychomotor performance including simulated driving tests, reaction times, verbal recall, auditory reaction times, card sorting and critical flicker fusion and many other tests (see Hindmarch, 1980); and more recently Lader and his associates have used the Bexley–Maudsley automated psychological screening (Acker and Acker, 1982), which provides a computerized system of administering the Little Men test, an adapted Wisconsin card-sorting test and spatial recognition test (Lader, 1987).

Measures of the acute effects of other drugs have not been investigated to the same extent. In recent reviews of the subject of impairment of driving competence due to drugs other than alcohol (Simpson *et al.*, 1984; Simpson, 1987) attention has been drawn to the possible widespread impairment due to cannabis, which was found in the blood of 85% of road traffic victims (Simpson, 1986). For a review of work examining the possible influence of illicit and prescribed opiates on road traffic accidents see Chesher (1985). Use of cannabis by special groups such as airline pilots has been the subject of concern and study (Blaine *et al.*, 1976; Janowsky *et al.*, 1976). These studies have involved use of a flight simulator with measurement of accuracy of response to various situations after smoking active drug or placebo. More recently, Yesavage *et al.* (1985) have described significant impairment in several measures on a flight simulator 24 hours after smoking a cannabis cigarette, despite the subject's reporting no awareness of impaired performance.

ASSESSMENT OF WITHDRAWAL

Assessing withdrawal severity is vital for the safe and effective management of drug withdrawal (or detoxification) and for research into methods of achieving this. Detoxification is best regarded as a two-stage procedure (Strang, 1987). The first stage involves establishing the minimum daily dose necessary to reduce withdrawal symptoms to a manageable level; and the second then involves steady reduction of this individual 100% starting dose. The first stage needs measurement of withdrawal distress—yet the measurement of this state is often not systematic, leading to possible errors of under-

or over-prescribing. The former may lead to grand mal convulsions and delirium tremens in alcohol, barbiturates or chlormethiazole withdrawal—each carrying a small but significant risk of fatality (Orford and Warman, 1986).

Severity of withdrawal reactions on drug cessation can be predicted by a number of factors. Obviously quantity and frequency of recent intake are most important; for example, Gross *et al.* (1975) have demonstrated how continuous and very high blood alcohol levels are needed for delirium tements to be part of the withdrawal response. With some of the drugs of dependence with shorter half-lives (e.g. heroin and alcohol) it is usually possible to assess likely withdrawal severity by enquiring about early morning withdrawal symptoms (or those upon waking after longest period of sleep) when drug levels are at their lowest. Thus assessments of degree of drug dependence (see later) will assist in predicting withdrawal severity. It should be noted that drugs with longer half-lives (e.g. methadone, diazepam) will normally produce more protracted withdrawal reactions, which are slower to develop and hence not usually apparent during periods of active usage. Also very heavy alcohol or drug binges may maintain drug levels high enough throughout a 24-hour period to mask any compensatory adaptive responses. Nevertheless, very high drug tolerance is also a good clue to subsequent withdrawal severity.

One complicating factor is the extent to which withdrawal symptoms occur due to such psychological processes as conditioning. Important recent work by Siegel and colleagues has demonstrated how anticipatory compensatory responses to an expected drug challenge may avert a fatal drug overdose (Siegel, 1987). A common clinical manifestation of the power of such conditioning processes is the exaggeration of withdrawal distress in a drug user who learns their supply has suddenly run out.

Despite the increasing trend towards multiple-substance abuse the only well-researched measures of withdrawal severity are intended to be substance-specific.

Kolb and Himmselsbach (1938) described a quantitative method for monitoring opiate withdrawal. This consists of judging the presence or absence of yawning, lacrimation, rhinorrhoea, perspiration (1 point for each); anorexia, goose-flesh, dilated pupils, tremor (3 points each); restlessness and emesis (5 points each). In addition, 1 point was added to the total for the following signs: fever, each 0.1°C rise; hyperpnoea, each respiration per minute increase; systolic blood pressure, each 2 mmHg rise up to 30 mm; weight, each pound loss. An advantage of this method is its objective nature, although judgement of the presence or absence of the signs mentioned above is subject to considerable variation. Moreover, for measuring the latter exact signs one needs a stable baseline, which may not always be available.

The Opiate Withdrawal Scale (OWS; Bradley *et al.*, 1987) was developed initially to evaluate electrostimulation (Gossop *et al.*, 1984) as a treatment for withdrawal. Since then it has been used to chart the course of withdrawal symptoms during a methadone detoxification schedule (Gossop *et al.*, 1987a), in a comparison of 10- and 21-day methadone detoxification (Gossop *et al.*, 1989), and it has enabled the investigation of psychological factors which are related to the intensity of withdrawal distress (Phillips *et al.*, 1986). The scale consists of 32 withdrawal symptoms and each symptom is rated on a four-point scale. A total score is obtained by adding up the item scores. The result can be adequately represented by a single factor of severity. It shows criterion validity in that during the opiate withdrawal phase the scores are significantly elevated and return to normal in the weeks following cessation of opiate use. Good discriminative efficiency is apparent in that the scale differentiates between addicts during the withdrawal phase and post withdrawal; in addition, the scores obtained by addicts in withdrawal differ significantly from those obtained in a non-addict sample. There is good agreement with nurses' observations of withdrawal at high levels of distress, but at low to moderate levels of symptoms there is poor agreement. This poor agreement does not seem to be due to a deficiency of the OWS; instead it appears to reflect insensitivity of the observer ratings at low levels of distress.

A matching pair of rating scales for measuring signs and symptoms of opiate withdrawal have been described by Handelsman *et al.* (1987). The Subjective Opiate Withdrawal Scale (SOWS) contains 16 symptoms, which the patient rates on a five-point scale. The Objective Opiate Withdrawal Scale (OOWS) contains 13 physically observable signs, which the observer rates as present or absent based on observations over a fixed time period. Handelsman *et al.* have recently reported on the good inter-rater reliability of the OOWS and good intra-subject reliability over time for both scales in both controls and in addicts, and they have reported on the validity and reliability of these scales as indicators of the severity of the opiate withdrawal syndrome.

The Addiction Research Centre Inventory (ARCI) developed withdrawal scales from a set of 550 items. These were subsequently subdivided into strong opiate withdrawal scales and weak opiate withdrawal scales (Haertzen, 1965; Haertzen and Meketon, 1968; Haertzen *et al.*, 1970).

Murphy *et al.* (1983) have described a shortened, modified version of an alcohol withdrawal assessment scale originally developed by Gross *et al.* (1973). The new scale is called the Selected Symptom Check-list and should be completed by experienced medical or nursing staff. On the basis of clinical interview and observation, ratings are made by the clinician of orientation, level of consciousness, agitation, sweating, tremor, gastrointestinal appetite and sleep disturbance. The presence or absence of hallucinations and convulsions are also noted and patients rate their desire for a drink. Individual items and/or the total scores can be used to chart changes in symptom severity throughout the withdrawal period and can produce data of research quality.

ASSESSMENT OF CURRENT DRUG USE

Use of a drug will have different meanings to different individuals, and to the same individual at different points in time. This drug use may be experimental, recreational or compulsive. Experimental drug use refers to the initial use of the substance, is prompted by curiosity and is likely to be a peer-group activity. It is a time-limited behaviour and once the curiosity has been satisfied the individual will either refrain from further use or will make a decision on the basis of knowledge and experience to use the drug in order to obtain an identifiable positive effect. This recreational use may be intermittent or regular. From a group of recreational users, some will come to use the drug as a way of reducing a negative effect—reducing physical or emotional discomfort which may have an origin outside the use of the drug or may be related to the drug use itself. Ongoing use of the drug becomes increasingly important and the individual perceives less choice. This loss of control appears to be a key element of dependence (Russell, 1976). These three terms should not be regarded as measures of the dangerousness of the drug use. Indeed, it may be that the initial experimental period of drug use may be particularly dangerous due to the probable low level of knowledge and experience of the individual drug-taker and his peer group.

Current drug use may be evidenced by signs of intoxication. Alternatively, signs and symptoms of drug withdrawal may be evident if dependence on the drug has developed; and these symptoms may be physical if the drug is from a group which is associated with potential for development of physical dependence—mainly sedative drugs such as alcohol, barbiturates, benzodiazepines and opiates. In addition there may be stigmata of current or past drug use. This evidence may be available from physical examination (e.g. hepatomegaly, venepuncture marks, dilated or pinpoint pupils) or by psychometric testing or following laboratory or other special investigation.

Routine Clinical Enquiries and Case Record Searches

Studies which depend on data drawn from search or examination of clinical case-notes are hampered by widespread failure to record the appropriate information. Barrison *et al.* (1980) found that alcohol consumption was not recorded for 39% of patients seen by junior hospital doctors; and Farrell and David (1988) found that junior psychiatrists failed to make any comment on alcohol consumption in 21% of their patients, and only recorded quantifiable information in 30% of patients. The illicit nature of some drug use seems to blind the interviewer and results in a failure to enquire about more than the substance of use, with the result that data are lost on the pattern of use—frequency, amount, source and route(s) of use. While brief screening questionnaires such as the CAGE questionnaire (Mayfield *et al.*, 1974) are often used in hospital and primary health care practice (Babor *et al.*, 1986) such instruments are not used for collection of data regarding other drugs.

The identification of HIV infection in injecting drug users has increased awareness of the risks associated with intravenous drug use and the sharing of equipment. Simple questionnaires about injecting and sexual habits of drug users have been used in several studies (e.g. Robertson *et al.*, 1986; Strang *et al.*, 1988; Morrison, 1989) to collect information on the extent of sharing and the 'at-risk' nature of the behaviours.

Laboratory Investigations

There are two widely used laboratory investigations with a degree of sensitivity to recent alcohol use that have been used successfully in major research studies. These are levels of γ-glutamyl transpeptidase (GGT) and mean cell volume (MCV) of red blood cells. Abnormal results are a GGT above 40 international units for women (55 for men) and a MCV of over 95 in women and 98 in men. Of the two tests, raised GGT readings tend to recover more quickly with a few days abstinence from alcohol.

Both these tests are best used in association with self-report measures of alcohol problems and consumption. On their own they will only detect two-thirds of problem drinkers. For example, Lloyd *et al.* (1982) found that only 61% of newly identified cases using a battery of tests had a raised GGT, and only a quarter had a raised MCV. Despite this less than perfect correlation with self-reported alcohol problems, one very good use of these blood tests is to confirm whether or not alcohol consumption has been reduced at post-treatment follow-up in subjects with previously raised tests.

Another ready indicator of an alcohol problem is an elevated blood alcohol level (BAL), especially in excess of 100 mg/100 ml blood and also in a patient showing few behavioural signs of intoxication, i.e. displaying high functional tolerance. The availability of relatively inexpensive and accurate hand-held breathalysers (e.g. the AE from Lion Laboratories, Cardiff) has led to their increasing use in research work. For example, one study of attenders at an Edinburgh casualty department found 32% to have BALs in excess of the legal limit (80% mg per 100 ml) (Holt *et al.*, 1980). Again, BAL readings are very useful additional measures of alcohol use, for example to disconfirm the self-report of the subject who claims total abstinence at follow-up.

Urine and blood samples may be used for laboratory investigation to detect the presence of the drugs themselves (and their metabolites), and to look for changes secondary to the drugs or the pattern of use. Despite evidence of high validity of self-reported drug use (Stimson and Oppenheimer, 1982; Wille, 1983; Gossop *et al.*, 1987b; Barnea *et al.*, 1987), the scarcity of comprehensive laboratory facilities for the testing of urine for drugs of abuse is a major handicap for studies of new clientele to a service, studies of their progress in treatment and rehabilitation, and follow-up studies. This testing may utilize one or more of several different methods. Most laboratories should be able to examine urine specimens using thin-layer chromatography (TLC) to detect the presence of a range of drugs, including opiates, amphetamines and barbiturates. However, confirmation of the particular drug within the group is likely to require experience as well as use of gas–liquid chromatography (GLC) and/or high-pressure liquid chromatography (HPLC), which are more expensive and require considerable skill and time.

Recently immunoassay techniques (such as the EMIT system) have been introduced, which are simple to use although expensive in reagent costs if many tests are required per specimen. Such immunoassay techniques should be backed up by confirmation from a laboratory with TLC, GLC and/or HPLC. The limitation of immunoassays is that they will fail to detect some drugs (such as the synthetic opiates dipipanone (Diconal), dextromoramide (Palfium) and buprenorphine (Temgesic) and will indicate use of an opiate such as heroin or morphine when only codeine has been taken. However, they have a valuable role in identifying some difficult-to-identify substances such as cocaine and cannabis. (For a summary of these approaches, see *Lancet* editorial, 1987.)

Urine provides a result from a larger window of time than blood, which would yield a snapshot result of that particular point in time. Drug testing of hair samples is being developed (Baumgartner *et al.*, 1979; Valente *et al.*, 1981) which could provide a valuable long-term result with approximate dating of positive findings according to their distance from the hair root. Despite the obvious limitation that urine results are largely qualitative, the non-invasive ease with which this body fluid is obtained is a distinct advantage, especially as venepuncture in an injecting drug addict with collapsed veins is often well-nigh impossible. (Use of the femoral vein for venepuncture should not be used except in emergencies, as many injecting drug addicts who use this vein originally learnt the technique from doctors.)

LSD cannot yet be identified for clinical or research purposes, although identification in forensic analysis is now possible. Interpretation of cannabis-positive results is difficult in view of the long period of excretion of this drug (up to several weeks after taking of the drug).

Use of such laboratory investigation requires a clear understanding of the significance of both positive and negative results—both of which may have implications for the management of ongoing treatment. A positive for methadone may result in termination of treatment from a drug-free rehabilitation hostel, while a negative for methadone may suggest irregular use or the selling of supplies and thus result in termination of treatment in a methadone maintenance or methadone detoxification programme.

Claims by the drug-taker that he cannot pass a urine specimen when requested should be regarded with suspicion. The drug-taker should be encouraged to drink plenty and remain until they have provided the specimen, as the offer of a specimen tomorrow may miss yesterday's drug use (or non-use). A degree of supervision of the passing of the urine specimen is commonly employed in drug clinics; alternatively the temperature of the returned urine specimen can be checked to ensure that it is at body temperature.

ASSESSING DEPENDENCE

The notion of alcohol and drug dependence has become increasingly important to the understanding and classification of drug problems (Edwards *et al.*, 1982). Important features of the concept of drug dependence include its existing on a continuum of severity, its independence from drug-related harm and drug consumption, and the twin role of learning and compensatory adaptive processes in its development (Hodgson and Stockwell, 1985).

Corresponding to the widespread interest in these concepts, numerous assessment devices have been developed, especially in the development of measures of alcohol dependence. For example, Chick has described a 30-minute interview with the Edinburgh Alcohol Dependence Scale (Chick, 1980a). Skinner and Horn (1984) has produced a manual for the use of a questionnaire called the Alcohol Dependence Scale, while Raistrick *et al.* (1983) have also developed a 15-item questionnaire specifically designed to assess severity of alcohol dependence.

The Severity of Alcohol Dependence Questionnaire (SADQ) is the earliest such scale and, to date, the most widely tested (Stockwell *et al.*, 1979, 1983). The SADQ is a 20-item self-completion questionnaire and concentrates on a 'recent month of heavy drinking'. Such aspects of dependence as signs of early morning withdrawal symptoms (psychological and physical), early morning relief drinking and rapidity of reinstatement of these after abstinence are assessed. While the SADQ has been criticized for failing to attempt to measure subtler aspects of the proposed 'alcohol dependence syndrome' (Orford, 1987), in fact other attempts to assess 'impaired control' of alcohol consumption by self-report have universally foundered (e.g. Chick, 1980a). The SADQ has been shown to have very high test–retest reliability and concurrent and predictive validity (Edwards, 1986). Specifically, a 2-week test–retest reliability coefficient was found to be 0.85 ($p<0.001$). Concurrent validity was demonstrated by the findings of a biserial correlation coefficient of 0.84 between SADQ and the clinical ratings of an experienced psychiatrist (Griffith Edwards, one of the originators of the concept of alcohol dependence). SADQ scores have also correlated with physicians' ratings of withdrawal severity and the quantity of medication prescribed (Stockwell *et al.*, 1979, 1983). Factor analytical studies have repeatedly demonstrated a single major factor in different clinical populations: 53% in one British study (Stockwell *et al.*, 1979) and 45% in an Irish sample (Meehan *et al.*, 1985).

The two major weaknesses of the SADQ are that it does not tap joint alcohol and other drug dependence, and that it only focuses on one rather recent period of drinking (Stockwell, 1986). Failure to assess for complementary substance abuse can also be attributed to the other measures of alcohol dependence, and also to measures designed specifically for opiate dependence.

Davison (1986) has written a very useful review of this and other alcohol dependence measures, including the Alcohol Dependence Scale or ADS (Skinner and Allen, 1983). This is an empirically derived scale, rather than devised on theoretical grounds, and comprises four factors of the larger 147-item Alcohol Use Inventory (Horn *et al.*, 1974): Obsessive-compulsive drinking, Loss of behavioural control, Psychoperceptual withdrawal symptoms and Psychophysical withdrawal symptoms. Skinner and Horn (1984) have produced a detailed manual describing the background to the 25-item ADS. While factor analysis of this scale reveals one major factor, this accounts for a far smaller proportion of the total variance than does the main factor of the SADQ. This is likely to be due to including items whose correlations with total score are as low as 0.35. Nonetheless, very high internal consistency reliability (alpha) coefficients have been calculated—including 0.92 and 0.94. A test–retest coefficient of 0.92 is also reported.

High ADS scorers are less likely to believe they can 'cut down to a few drinks a day' and are likely to be particularly heavy drinkers. In one study, two-thirds of low ADS scorers (mean 14.1 on earlier 29-item ADS) will reject a treatment goal of total abstinence (Sanchez-Craig, 1980).

Instruments for 'Alcoholism' Screening

The most widely used questionnaires of all in this field must surely be the CAGE (Mayfield *et al.*, 1974) and the Michigan Alcoholism Screening Test or MAST (Selzer, 1971). While both permit a range of scores, they are both based on earlier conceptions of 'alcoholism' rather than alcohol dependence. They both confuse dependence signs with alcohol-related disabilities and suggest cut-off points indicative of 'alcoholism' as a unitary condition.

The CAGE is thought to be particularly useful as a quick screening approach as it comprises only four non-threatening questions about drinking:

C—have you ever felt the need to *cut* down on your drinking?
A—have other people *annoyed* you by criticizing your drinking?

G—have you ever felt bad or *guilty* about your drinking?
E—have you ever had a drink (an 'eye-opener') first thing in the morning?

A positive score of two or more questions is deemed indicative of 'alcoholism'.

Although these questions fairly reliably distinguish groups who have been diagnosed 'alcoholic' from other clinical samples, they do also produce a number of false positives and individuals who no longer have an alcohol problem. Nonetheless its brevity and ease of use has meant it has been widely used in research studies, particularly for general hospital samples (Chick, 1987).

The MAST focuses more on alcohol-related disabilities and comes in ten-item (Selzer *et al.*, 1975) and 25-item versions. Many of its items enquire whether the respondent has *ever* had previous treatment episodes as a consequence of their drinking, for example AA, psychiatric hospital. As with the CAGE the time-frame of the questions is the individual's complete personal history—most questions are phrased 'have you ever?' In a recent study of individuals prosecuted for drunk-driving, the MAST successfully identified 86% of individuals considered by alcohol counsellors to have a significant problems, while the CAGE identified only 60%. The same study reported split-half reliability coefficients of 0.84 for the MAST and 0.71 for the CAGE (Mischke and Venneri, 1987).

The Severity of Opiate Dependence Questionnaire (SODQ) aims to measure *dependence* separately from problems arising from drug-taking. It consists of five main sections which assess:

1. Quantity and pattern of opiate use.
2. Physical symptoms of withdrawal.
3. Affective symptoms of withdrawal, including craving.
4. Withdrawal-relief drug-taking.
5. Speed of reinstatement of withdrawal symptoms after a period of abstinence.

The structure of the questionnaire was adequately represented by a single factor in a sample of US addicts; each section correlated very highly with the factor score (Sutherland *et al.*, 1986). This factor score correlated significantly with frequency of opiate use and with a subjective measure of dependence but not with quantity of drug use, nor did it relate to milestones in the user's drug career. In contrast, with a British sample two factors emerged: one measures withdrawal symptoms, while the other measures drug-taking to relieve withdrawal (Phillips *et al.*, 1987). In this sample the total SODQ score correlated with the frequency of opate use but not with any other index of severity. Further work is necessary to establish the validity and usefulness of this scale.

Fear of detoxification itself has been examined by Milby *et al.* (1987). In their Detoxification Fear Survey Schedule (DFSS) they purport to measure the negative emotional reactions to detoxification; and report that a pathological fear of detoxification exists in subgroups of the addict population and contributes to the poor success rate of many detoxification programmes.

Clinical. Drug treatment clinics have developed procedures for assessing the drug/dose requirements of addicts requesting drug treatment. Day attendance (Aylett, 1982; Ghodse *et al.*, 1987a) and brief in-patient admissions (Strang and Clark, in preparation) have been used in modifications of Jaffe's description of simple methadone dose assessment for US heroin addicts (Jaffe, 1980). This approach is best used in conjunction with systematic recording of subjective and objective evidence of drug effect as described elsewhere in this chapter (see 'Assessment of Withdrawal'). Such dose assessment should be preceded by observation of signs of drug withdrawal. The injectable opiate antagonist naloxone (Narcan) may sometimes be used to precipitate a full-blown opiate withdrawal syndrome, so as to confirm that physical dependence has been established. Naloxone eye-drops have been found to cause mydriasis in a high proportion of patients on methadone maintenance (Ghodse *et al.*, 1986), although concern has been expressed (Sanchez-Ramos and Senay, 1987) that there may be systemic absorption with a consequent general withdrawal syndrome.

ASSESSMENT FOR TREATMENT

There would be clear benefit from a procedure which identified suitability for a particular treatment or predicted compliance and outcome. However, Gossop found no evidence of predictive accuracy in a study of multidisciplinary screening of referrals to a treatment programme (Gossop and Connell, 1983); and little difference was found in the course of treatment for a cohort of drug addicts accepted with no selection procedure from those who went through a detailed assessment procedure (Strang and Connell, 1982). Motivation is not an all-or-nothing phenomenon, and it is probable that the interviewer/assessor is not merely observer but has an active influence on the extent of motivation to change (Miller, 1983). Factors such as the appearance and drug-using background of the interviewer have a marked impact on the information provided by a drug user (Davies and Baker., 1987).

Similarly, previous treatment contact may influence repeat presentation for help. In two studies (Eiser and Gossop, 1979; Bradley and Gossop, 1982), a 15-item attitude questionnaire revealed that addicts undergoing treatment tended to understand their own drug-taking in terms of being 'hooked' or 'sick'. New out-patients regarded themselves as being more 'hooked' and 'sick' than regular out-patients or in-patients. It was suggested that the unit's policy (e.g. emphasizing personal responsibility and control over drug-taking) may tend to counteract these attitudes in new patients. A more promising line of enquiry may involve the assessment of the drug-user with regard to suitability for a particular type of treatment.

Relapse prevention is a cognitive–behavioural approach which aims to reduce the risk of relapse to renewed drug use, following abstinence. Two key concepts are *high-risk situations*, and *coping strategies*. High-risk situations are situations or events which carry an increased risk of relapse; for example, being offered a drink, or feeling fed up and bored. Coping strategies are behaviours which the individual employs to cope with high-risk situations; for example, being assertive in refusing a drink, or taking up a hobby to minimize boredom. In the section that follows a number of techniques are mentioned. These are described in greater depth by Marlatt (1985).

Classification of High-risk Situations

Litman *et al.* (1979, 1983a and b) found that the situations surrounding relapse to alcohol abuse could be grouped into three main areas: unpleasant mood states, external events and euphoria, and lessened cognitive vigilance. The first two factors helped predict subsequent outcome. Cummings *et al.* (1980) suggested that relapses across a range of addictive problems could be classified under intrapersonal and interpersonal determinants. The former consisted of negative emotional states, negative physical states, positive emotional states, testing personal control, and urges and temptations. Interpersonal determinants consisted of conflict, social pressure and positive emotional states. This classification system is based on a detailed interview (see Marlatt, 1985).

While Marlatt classified each relapse episode into one relapse category, Bradley *et al.* (1989) reported 11 factors which were described by opiate addicts as having caused a lapse to renewed opiate use. A given lapse episode often contained a number of such factors. These were: cognitive, mood, external, interpersonal, leaving a protected environment, drug availability, drug-related cues, craving, priming and social pressure.

Assessing High-risk Situations

Self-monitoring

Self-monitoring requires the client to keep a record of drug taking, together with other information such as the time, antecedents or the context of drug use, and consequences (see McFall, 1977; Miller and Taylor, 1980). The client should carry this record with them and record the information at the time when the drug-taking, or the desire to do so, occurs. Marlatt (1985) discusses how these records can be used to construct a bar graph which reveals different types of drinking situations, for example being alone at home, in social settings, etc. By identifying a range of high-risk situations in advance the client can anticipate and plan what to do in these situations:

Time and date	Place and context	Antecedents: how were you feeling?	Behaviour: did you use/how much?	Consequences: what happened?

Self-monitoring may change the behaviour which is being monitored. In the case of drug or alcohol consumption it may result in a reduction in use. While this is a problem for a pure assessment measure, it is a bonus for treatment programmes. A further advantage of conducting such monitoring is that cooperation with it can provide an index of compliance with the treatment plan.

Direct Observation of Drug-taking

With alcohol abuse, some investigators have observed drinking behaviour in the natural setting such as home, bars or restaurants, and others have constructed settings to resemble naturalistic ones, such as research bars, with hidden video cameras for unobstrusive observation. In such settings there is the possibility of obtaining a more valid picture of the pattern of drug-taking. However, this method of assessment can also be reactive. While the setting may be natural, or may resemble the natural environment, the presence of the observer, or the subject's knowledge that he is being observed, can influence the behaviour which is being assessed, often resulting in an inhibition of drinking. Moreover, it can be expensive or time-consuming for the researcher or clinician to accompany the client to such a setting. Direct observation is not usually a viable option for illegal drug-taking.

Subjective Judgement of Risk

High-risk situations are described by subjects or supplied by the interviewer, and subjects judge how difficult it would be to experience the situation without drug-taking.

History of Past Relapse Situations

Subjects are asked what were the antecedents and concomitants of lapses in the past. What events/moods/places/people appeared influential in provoking the individual to use drugs again?

In an in-patient setting where there is little access to the normal environment, one may have to rely on the latter two methods of assessment, although self-monitoring of craving can also be used. As the client begins the 're-entry' phase, it is often helpful to assess in advance what high-risk situations are likely to occur. The assessment of such situations must allow for the fact that they can range from discrete stimuli, such as seeing someone 'stoned', to broader categories, such as living in an area where many friends and acquaintances are drug users.

Assessment of Coping Strategies

The aim here is to find out what response the individual employs when in a high-risk situation, and to assess its effectiveness in reducing the risk of drug use. The same basic techniques as used to assess high-risk situations may be employed, i.e. self-monitoring, direct observation, subjective judgements, history of past coping responses. It can be helpful to enlist the support of friends and relatives in providing information.

An example of a structured subjective judgement method is the Situational Competency Test (SCT; Chaney *et al.*, 1978). A high-risk situation is described orally and the subject says what he would do in that situation. The original version of the SCT presented 16 different situations from four categories of high-risk situations; frustration and anger, interpersonal temptation, negative emotional states and intrapersonal temptation. Chaney and colleagues measured four indices: response latency, duration of response, compliance and specification of new behaviour. Clients can also be asked how well they believe they will cope with the situation, a measure of self-efficacy in the situation. A questionnaire version of the test may be given, where subjects read descriptions of high-risk situations and describe in writing how they would respond. A multiple-choice format may also be used for subjects' responses. Of course such written tests cannot be used with poor literacy. Therefore, such clients should be screened out, before using a test relying on reading and writing ability.

Litman and her colleagues have devised the Coping Behaviours Inventory (CBI) and the Effectiveness of Coping Behaviours Inventory (ECBI) for more systematic study of alcoholics (Litman *et al.*, 1983a, 1984). They found that a similar factor structure was evident with both inventories, with four factors accounting for 59% of the variance: 'positive thinking', 'negative thinking', 'avoidance/distraction' and 'seeking social supports'. The intake factor scores for 'positive thinking' and 'avoidance/distraction' on the ECBI (but not the CBI) discriminated between subsequent relapsers and survivors when examined 6–12 months later. In a related study, Litman *et al.* (1983b) found that the total score on their 25-item Relapse Precipitants Inventory

(RPI) and the factor scores on 'Unpleasant mood states' and 'External events and euphoria' significantly discriminated between relapsers and survivors.

Another very useful instrument for assessing an individual's own perceived ability to cope in high-risk situation—or their degree of 'self-efficacy'—is the Situational Confidence Questionnaire (Annis, 1986). This 100-item self-completion questionnaire provides clients' ratings for how well they believe they can cope with situations in one of two categories: 'Personal' and 'Interpersonal'. The former includes emotional states and temptations while the latter covers the areas of social situations and relationships.

Role-playing can be a very powerful way of assessing clients' coping responses. When the technique has been explained to the patient and his permission obtained, the therapist, or a fellow drug abuser, will recreate a high-risk situation, for example offering the patient a drink. The patient's responses are noted or recorded on video- or audiotape. Discussion and re-examination of the response can enable the strengths and weaknesses of different coping strategies to be evaluated. This technique has the advantage that actual behaviour is elicited, rather than statements about intended behaviour, and there is the possibility of obtaining a more valid picture of the behaviour that would occur in a real situation. However, some role plays may appear artificial to the patient, and sometimes the context within which the role play takes place (e.g. in a hospital) may greatly influence the response, so that ecological validity can be questionable. Such issues should be discussed in order that discrepancies between responses in the role play and in real life can be determined.

Assessment of Coping Resources

Coping resources are existing factors such as environment, occupation, social network, leisure activities or beliefs which increase the individual's capacity to cope, for example family support, living in a half-way house, commitment to a healthy lifestyle. At this stage, such resources are most commonly assessed by semi-structured interview.

Psychophysiological and Subjective Assessment of Craving

A number of investigators (e.g. O'Brien *et al.*, 1974) have investigated craving by exposing drug abusers to drug-related cues, such as slides or videotapes of drug-taking, or objects commonly used in drug-taking, such as syringes and needles. Many drug abusers show increased desire to use drugs, accompanied by psychophysiological changes. Recent UK papers have described highly individualized case studies looking at extinction with cue exposure and response prevention (Bradley and Moorey, 1988) and changes in cue vulnerability following exposure (Fuller and Strang, submitted for publication) as well as describing the psychophysiological approach adopted (Legarda *et al.*, in press). These investigations are individually designed for specific research purposes and, as yet, there is no standardized or routine form for this assessment.

Assessment of self-reported craving on a simple numerical scale, ranging from 0 (none) to 10 (the maximum you have ever felt), is acceptable to most patients. A variety of such scales are used, often with 8, 10 or 100 as the maximum. These scales are widely used in behavioural work on anxiety and have been found to be useful in determining hierarchies of anxiety-provoking situations and in ensuring that the pace of exposure treatment and the duration of sessions are tailored to the individual patient's needs. Likewise, such scales are used, for similar purposes, in experimental applications of exposure treatment to drug abuse (Childress *et al.*, 1984). In conducting exposure, it can be helpful to select the initial exposure stimulus so that the patient initially experiences a moderate level of craving, say 4–7 on a 0–10 scale. If too high a level is produced initially, the patient may be distressed or may not be able to resist using the drug; on the other hand, if the initial level is too low, many more exposure sessions will probably be necessary in order to deal with the range of relevant stimuli. As in the use of exposure with anxiety, it appears helpful to end an exposure session when the craving level has reduced to a low level (0–3). Ending the session when craving is high can lead to the patient's viewing the session as a failure, and may not be optimal in allowing extinction of craving to take place.

Meyer and Mirin (1979) used a visual analogue scale, one end representing no craving while the other represented maximum craving. Subjects make a mark on the line to represent the degree of craving experienced. This proved satisfactory in their investigations.

Psychophysiological assessment is complex, requiring the use of satisfactory transducers or electrodes, good-quality amplifiers and a permanent recording device, such as polygraph or computer disk. It is not appropriate to discuss the complexity of these measures here; instead, the interested reader may refer to Martin and Venables (1980). The most common indices used in investigations of drug and alcohol abuse are heart rate, skin conductance, skin temperature, respiration rate and muscle activity. Individual measures are often selected because they are affected by the drug or by withdrawal from the drug. Fuller and Strang (submitted for publication) have reported on the poor sensitivity and specificity of the base level itself in measurements of galvanic skin response (GSR). Instead, they found greater value in study of the number of spike responses and skin conductance response amplitude. Use of a GSR machine with automated back-off and shifting baseline was necessary so as to permit extraction of these data.

ASSESSMENT OF SUCCESS

'But what is the success rate?' How often this question is asked of drug treatment programmes, and how lacking in detail the enquirer becomes when asked 'What do you mean by success?' Even something as straightforwardly medical as the prescribing of methadone to heroin addicts is not straightforward after all. In a low-threshold methadone outreach programme, one important measure of success may be the percentage capture rate of the population of heroin users in the community—the degree of penetration of the potential market. Once contact has been established with a heroin addict, then another measure of the success of a methadone-prescribing programme may be the retention rate in treatment. Even if the heroin addict has been contacted and engaged in treatment, the enquirer may wish to look at the extent of on-going use of other drugs or of continued high-risk behaviour in this methadone-prescribed group. Finally, the throughput of the treatment programme may be examined—the proportion who have been through the methadone-prescribing stage and on to a drug-free state. Each of these are valid treatment goals for different components of an overall service; but study of the effectiveness of a particular component must be preceded by an identification of the actual treatment goals and the relevant measures of outcome. Several recent studies (Gossop *et al.*, 1987b; Strang *et al.*, 1987; Ghodse *et al.*, 1987b) have demonstrated the reduction that may occur in the 'at-risk' nature of on-going drug use for drug users who in simple terms would be regarded as treatment failures.

Few studies in the drug and alcohol field have included an untreated control group, and so special care must be taken in attributing an observed change to the studied intervention. The introduction of measurements will itself have an impact on the behaviour being studied, in addition to which measurement of treatment outcome must take note of the probable natural untreated outcome.

Perhaps the measure should be the proportion who become totally drug- and alcohol-free; perhaps free of all drugs except alcohol and/or cannabis; perhaps free of all illicit drugs; perhaps free of the identified problem drug(s); perhaps no longer using regularly or in a dependent manner; perhaps no longer using a high-risk route or continuing with other high-risk behaviours. Each of these may be an appropriate goal of different types of intervention, and may be the subject of enquiry of different studies. In attempting to achieve the called-for partnership between research and clinical initiatives (Edwards and Busch, 1981), the researcher may find that the clinical service or drug-using population under study may hold several different treatment goals concurrently. However, without preliminary clarification of the goals and of the purpose of the enquiry, the eventual conclusion is likely to become bogged down with resulting apologies and disclaimers.

REFERENCES

Acker, W. and Acker, C. (1982). *Bexley-Maudsley Automated Psychological Screening*. NFER—Nelson, Windsor.

Anderson, P. (1987). Early intervention in general practice. In *Helping the Problem Drinker: New Initiatives in Community Care* (T. Stockwell and S. Clement, eds), Croom Helm, London.

Annis, H. M. (1986). A relapse prevention model for treatment of alcoholics. In *Treatment Addictive Behaviours: Processes of Change*, W. E. Miller and N. Heather, eds), Plenum Press, New York, pp. 407–434.

Aranko, K., Mattila, M. J. and Bordignon, D. (1985). Psychomotor effects of alprazolam and diazepine during acute and sub-acute treatment, and during the follow-up phase. *Acta Pharmacol. Toxicol.* **56**, 364–372.

Aylett, P. (1982). Methadone dose assessment in heroin addiction. *Int. J. of Addict.* **17**, 1329–1336.

Babor, T. F., Ritson, E. B. and Hodgson, R. J. (1986). Alcohol related problems in the primary health care setting: a review of early intervention strategies. *Br. J. Addict.* **81**, 23–46.

Barnea, Z., Rahav, G. and Teichman, M. (1987). The reliability and consistency of self reports on substance use in a longitudinal study. *Br. J. Addict.* **82**, 891–898.

Barrison, I. G., Viola, L. and Murray-Lyon, I. M. (1980). Do housemen take an adequate drinking history? *Br. Med. J.* **281**, 1040.

Baumgartner, A. M., Jones, P. F., Baumgartner, A. W. and Black, T. C. (1979). Radioimmunoassay of hair for determining opiate abuse histories. *J. Nucl. Med.* **20**, 748.

Blaine, J. D., Meacham, M. P., Janowsky, D. S., *et al.* (1976). Marijuana smoking and simulated flying performance. In Braude, M. C. and Szara, S. (eds) *Pharmacology of Marijuana* (M. C. Braude and S. Szara, eds), Raven Press, New York.

Bradley, B. and Gossop, M. (1982). Differences in attitudes towards drug taking among drug addicts: implications for treatment. *Drug Alcohol Depend.* **10**, 361–366.

Bradley, B. P. and Moorey, S. (1988). Extinction of craving during exposure to drug-related cues: three single case reports. *Behav. Psychother.* **16**, 45–56.

Bradley, B., Gossop, M., Phillips, G. and Legarda, J. (1987). The development of an opiate withdrawal scale (OWS). *Br. J. Addict.* **82**, 1139–1142.

Bradley, B.P., Phillips, G., Green, L. and Gossop, M. (1989), Circumstances surrounding the initial lapse to opiate use following detoxfication, *Br. J. Psychiatry* **154**, 354–9.

Busto, V., Simpkins, J., Sellers, E. M., Sisson, B. and Segal, R. (1983). Objective determination of Benzodiazepine use and abuse in alcoholics. *Br. J. Addict.* **74**, 415–428.

Chaney, E., O'Leary, M. and Marlatt, G. A. (1978). Skill training with alcoholics. *J. Consult. Clin. Psychol.* **46**, 1092–1104.

Chesher, G. B. (1985). The influence of analgesic drugs in road crashes. *Accid. Anal. Prevent.* **17**, 303–309.

Chick, J. (1980a). Alcohol dependence: methodological issues in its measurement; reliability of the criteria. *Br. J. Addict.* **75**, 175–186.

Chick, J. (1980b). Is there a unidimensional alcohol dependence syndrome? *Br. J. Addict.* **75**, 265–280.

Chick, J. (1987). Early intervention in the general hospital. In Stockwell, T. and Clement S. (eds) *Helping the Problem Drinker: New Initiatives in Community Care* (T. Stockwell and S. Clement, eds), Croom Helm, London.

Childress, R. McLellan, A. T. and O'Brien, C. P. (1984). Assessment and extinction of conditioned withdrawal-like responses in an integrated treatment for opiate dependence. *NIDA Research Monograph* No. 55. National Institute of Drug Abuse, Washington.

Cummings, C., Gordon, J. R. and Marlatt, G. A. (1980). Relapse: strategies of prevention and prediction. In *The Addictive Behaviours* (W. R. Miller, ed.), Pergamon Press, Oxford.

Davies, J. B. and Baker, R. (1987). The impact of self-presentation and interviewer bias effect on self-reported heroin use. *Br. J. Addict.* **82**, 907–912.

Davison, R. (1986). Assessment of the alcohol dependence syndrome: a review of self-screening questionnaires. *Br. J. Clin. Psychol.* **26**, 243–256.

Department of Health and Social Security (1985) *Drug Misuse: Prevalence and Service Provision*, DHSS, London.

Donmall, M. C., Webster, A. J. K., Strang, J. and Tantam, D. (1988). Compliance by medical practitioners with two systems of reporting of drug addiction: the Home Office Addicts Index compared with an anonymised Regional database (in preparation).

Duffy, J. and Waterton, J. (1984). Under-reporting of alcohol consumption in sample surveys: the effect of computer interviewing in fieldwork. *Br. J. Addict.* **3**, 303–308.

Editorial (1987). Screening for drugs of abuse. *Lancet* **(i)** 365–366.

Edwards, G. (1981). The Home Office Index as a basic monitoring system. In *Drug Problems in Britain: A Review of Ten Years* (G. Edwards and C. Busch, eds), Academic Press, London.

Edwards, G. (1986). The alcohol dependence syndrome: a concept as stimulus to enquiry. *Br. J. Addict.* **81**, 171–183.

Edwards, G. and Busch, C. (eds) (1981). The partnership between research and policy. In *Drug Problems in Britain: A Review of Ten Years*. Academic Press, London.

Edwards, G., Arif, A. and Hodgson, R. (1982). Nomenclature and classification of drug and alcohol related problems: a shortened version of a WHO memorandum. *Br. J. Addict.* **77**, 287–306.

Eiser, J. R. and Gossop, M. R. (1979). 'Hooked' or 'sick': addicts' perceptions of their addition. *Addict. Behav.* **4**, 185–191.

Farrell, M. P. and David, A. S. (1988). Do psychiatric registrars take a proper drinking history? *Br. Med. J.* **296**, 395–6.

Fuller, J. and Strang, J. (1988). Cue exposure as an assessment technique in the management of the heroin addict (submitted for publication).

Ghodse, A. H., Bewley, T. H., Kearney, M. K. and Smith, S. E. (1986). Mydriatic response to topical naloxone in opiate abusers. *Br. J. Psychiatry* **148**, 44–46.

Ghodse, A. H., London, M., Bewley, T. H. and Bhat, A. V. (1987a). In-patient treatment for drug abuse. *Br. J. Psychiatry* **151**, 72–75.

Ghodse, A. H., Tregenza, G. and Li, M. (1987b). Effect of fear of AIDS on sharing of injection equipment among drug abusers. *Br. Med. J.* **295**, 698–699.

Gossop, M. and Connell, P. H. (1983). Drug dependence: who gets treated. *Int. J. Addict.* **18**, 99–109.

Gossop, M., Bradley, B., Strang, J. and Connell, P. H. (1984). The clinical effectiveness of electrostimulation vs oral methadone in managing opiate withdrawal. *Br. J. Psychiatry* **144**, 203–208.

Gossop, M., Bradley, B. and Phillips, G. (1987a). An investigation of withdrawal symptoms shown by opiate addicts during and subsequent to a 21-day inpatient methadone detoxification procedure. *Addict. Behav.* **12**, 1–6.

Gossop, M., Green, L., Phillips, G. and Bradley, B. (1987b). What happens to opiate addicts immediately after treatment: a prospective follow-up study. *Br. Med. J.* **294**, 1377–1380.

Gossop, M., Griffiths, P. and Strang, J. (1988). Chasing the Dragon: characteristics of heroin chasers. *Br. J. Addict.* **83**, 1159–1162.

Gossop, M. Griffiths, P., Bradley, B. and Strang, J. (1989). Opiate withdrawal symptoms in response to 10 day and 21 day methadone withdrawal programmes. *Brit. J. Psychiat* **154**, 360–363.

Gross, M., Lewis, E. and Nagareijan, M. A. (1973). An improved quantitative system for assessing acute alcohol psychoses and related states (TSA and SSA). In *Alcohol Intoxication and Withdrawal Experimental Studies* (M. M. Gross, ed.), Plenum Press, New York.

Gross, M., Kierszenbaum, H., Lewis, E. and Lee, Y. (1975). Desire to drink—relationship to age, blood alcohol concentration and severity of withdrawal syndrome on admission for detoxification. National Council on Alcoholism, Milwaukee, Wisconsin.

Haertzen, C. A. (1965). Addiction Research Centre Inventory (ARCI): development of a general drug assessment scale. *J. Nerv.* **141**, 300–307.

Haertzen, C. A. and Meketon, M. J. (1968). Opiate withdrawal as measured by Addiction Research Centre Inventory. *Dis. Nervous System* **29**, 450–455.

Haertzen, C. A., Meketon, M. J. and Hooks, N. T. (1970). Subjective experiences produced by the withdrawal of opiates. *Br. J. Addict.* **65**, 245–255.

Handelsman, L., Cochrane, K. J., Aronson, M. J., Ness, R., Rubinstein, K. J. and Kanof, P. D. (1987). Two new rating scales for opiate withdrawal. *Am. J. Drug Alcohol Abuse* **13**, 293–308.

Hartnoll, R., Bryer, S., Lewis, R. and Mitchison, M. (1985). Estimating the prevalence of opioid dependence. *Lancet* **i**, 203–205.

Haw, S. (1985). *Drug Problems in Greater Glasgow*, SCODA, London.

Hindmarch, I. (1980). Psychomotor function and psychoactive drugs. *Br. J. Clin. Pharmacol.* **10**, 189–209.

Hodgson, R. and Stockwell, T. (1985). The theoretical and empirical basis of the Alcohol Dependence Construct. In *The Misuse of Alcohol: Current Issues in Dependence, Treatment and Prevention* (N. Heather, ed.), Croom Helm, London.

Holt, S., Stewart, I. C., Dixon, J. M. J., Elton, R. A., Taylor, T. V. and Little, K. (1980). Alcohol and the emergency service patient. *Br. Med. J.* **281**, 638–640.

Horn, J. L., Wanberg, K. and Adams, S. G. (1974). Diagnosis of alcoholism. *Q. J. Studies Alcohol* **35**, 147–175.

Jaffe, J. H. (1980). Drug addiction and drug abuse. In *The Pharmacological Basis of Therapeutics*, 6th edn (A. G. Gilman *et al.*, eds), Macmillan, New York, pp. 535–584.

Janowsky, D. S., Meacham, M. P., Blaine, J. D., Schoor, M. and Bozzetti, L. (1976). Marijuana effects on simulated flying ability. *Am. J. Psychiatry* **133**, 384–388.

Kolb, L. and Himmselsbach, C. K. (1938). Clinical studies of drug addiction III. *Am. J. Psychiatry* **94**, 759–799.

Lader, M. H. (1983). Benzodiazepines, psychological functioning and dementia. In *Benzodiazepines Divided* (M. R. Trimble, ed.), Wiley, Chichester, pp. 309–325.

Lader, M. H. (1987). Long-term benzodiazepine use and psychological functioning. In *The Benzodiazepines in Current Clinical Practice*, (H. Freeman and Y. Rue, eds), Royal Society of Medicine, London, pp. 55–69.

Legarda, J. J., Bradley, B. P. and Sartory, G. (1987). Subjective and psychophysiological effects of drug-related cues in drug users. *J. Psychophysiol.* **1**, 393–400.

Levy, B. (1985). *Prevalence of Abuse of Substances in the Brighton Area Health Authority*, Drug Dependency Clinic, Brighton.

Litman, G. K., Eiser, J. R., Rawson, N. S. B. and Oppenheim, N. A. (1979). Differences in relapse precipitants and coping behaviours between alcohol relapsers and survivors. *Behav. Res. Ther.* **17**, 89–94.

Litman, G. K., Stapleton, J., Oppenheim, A. N. and Peleg, M. (1983a). An instrument for measuring coping behaviours in hospitalised alcoholics: implications for relapse prevention treatment. *Br. J. Addict.* **78**, 269–276.

Litman, G. K., Stapleton, J., Oppenheim, A. N., Peleg, M. and Jackson, P. (1983b). Situations related to alcoholism relapse. *Br. J. Addict.* **78**, 381–389.

Litman, G. K., Stapleton, J., Oppenheim, A. N. and Peleg, M. (1984). The relationship between coping behaviours, their effectiveness and alcoholism relapse and survival. *Br. J. Addict.* **79**, 283–291.

Lloyd, G., Chick, J. and Crombie, E. (1982). Screening for problem drinkers among medical in-patients. *Drug Alcohol Depend.* **10**, 355–359.

Lucas, R. W., Mullin, P. J., Luna, C. B. X. and McInroy, D. C. (1977). Psychiatrists and a computer as interrogators of patients with alcohol-related illnesses: a comparison. *Br. J. Psychiatry* **131**, 160–167.

Marlatt, G. A. (1985). Relapse prevention: theoretical rationale and overview of the model. In *Relapse Prevention* (G. A. Marlatt and J. R. Gordon, eds), Guilford Press, New York.

Martin, I. and Venables, P. H. (1980). *Techniques in Psychophysiology*, Wiley, Chichester.

Mayfield, D., McLeod, G. and Hall, P. (1974). The CAGE questionnaire: validation of a new alcoholism screening instrument. *Am. J. Psychiatry* **131**, 1121–1123.

McFall, R. M. (1977). *Behavioural Training: a Skill-acquisition Approach in Clinical Problems*, General Learning Press, Morristown, New Jersey.

Meehan, J. P., Webb, M. and Unwin, A. (1985). The Severity of Alcohol Dependence Questionnaire (SADQ) in a sample of Irish problem drinkers. *Br. J. Addict.* **80**, 57–64.

Meyer, R. E. and Mirin, S. M. (1979). The *Heroin Stimulus*, Plenum Press, New York.

Milby, J. B., Gurwitch, R. H., Hohmann, A. A. and Wiebe, D. J. (1987). Assessing pathological detoxification fear among methadone maintenance patients: the DFSS. *J. Clin. Psychol.* **43**, 528–538.

Miller, W. R. (1983). Motivational interviewing with problem drinkers. *Behav. Psychother.* **11**, 147–172.

Miller, W. and Taylor, C. (1980). Relative effectiveness of bibliotherapy: individual and group self-control training in the treatment of problem drinkers. *Addict. Behav.* **5**, 13–24.

Mischke, H. D. and Venneri, R. L. (1987). Reliability and validity of the MAST, Mortimer–Fitkins Questionnaire and CAGE in DWI Assessment. *J. Stud. Alcohol* **48**, 492–501.

Morrison, V. (1989). Psychoactive substance use-related behaviours of 135 regular illicit drug users in Scotland. *Drug and Alcohol Dependence* (in press).

Murphy, D. J., Shaw, G. K. and Clarke, I. (1983). Tiapride and chlormethiazole in alcohol withdrawal: a double blind trial. *Alcohol Alcohol.* **18**, 227–237.

O'Brien, C. P., Chaddock, B., Woodey, G. and Greenstein, R. (1974). Systematic extinction of addiction-associated rituals using narcotic antagonists. *Psychosom. Med.* **36**, 458.

Orford, J. (1987). Is controlled drinking possible for the severely dependent drinker? A reply to Horn and Stockwell. *Br. J. Addict* **82** (3), 250–252.

Orford, J. and Warman, T. (1986). Alcohol detoxification services: a review. Paper prepared for the DHSS Addictions and Homelessness Research Liaison Group.

Parker, J., Pool, Y., Rawle, R. and Gay, M. (1988). Monitoring problem drug use in Bristol. *Br. J. Psychiatry* **152**, 212–221.

Phillips, G. T., Gossop, M. and Bradley, B. (1986). The influence of psychological factors on the opiate withdrawal syndrome. *Br. J. Psychiatry* **149**, 235–238.

Phillips, G. T., Gossop, M. R., Edwards, G., Sutherland, G., Taylor, C. and Strang, J. (1987). The application of the SODQ to the measurement of the severity of opiate dependence in a British sample. *Br. J. Addict.* **82**, 691–699.

Plant, M. (1987). *Drugs in Perspective*, Hodder & Stoughton, London.

Raistrick, D., Dunbar, G. and Davidson, R. (1983). Developments of a questionnaire to measure alcohol dependence. *Br. J. Addict.* **78**, 89–96.

Robertson, J. R., Bucknall, A. B. V. and Wiggins, P. (1986). Regional variations in HIV antibody seroposivity in British intravenous drug users. *Lancet* **(i)** 1435.

Russell, M. A. H. (1976). What is dependence? In *Drugs and Drug Dependence* (G. Edwards *et al.*, eds), Saxon House/Lexington Books, London, pp. 182–187.

Sanchez-Craig, M. (1980). Random assignment to abstinence or controlled drinking in a cognitive behaviour programme: short-term effects on drinking behaviour. *Addict. Behav.* **5**, 35–39.

Sanchez-Ramos, J. R. and Senay, E. C. (1987). Ophthalmic Naloxone elicits abstinence in opioid dependent subjects. *Br. J. Addict.* **82**, 313–315.

Selzer, M. L. (1971). The Michigan Alcoholism Screening Test: the quest for a new diagnostic instrument. *Am. J. Psychiatry* **127**, 1653–1658.

Selzer, M. L., Vinokur, A. and van Rooijen, L. (1975). A self-administered Short Michigan Alcoholism Screening Test (SMAST). *J. Stud. Alcohol* **36**, 117–126.

Siegel, S. (1987). Drug anticipation and drug tolerance. In *The Psychopharmacology of Addiction* (M. H. Lader, ed.), British Association for Psychopharmacology Monographs, London.

Simpson, H. M. (1986). Epidemiology of road accidents involving marijuana. *Alcohol, Drugs Driv.* **2**, 15–30.

Simpson, H. M. (1987). Young drivers, alcohol and drug impairment: magnitude, characteristics and significance of the problem. In *Young Drivers Impaired by Alcohol and other Drugs* (T. Benjamin, ed.), Royal Society of Medicine, London, pp. 1–7.

Simpson, H. M., Mayhew, D. R. and Warren, R. A. (1984). Epidemiology of road accidents involving young adults: alcohol, drugs and other factors. *Drug Alcohol Depend.* **10**, 35–63.

Skinner, H. A. and Allen, B. A. (1983). Alcohol dependence scale, measurement and validation. *J. Abnorm. Psychol.* **91**, 199–209.

Skinner, H. and Goldberg, A. (1986). Evidence for a drug dependence syndrome among narcotic users. *Br. J. Addict.* **81**, 479–484.

Skinner, H. and Horn, J. L. (1984). *The Alcohol Dependence Scale (ADS) User's Guide*, Addiction Research Foundation, Toronto.

Stimson, G. V. (1987). British drug policies in the 1980s: a preliminary analysis and suggestions for research. *Br. J. Addict.* **82**, 477–488.

Stimson, G. V. and Oppenheimer, E. (1982). *Heroin Addiction Treatment and Control in Britain*, Tavistock Publications, London.

Stockwell, T. (1986). What I'd still like to know: cracking an old chestnut—is con-

trolled drinking possible for someone who has been severely alcohol dependent? *Br. J. Addict.* **81**, 455–456.
Stockwell, T. R., Hodgson, R. J., Edwards, G., Taylor, C. and Rankin, H. (1979). The development of a questionnaire to measure severity of alcohol dependence. *Br. J. Addict.* **74**, 79–87.
Stockwell, T., Hodgson, R. and Rankin, H. (1982). Alcohol dependence beliefs and the priming effect. *Behav. Res. Ther.* **20**, 513–522.
Stockwell, T., Murphy, D. and Hodgson, R. (1983). The severity of alcohol dependence questionnaire: its use, reliability and validity. *Br. J. Addict.* **78**, 145–155.
Stockwell, T., Sutherland, G. and Edwards, G. (1984). Impact of a new alcohol-sensitizing agent (nitrefazole) on craving in severely dependent alcoholics. *Br. J. Addict.* **79**, 403–409.
Strang, J. (1987). Drug abuse and drug dependence. *Med. Internat.* **2**, 1801–1807.
Strang, J. (1989). A model service: turning the generalist onto drugs. In *Drugs and British Society*, (S. McGregor, ed.), Routledge/Tavistock, London, pp. 143–170.
Strang, J. and Clark, M. (1989). Dose estimation in heroin addicts during three day assessment admissions (in preparation).
Strang, J. and Connell, P. H. (1982). Assessment of an urgent admission procedure to an inpatient drug dependence unit. *Br. J. Addict.* **77**, 311–318.
Strang, J. and Shah, A. (1985). Notification of addicts and the medical practitioner—an evaluation of the system. *Br. J. Psychiatry* **147**, 194–198.
Strang, J., Heathcote, S. and Watson, P. (1987). Habit moderation in injecting drug addicts. *Health Trends* **19**, 16–18.
Strang, J., Johns, A. and Hunt, S. (1988). Syringe exchange schemes. *Br. Med. J.* **297**, 200.
Sutherland, G., Edwards, G., Taylor, C., Phillips, G., Gossop, M. and Brady R. (1986). The measurement of opiate dependence. *Br. J. Addict.* **81**, 485–494.
Topham, A. (1983). Alcohol dependence and craving. Unpublished PhD thesis, Institute of Psychiatry, University of London.
Valente, D., Cassine, M., Pigliabochi, M. and Vansetti, G. (1981). Hair as the sample in assessing morphine and cocaine addiction. *Clin. Chem.* **27**, 1952–1953.
Wallace, P. and Haines, A. (1985). Use of a questionnaire in general practice to increase the recognition of patients with excessive alcohol consumption. *Br. Med. J.* **290**, 1949–1953.
Wille, R. (1983). Britain: ways of coming off heroin. In: *Drug Use and Misuse—Cultural Perspectives* (G. Edwards *et al.*, eds), World Health Organization and Croom Helm, Beckenham, pp. 139–147.
Yesavage, J. A., Leirer, V. O., Denari, M. and Hollister, L. E. (1985). Carry-over effects of marijuana intoxication on aircraft pilot performance: a preliminary report. *Am. J. Psychiatry* **142**, 1325–1329.

The Instruments of Psychiatric Research
Edited by C. Thompson

CHAPTER 10

Personality disorders

Brian Ferguson[1] and Peter Tyrer[2]
[1]*Department of Psychiatry, Mapperley Hospital, Nottingham, UK*

[2]*Department of Psychiatry, St Mary's Hospital, London, UK*

INTRODUCTION

The categorical assessment of personality has been hampered by poor reliability between raters (Walton and Presly, 1973) to the extent that until recently some researchers doubted that standardized assessments could ever be carried out. Over the past few years a considerable number of new instruments have been developed which have been more successful in gaining acceptance by both researchers and clinicians, although many are still in the early stages of testing. This review will focus primarily on standardized procedures which yield categorical diagnoses, mentioning some of their strengths and weaknesses. This should enable the reader to select an instrument for closer scrutiny before incorporating it in a research protocol. It is worthwhile repeating a few principles at the outset which will impinge on the selection process depending on individual requirements of each project.

GENERAL PRINCIPLES OF PERSONALITY ASSESSMENT

In general personality disorder assessments have adopted one of two formats. The first is that of a self-rating questionnaire where the subject answers a series of questions, usually along a forced choice yes or no basis. When used alone a so-called 'lie scale' is incorporated so that any inconsistencies in the replies can be picked up. If well constructed these tests have been shown to have good reliability and have been the basis of most dimensional assessments of personality, for example the Cattell-16 Personality Factor Questionnaire and the Minnesota Multi-phasic Personality Inventory. Their value in categorical diagnosis has not been as well established and standardization has usually been achieved by the use of structured interviews. The earlier structured interviews had poor reliability, but more recent attempts have led to improvement in this area through expansion and better definition of the test items, thereby reducing the level of judgement required by the interviewer. A few procedures combine both approaches (e.g. SCID-II) using positive replies on the subject questionnaire to identify areas for clarification in a subsequent interview. Because of the nature of some of the phenomena in DSM-III-R (American Psychiatric Association, 1987), it is also pertinent to rate some items of observed behaviour during the interview itself.

Although there has been a lot of criticism from the situationists (Mischel, 1968) questioning the permanence of personality attributes, most clinicians would accept that personality disorder reflects long-standing ingrained, maladaptive patterns of behaviour (World Health Organization, 1978). Unfortunately the results of some personality assessments have been shown to be subject to serious distortion by the subject's mental state at the time of the assessment. The common mood changes of anxiety and depression have both been shown to affect personality assessment, so that personality status apparently changes when the symptoms improve (Hirschfeld *et al.*, 1983; Reich *et al.*, 1986). As a result of this factor the evaluation of mental state in terms of an Axis-I diagnosis is now considered to be mandatory in most studies prior to assessing any underlying personality disorder.

The source of information to be analysed is also important. By definition subjects are disordered in a way that might be likely to interfere with an adequate assessment (Tyrer and Ferguson, 1987). An informant who knows the subject well may be more useful in cases where the subjective information required is minimal. Some of the instruments to be described are only available at present in a subject format (PDE, SCID-II, MCMI) and will therefore have their disadvantages in particular settings. Others also have an informant version which may be used either alone (PAS, SAP) or in combination (PAS, SIDP) with the subject version.

As with all investigations of this nature the attitude of the test taker to the test will be very important, even to the extent of invalidating the results if completely ignored. Considerably more research needs to be carried out in this area in respect of categorical diagnosis, particularly as many of the severely disordered subjects reside in institutions which may exert significant overt and more subtle pressures on respondents (Goffman, 1961).

The two major international classifications, ICD-10 and DSM-III-R, have clear differences in their approach despite their common origins. As a result most standardized instruments yield diagnoses of either one or the other classification. Increasingly, however, there has been a tendency to develop question contents in a way that allows diagnosis in both systems, a move which hopefully will help to resolve many of the confused areas where overlap and discrepancy occur. The two international systems involve acceptance of certain basic assumptions on the nature of the individual disorders which may not be universally shared. An alternative empirically based diagnostic system has been developed by Tyrer and Alexander (1979) and will also be described. This has been modified recently so that if necessary diagnoses can be derived for all three classifications (Tyrer *et al.*, 1988).

Too frequently personality researchers embark on studies without being fully aware of the training requirements of the instruments being used. Because of the necessity of distinguishing between present state and more long-term aspects of personality function it is usually recommended that the assessor have adequate clinical experience backed by a training in psychiatry or psychology. Other workers, for example psychiatric social workers and lay interviewers, will require more extensive training and may even then be only able to use some of the more highly structured interviews. Because many of these assessment procedures are still at an early stage the authors frequently recommend training at the centre where they were developed. For others it is possible to get detailed instructions for training, including video- and audiotaped interviews using established raters. In general, because of the fluid state of the art it is wise to contact original sources for the latest advice on training and procedures for establishing satisfactory inter-rater reliability with that particular instrument.

INSTRUMENTS FOR DIAGNOSIS OF PERSONALITY DISORDER ACCORDING TO THE INTERNATIONAL CLASSIFICATION OF DISEASES (ICD)

Standardized Assessment of Personality (SAP)

The SAP was developed by Mann and colleagues from the Institute of Psychiatry (Mann *et al.*, 1981). It is probably the least structured, being specifically designed to match the usual psychiatric interview in a clinical context. An informant is chosen and invited to talk about the personality of the index subject at a time when he or she was well. If this is not productive seven standard questions are asked, covering usual mood and behaviour. If abnormal traits emerge in the form of predefined descriptive terms, for example 'shy', 'house-proud', the interviewer evaluates the significance of the relevant personality features.

The interview itself takes approximately 10 minutes to complete and yields the ICD diagnoses with the addition of two extra descriptive types: the anxious and the self-conscious. Two grades are possible for each type.

Weighted kappa values for inter-rater reliability have been established for the most common disorders according to this scheme (N=24); cyclothymic (κ_w=0.85), self-conscious (κ_w=0.67), anxious (κ_w=0.61) and obsessional (κ_w=0.60). Because of the loose structure inherent in this system a considerable degree of judgement is required by the interviewer at the stage of evaluation, and training in its use is therefore essential if reliability between raters is to carry through to other centres. It has been administered to psychiatric out-patient and general practice populations (Mann *et al.*, 1981) and it has also been applied in a mental handicap setting (Ballinger and Reid, 1987). Serious methodological questions arise in this group, however, in view of the fact that their study made use of trained nursing staff as sources of the personality descriptions, and it is to be expected that profiles obtained in this way would be situation-determined (i.e. the institution) despite a high level of professionalism among staff. Those thinking of using the SAP should get in touch with its originator, Professor Mann, at the Institute of Psychiatry, London, to discuss training procedures.

INSTRUMENTS USED FOR SPECIFIC DSM-III-R PERSONALITY DISORDERS

Borderline Personality Disorder

The present concept of borderline personality disorder has many of its roots in the psychoanalytical tradition and it is not surprising that one of the more influential methods of standardized diagnosis has been the structured interviewing technique of Otto Kernberg (1981). It relies heavily on the patient's presentation during the course of one cross-sectional interview and has been likened to an ordinary clinical diagnosis which would only be safe in the hands of an expert (Reich and Frances, 1984). Fortunately a variety of other instruments are available for use which would be more suitable for non-analytical research in larger populations.

Diagnostic Interview for Borderlines (DIB)

The diagnostic interview for borderlines was derived in part from an analysis of the literature covering various concepts of borderline personality over a 50-year period (Gunderson and Singer, 1975). Five content areas cover social adaptation, impulse/action patterns, affects, psychosis and interpersonal relationships. Each of these areas in turn are scored on a series of statements by an interviewer who bases his evaluation on subjects' replies to structured questions, lists of defined behaviours and phenomena observed during the course of the interview (165 items in all). Units of information are synthesized into a clinical impression and a pyramidal scoring system used to obtain an overall diagnostic score. A cut-off point above seven is considered to be indicative of the presence of borderline disorder.

The instrument differs in its orientation from the DSM-III description of borderline, which regards psychotic episodes as optional in the diagnosis, whereas Gunderson feels they are 'central defining features'. It has now been widely used in a variety of studies. Kolb and Gunderson (1980) have demonstrated good inter-rater reliabilities (intraclass R = 0.60–1.00) in respect of individual statements within the instrument and it has been shown to discriminate well between borderline, neurotic depressives and schizophrenic patients (Gunderson and Kolb, 1978). The overall reliability between raters is in the region of kappa coefficient 0.62–0.78 (Kroll *et al.*, 1981). Although many studies have examined the validity of the borderline concept as a distinct 'disease entity' the subject remains clouded in controversy (Goldberg and Shultz, 1984).

Borderline and Schizotypal Disorders

Schedule for Interviewing Borderlines (SIB)

This instrument, developed by Baron and his colleagues, is capable of making the DSM-III specific schizotypal and borderline personality disorder diagnosis (Baron, 1981). There are 70 items, each of which is rated on a five-point scale, and the interview takes just under an hour to administer. Joint interviews have yielded kappa reliabilities of 0.71 for schizotypal symptoms (Jacobsberg *et al.*, 1986).

PERSONALITY ASSESSMENT INSTRUMENTS CAPABLE OF MAKING ALL DSM-III DISORDER DIAGNOSES

Structured Interview for DSM-III Personality (SID-P)

The SID-P was developed by the Iowa group led by Pfohl *et al.* and takes the form of a semi-structured interview administered by trained personnel. (Pfohl *et al.*, 1983) Knowledge of present mental state through determination of an Axis-I diagnosis is mandatory but may be carried out separately. Information from subject, informant and other available sources including hospital charts is utilized and where discrepancies arise the interviewer uses clinical judgement to decide which is likely to be more valid. It takes approximately 60 minutes to administer, with another 30 minutes allowed for the informant interview. Where change in personality appears to have occurred the predominant attributes of the previous 5 years are evaluated.

The instrument covers 16 areas of personal functioning in a 60-item interview, with three predetermined anchor points in each dimension. When all the sections have been rated the replies are transcribed to a summary sheet which organizes the criteria in terms of specific DSM-III personality disorders. A positive diagnosis is then made if sufficient criteria summate to pass the threshold for that disorder. Inter-rater reliabilities for joint interviews of in-patients (κ_w) are as follows: 0.90 for dependent personality, 0.85 for borderline, 0.75 for histrionic, 0.62 for schizotypal, 0.45 for avoidant personality disorder. The instrument has also been found to be of value in assessing out-patient groups (Reich, 1987).

Personality Disorder Examination (PDE)

Developed by Loranger *et al.* (1985), the PDE is a highly structured interview which requires training in its use. Considerable efforts are made within its structure to reduce judgements made by the assessor, and the present available version is designed to diagnose specific DSM-III-R personality disorder. For that reason much of the wording of the 359 items closely parallels the descriptive accounts of personality disorder covered by the DSM-III-R manual. Most questions therefore directly examine negative traits, a feature that may lead to resistance among a proportion of respondents. It takes between 2 and 2½ hours to administer and covers five areas of functioning: work, self, interpersonal relations, affects and impulse control. In addition there is a section which rates behaviour observed during the interview with a set of exclusion criteria, preventing certain diagnoses being made if some of the major clinical syndromes are present. Each item is rated on a three-point scale depending on whether it is absent or clinically significant, the intermediate level indicating doubtful current significance.

The PDE is still undergoing revision in order to enable it to provide equivalent ICD diagnoses. Initial reliability studies have been encouraging and a large international comparability study is under way which will look further at these issues of reliability and validity. Its length and present North American orientation, however, may limit its application in other countries.

Structured Clinical Interview for DSM-III-R Personality Disorders (SCID-II)

The SCID-II developed by Spitzer *et al.* (1987) is the latest in a line of diagnostic interviews developed by the New York group, although it is the first such interview to focus on Axis-II. Again it is recommended that a present mental state diagnosis is made and this is usually done with the SCID-I prior to the personality assessment. It is preceded by completion of the Personality Disorder Questionnaire, in which the subject is presented with a dichotomous yes/no choice. A reasonable reading level is required although the respondent is instructed to leave questions blank if they are not understood. The SCID-II interview then focuses on the questions to which the subject has given a positive reply. A series of six standard stem questions are available in order to obtain a precise account of the way in which these items manifest themselves in the person's usual life. The interview goes through each of the DSM-III-R personality disorder classes in turn in a format similar to SCID-I. Opportunity exists for the interviewer to clarify negative or unanswered items and clinical judgement is expected where inconsistencies arise. Limited training is offered by the Biometrics Research Department of the New York State Psychiatric Institute and may involve attendance at workshops or review of audiotapes.

Personality Assessment Schedule (PAS)

The PAS was developed by Tyrer and Alexander (1979) using an agnostic empirically orientated approach. They distilled information on personality disorder from the literature and clinical sources and came up with the series of 28 personality dimensions based on the premise that personality disorder assumes clinical significance only when it is accompanied by some level of social disruption. Following their initial analysis the number of items was reduced to 24 owing to the high correlation between some of them. Each is therefore measured on a well-delineated nine-point scale, the score depending on the degree of social impairment produced by the characteristic in question.

The initial study (Tyrer and Alexander, 1979) was carried out on 130 patients and used factor and cluster analytical procedures to identify five discrete personality categories: sociopathic, passive dependent, anankastic, schizoid and a normal group. A further nine subgroups have been identified including explosive, sensitive aggressive, histrionic, asthenic, anxious, paranoid, hypochondriacal, dysthymic and avoidant. Once the 24 ratings are complete a brief computer program calculates the score for each of these 13 categories and predefined cut-off points are used to decide if personality disorder is present. Manual analysis is also possible and with the aid of a pocket calculator takes about 5 minutes. Three levels of severity exist: personality difficulty, personality disorder and severe personality disorder. Mixed classification is allowed and uses a hierarchical procedure to decide which category should be pre-eminent.

Using the computer-generated results it is possible to obtain personality profiles of individuals and of groups in addition to the categorical diagnoses according to the scheme above. ICD-10 equivalent diagnoses can also be made and recently the instrument has been modified to yield DSM-III-R diagnoses, although these are not derived from strict operational criteria and cannot be regarded as strictly equivalent (Tyrer *et al.*, 1988).

The PAS has now been used to assess the personality attributes of over a thousand cases, including psychiatric out-patients (Tyrer *et al.*, 1983a), in-patients, general practice attenders and normal groups (Casey *et al.*, 1984), forensic (Mbatia and Tyrer, 1988) and alcoholic populations (Griggs and Tyrer, 1981) Inter-rater (R_1=0.547–0.605) and temporal reliability are satisfactory (Tyrer *et al.*, 1984, 1983b). It can be administered to a subject, informant or in combination with both and takes approximately 30–45 minutes to complete. Training is by means of videotaped interviews obtained from the authors, with occasional seminars when the demand is sufficient.

Millon Clinical Multi-axial Inventory (MCMI)

This instrument, developed by Theodore Millon (1984), has been in use for a number of years and consists of a self-administered questionnaire scored by computer. It has 175 items and takes approximately 25 minutes to complete. The results are forwarded either by post or computer link to the National Computer System in Minneapolis for analysis, or alternatively assessment and scoring software is available. It consists of 20 clinical scales made up of eight basic personality 'patterns' or disorder, three pathological personality disorders and nine clinical syndromes. As a result of this format some doubt may exist as to its ability to distinguish between present mental state and more long-standing personality attributes. There are two additional features of note: a weight factor which suppresses the distorting effect of self-defensiveness or self-depreciation and a validity index which helps detect those who are unable to cooperate. The diagnostic criteria utilized in MCMI differ from those incorporated in DSM-III-R but the instrument allows a tentative DSM-III multi-axial diagnosis to be made, which needs to be checked against objective interview and historical data. The results include an individual profile report, a clinical interpretative report in narrative style and a third report oriented towards a forensic setting. The interpretative account based on standardized norms of a sample of 1591 out-patients necessarily has limited value in research settings. A new revised version, the MCMI-II, has recently been published and is said to be capable of making specific DSM-III-R diagnoses, but reliability data are not yet available.

EPIDEMIOLOGICAL STUDIES

In general it has been hard to develop personality assessment interviews which can be used in community studies because of the complexities of the concepts involved and the need to use lay interviewers. One exception has been the category of antisocial personality disorder of DSM-III-R, largely because the diagnosis is made on the basis of behaviour patterns which can be objectively determined without requiring specialized clinical judgement. It has, therefore, been possible to incorporate this category into the National

Institute of Mental Health Diagnostic Interview Schedule (NIMH–DIS). This instrument, developed by Lee Robins for epidemiological work, can be used by lay interviewers as it has an acceptable test–retest reliability for antisocial personality disorder (κ=0.63) (Robins, *et al.*, 1981).

Attempts have been made to modify other Axis-I schedules to measure specific personality disorders, with variable degrees of success. Loranger *et al.* (1985) used modified versions of the Schedule for Affective Disorders and Schizophrenia (SADS) to yield borderline personality diagnosis, comparing it with the DIB for reference. They concluded that the disparity between the SADS and DIB system of diagnoses was sufficient to question whether they were measuring the same concepts. The SADS can, however, be used to diagnose antisocial personality disorder, although again the Research Diagnostic Criteria (RDC) on which it is based differs slightly from the DSM-III account. Joint interview reliability with the SADS has been reported as κ=0.72.

A recent approach towards the problems of standardizing personality assessment has proved encouraging, although a specific measuring instrument has not yet emerged. Livesley has explored a number of behavioural criteria which were found to be highly equated with clinical concepts of the individual personality disorders held by practising psychiatrists, with the possible exception of the borderline category (Livesley, 1986; Livesley and Jackson, 1986). Since such criteria are liable to be more objective than some of the present inferential ones it is to be hoped that an instrument based on such principles could lead to improved reliability without loss of validity.

The instruments available for assessing personality disorder are summarized in Table 1. Compared with 15 years ago they represent a major advance but are still woefully lacking in many important respects. The assessment of personality disorder, to borrow from Groucho Marks in one of his films, 'has raised itself up from nothing to a state of absolute poverty'. The best that can be said about most of the instruments is that they are a reasonably good reflection of the descriptions of personality disorder in current classifications. Whether these descriptions, particularly those in DSM-III, are good ones is quite another matter. The operational criteria of DSM-III are the 'gold standard' by which all the American instruments are compared. However, much of them may be fool's gold as only the criteria for antisocial personality disorder and, to a lesser extent, borderline personality disorder, have been properly researched. There is also a considerable degree of overlap between the different personality disorders in both ICD and DSM-III classifications and it is quite possible to obtain a diagnosis of six or seven simultaneous personality disorders in one individual. This can be very confusing for the research worker, and the attractions of a dimensional system of classification, in which all individuals have a personality score for each of the main group-

Table 1. Rating instruments for personality disorder

Instrument	Source	Key reference concerning use	Subject or informant	Main use
Diagnostic Interview for Borderlines (DIB)	J. G. Gunderson, Psychosocial Research Programme, McLean Hospital, 115 Mill Street, Belmont, MA 02178, USA	Gunderson and Kolb (1978)	Subject	Diagnosis of borderline personality disorder
Schedule for Interviewing Borderlines (SIB)	M. Baron, New York State Psychiatric Institute, New York 10032, USA	Jacobsberg *et al.* (1986)	Subject	Diagnosis of borderline and schizotypal personality disorder
Personality Assessment Schedule (PAS)	P. Tyrer Mapperley Hospital, Nottingham, NC3 6AA, UK	Tyrer and Alexander (1979)	Subject or informant (informant preferred)	Diagnosis of personality disorders (equivalent to ICD-10 and DSM-III-R) and recording of key trait dimensional scores
Standardized Assessment of Personality (SAP)	A. Mann, Academic Department of Psychiatry, Royal Free Hospital, London NW3, UK	Mann *et al.* (1981)	Informant	Classification of personality disorder according to ICD-9 categories (with two additional diagnoses)

Millon Clinical Multiaxial Inventory (MCMI)	T. Millon, c/o National Computer Systems, PO Box 1416, Minneapolis, MN 55440, USA	Millon (1981)	Subject	Classification of personality disorder according to Millon's scheme, but conversion to DSM-III-R also possible
Structured Interview for DSM-III Personality Disorder (SID-P)	B. Pfohl, Department of Psychiatry, University of Iowa Hospitals and Clinics, 500 Newton Road, Iowa City, IA 52242, USA	Stangl *et al.* (1985)	Subject	Diagnosis of DSM-III personality disorders
Structured Clinical Interview for DSM-III and DSM-III-R (SCID-II)	R. Spitzer, Biometrics Research, New York State Psychiatric Institute, 722 West 168th Street, New York 10032, USA	None available (instrument constantly being updated)	Subject	Diagnosis of DSM-III and DSM-III-R personality disorders
Personality Disorder Questionnaire (PDQ)	As for SCID-II	Reich (1987)	Subject (self-rated)	Diagnosis of DSM-III personality disorders

ings, is considerable. Such 'key trait' scores are derived from the PAS and have proved to be valuable measures (Seivewright, 1987).

Despite the deficiencies of current diagnosis and assessment of personality disorder, it is extremely important for the research worker not to forget this area of classification. Even with our imperfect measures, personality disorder has a major influence on outcome of psychiatric disorder (Tyrer *et al.*, 1983a) and is likely to attract increasing interest as assessment procedures improve.

REFERENCES

American Psychiatric Association (1987). *Diagnostic and statistical Manual of Mental Disorders*, 3rd edn, revised, American Psychiatric Association, Washington, DC.

Ballinger, B. and Reid, A. (1987). A standardized assessment of personality in mental handicaps. *Br. J. Psychiatry* **150**, 108–109.

Baron, M. (1981). *Schedule for Interviewing Borderlines*, New York State Psychiatric Institute, New York.

Baron, M., Asnis, L. and Gruen, R. (1981). Schedule of interviewing schizotypal personalities: a diagnostic interview for schizotypal features. *Psychiatr. Res.* **4**, 213–228.

Casey, P. R., Dillon, S. and Tyrer, P. (1984). The diagnostic status of patients with conspicuous psychiatric morbidity in primary care. *Psychol. Med.* **14**, 637–681.

Goffman, E. (1961). *Asylums*, Anchor Books, Garden City, New York.

Goldberg, S. and Schultz, S. (1984). Bordeline personality disorder: new findings on pharmacotherapy. *Psychopharmacol. Bull.* **20**, 554–560.

Griggs, S. M. and Tyrer, P. J. (1981). Personality disorder, social adjustment and treatment outcome in alcoholics. *J. Stud. Alcohol* **42**, 802–805.

Gunderson, J. G. and Kolb, J. E. (1978). Discriminating features of borderline patients. *Am. J. Psychiatry* **135**, 792–796.

Gunderson, J. G. and Singer, M. T. (1975). Defining borderline patients: an overview. *Am. J. Psychiatry* **132**, 1–10.

Hirschfeld, R. M. A., Klerman, G. L., Clayton, P. J. *et al.* (1983). Assessing personality: effects of the depressive state on trait measurement. *Am. J. Psychiatry* **140**, 695–699.

Jacobsberg, L. B., Hymiortz, P., Barasch, A. and Francis, A. (1986). Symptoms of schizotypal personality disorder. *Am. J. Psychiatry* **143**, 1222–1227.

Kernberg, O. F. (1981). Structural interviewing. *Psychiatric Clin. North Am.* **4**, 169–195.

Kolb, J. and Gunderson, J. G. (1980). Diagnosing borderline patients with a semi-structured interview. *Arch. Gen. Psychiatry* **37**, 37–40.

Kroll, J., Pyle, R., Zander, J., Martin, K., Lori, S. and Sines, L. (1981). *Schizophr. Bull.* **7**, 165–173.

Livesley, W. J. and Jackson D. N. (1986). The internal consistency and factorial structure of behaviours judged to be associated with DSM-III personality disorders. *Am. J. Psychiatry* **143**, 1473–1474.

Loranger, A. W., Susman, V. L., Oldham, J. M. and Russakoff, L. M. (1985). Personality disorder examination (PDE). A structured interview for DSM-III-R and ICD-9 personality disorders. WHO/ADAMHA pilot version, 1985. New York Hospital—Cornell Medical Center, Westchester Division, White Plains, New York.

Mann, A. H., Jenkins, R., Cutting, J. C. and Cowen, P. J. (1981). The development and use of a standardized assessment of abnormal personality. *Psychol. Med.* **11**, 839–847.

Mbatia, J. and Tyrer, P. (1988). Personality disorder in a special hospital. In *Personality Disorder: Diagnosis, Management and Course* (P. Tyrer, ed.), John Wright, Bristol.

Millon, T. (1981). *Disorders of Personality: Axis II*, Wiley, New York.

Millon, T. (1984). *The Millon Clinical Multiaxial Inventory*, National Computer Systems, PO Box 1416, Minneapolis.

Mischel, W. (1968). *Personality and Assessment*, Wiley, New York.

Pfohl, B., Stangl, D. and Zimmerman, M. (1983). *Structured Interview for DSM-III Personality SIDP*, Department of Psychiatry, University of Iowa.

Reich, J. H. (1987). Instruments measuring DSM-III and DSM-III-R personality disorders. *J. Pers. Disord.* **1**, 220–240.

Reich, J. and Frances, A. (1984). The structural interview method for diagnosing borderline disorders: a critique. *Psychiatr. Q.* **56**, 229–235.

Reich, J., Noyes, R., Caryell, W. and O'Gorman, T. (1986). The effect of state anxiety on personality measurement. *Am. J. Psychiatry* **143**, 760–763.

Robins, L., Helzer, J., Crangham, J. *et al.* (1981). National Institute of Mental Health. Diagnostic interview schedule: its history characteristics and validity. *Arch. Gen. Psychiatry* **38**, 381–389.

Seivewright, N. (1987). Relationship between life events and personality disorder. *Stress Med.* **3**, 163–168.

Spitzer, R. L., Williams, J. and Gibbon, M. (1987). *Structured Clinical Interview for DSM-III-R (SCID-II).* Biometric Research, New York State Psychiatric Institute, New York.

Stangl, D., Pfohl, B., Zimmerman, M., Bowers, W. and Carenthal, C. (1985). Structured interview for DSM-III personality disorders. *Arch. Gen. Psychiatry* **42**, 591–596.

Tyrer, P. and Alexander, J. (1979). Classification of personality disorder. *Br. J. Psychiatry* **135**, 163–167.

Tyrer, P. and Ferguson, B. (1987). Problems in the classification of personality disorder. *Psychol. Med.* **17**, 15–20.

Tyrer, P., Casey, P. and Gall, J. (1983a). Relationship between neurosis and personality disorder. *Br. J. Psychiatry* **142**, 404–408.

Tyrer, P., Strauss, J. and Cicchetti, D. (1983b). Temporal reliability of personality in psychiatric patients. *Psychol. Med.* **13**, 393–398.

Tyrer, P., Cicchetti, D. V., Casey, P. R., Fitzpatrick, K., Oliver, R., Balter, A., Giller, E. and Harkness, L. (1984). Cross national reliability study of a schedule for assessing personality disorders. *J. Nerv. Ment. Dis.* **172**, 718–721.

Tyrer, P., Ferguson, B. and Alexander, J. (1988). Personality Assessment Schedule (4th edition). In *Personality Disorder: Diagnosis, Management and Course*, John Wright, Bristol.

Walton, H. J. and Presly, A. S. (1973). Use of a category system in the diagnosis of abnormal personality. *Br. J. Psychiatry* **122**, 259–268.

World Health Organization (1978). *Mental Disorders: Glossary and Guide to the Classification in Accordance with the Ninth Revision of the International Classification of Diseases*, World Health Organization, Geneva.

The Instruments of Psychiatric Research
Edited by C. Thompson

CHAPTER 11

Social psychiatry

TRAOLACH S. BRUGHA
*Department of Psychiatry,
Leicester Royal Infirmary,
Leicester, UK*

INTRODUCTION

The aim of social psychiatry is to study the relationship between the social environment and the mental health of the individual person. Social psychiatry is therefore an extension of social medicine and like it requires of those who intend to use its measures a sound knowledge of the methods of epidemiology (Alderson, 1983). In order to achieve this aim it has been necessary to measure both the social and psychological (including the clinical) characteristics of the person as well as those of others in the social environment of which he or she is a part. Accordingly, sociology and psychology are the principal sciences from which many of the measurement techniques of social psychiatry are derived.

Social psychiatry is a term that encompasses a broad field within psychiatry. Other chapters in this book will focus on some specific aspects of social and psychological functioning within psychiatry, for example in relation to children, adolescents and the elderly. Accordingly, some measures that have been devised for use in these other areas, such as those that assess the behaviour and social functioning of children when observed by teachers and parents, will not be covered in this chapter. Similarly, as this book provides a comprehensive overview of clinical instruments in use in psychiatric research, this fundamental part of the methodology of social and epidemiological psychiatry will not be referred to any further here, except when it is necessary to the discussion of a particular topic—for example, in relation to measures of abnormal behaviour used in studies of long-term patients in psychiatric institutional settings (Sturt and Wykes, 1987).

As this chapter can only provide an introductory glimpse of a large and very diverse area of research instrumentation, it is important to consider some conceptual and methodological issues before discussing the details of specific measures. Care and thought need to be given to choosing an instrument. It should also be borne in mind that research workers who are new to social psychiatry are particularly prone to devising new and ad hoc measures. There are probably a number of reasons for this: often there is no obvious and reliable instrument available for the measurement of the construct to be studied; much research is carried out by sociologists and psychologists who may not be very familiar with the more worthy technical achievements of well-established social psychiatry research groups. Unfortunately, the decision to devise one's own measure can sometimes be unnecessary and indeed unwise. An important function of this book and this chapter is to save intending research workers the wasteful labour of 're-inventing the wheel'. Unfortunately, a significant volume of research in this field is marred by the uncertainty of findings based on hastily devised measures of unknown reliability and validity that are unlikely to be used on more than one occasion.

Whilst the importance of methodological issues may be obvious, one should also take care that equal consideration is devoted to questioning the theoretical assumptions that underpin the intended purpose of a particular measure. The next section will discuss this point in relation to the field as a whole, citing examples of specific, well-developed instruments from the areas covered. The chapter will then be rounded off with a more detailed discussion of two categories of instruments—measures of adversity (i.e. life events) and of social support—both of which are of considerable interest to social psychiatry research at the present time.

CONCEPTUAL ISSUES

If there is one single concept that underpins all social psychiatry research it is that of an individual person constantly in a state of interaction with the social and physical environment, whose mental and physical well-being depends on the availability of both physical and psychosocial (environmental) resources (whilst minimizing the cost to that individual arising from the demands of their environment). Although effective research in social psychiatry depends on a clear-cut separation of those factors that reflect the social environment from those that deal with the characteristics (especially the psychological characteristics) of the person being studied, the successful achievement of this division can give rise to considerable difficulties in practice. Perhaps the best example of this was the recognition of the need to develop a measure of environmental stress that was not contaminated by the measure of psychopathology used in the same research. Brown and his colleagues (1975, 1978) developed the concept of 'independence' in their life event rating scales in order to allow the research worker to take into account and attempt to exclude the possibility that the subject's psychiatric symptoms might distort the stress measurement instrument.

We can now consider three separate concepts, which can be thought of as potentially distinct groups of variables, which may be helpful to us in attempting to categorize the instruments of social psychiatry. These are:

1. The individual's capacity to function.
2. The social and physical resources that we can identify and measure in the environment.
3. The potentially stressful demands of the environment on the person.

These will now be discussed in further detail, with examples of the more notable and highly developed measures that have been devised in each area. Only those instruments that have been consistently shown to be reliable and useful will be mentioned.

Measures of Individual Capacity

The capacity to function or adapt to environmental demands can be thought of as depending on the person's developmental level, on learning and on the impairment of capacity that results from physical or psychiatric illness. The Handicaps, Behaviour and Skills (HBS) structured interview schedule (Wing and Gould, 1978) was designed to assess developmental skills in mentally retarded individuals by eliciting information from parents and professional informants. Similarly, the MRC Social Role Performance Schedule (SRP; Hurry and Sturt, 1981; Sturt and Wyke, 1987) was designed to gather information during an interview with an informant concerning the social performance of the individual in eight areas of social role functioning.

Whilst both the HBS and SRP have been carefully designed in order to focus on the abilities of the individual being assessed, it would be unwise to suppose that the expression of these abilities is not capable of being influenced by external factors such as cultural expectations and norms and restrictions on the availability of opportunities to demonstrate skills. A new method for assessing the needs of the long-term mentally ill (Brewin *et al.*, 1987), which drew on experience in the use of the SRP, has therefore been designed to take into account whether the subject has had an opportunity to exercise a skill. Clearly this may be very important in studies carried out in highly restricted environments traditionally associated with poorly managed and resourced long-stay institutions. For example, one cannot rate a subject's ability to use public transport if he is not permitted to leave the hospital, hostel or other institution. A more subtle example arises in transcultural psychiatric research: for example, in deciding whether an adult male of normal intelligence can prepare a cooked meal it is necessary to consider whether he belongs to a society in which it is ruled that men are only permitted to engage in such behaviour if they are employed as cooks in a restaurant or hotel!

A number of useful reviews of measures of social functioning have appeared in recent years (Weissman, 1975; Sturt and Wyke, 1987; Weissman *et al.*, 1981; Platt, 1985). These provide a more detailed view of the theoretical and technical issues, together with details of other related instruments. A similar and well-evaluated, combined package of such measures, covering the dimensions of disturbed behaviour, social performance and effects (burden) on the patient's household, is the Social Behaviour Assessment Schedule (SBAS) (Platt, *et al.*, 1980).

Measures of Environmental Social Resources

There are many ways of considering the environmental and social resources available to an individual and, once again, it may not be easy to delineate those that are purely a function of the external world from those that represent an extension of the person's own influence on the world around them. These 'resources' can include social and cultural status (social class, profession, ethnic origins and age), educational level achieved, personal wealth and consequently the quality of the person's home and work environment, and finally a more abstract concept of comparatively recent development: social support (see below). The measurement of social class (Goldthorpe and Hope, 1974; Dohrenwend and Dohrenwend, 1969) is a huge topic that cannot be taken any further here; nor is it possible to do more than mention the important topics of race, migration and related issues pertinent to transcultural psychiatry (Cox, 1986).

A variety of ways of assessing the quality of the social and physical environment, whether in the community or in institutions, have been developed under the umbrella of a number of academic disciplines: these have included the measurement of the quality of the urban environment by sociologists (Webb, 1984) and geographers (Smith, 1984). Another useful approach is to make use of existing gradings of the social and economic qualities of defined administrative areas, either directly from census data or by means of a systematically devised scale of underprivileged areas such as the Jarman Index (Jarman, 1983). The quality of institutional settings has been assessed by instruments that take into account the range of facilities and material resources available to the occupants, and the policies and practices of the managers and staff in such settings. A notable example of an instrument that has been developed over a number of years and used in many studies is the Hospital and Hostel Practices Profile (HHPP) (Wyke, 1982). The Management Practices Questionnaire (MPQ; Garrety and Morris, 1984) is a similar measure designed to identify management practices on a continuum of 'resident-oriented' to 'institutionally oriented' care.

The topic of social support earns a special mention both because of the keen and growing interest in it and because of the considerable technical challenges that its measurement poses (Brugha, 1988). Within this term one can include a wide range of measures that assess the quality of personal relationships such as marriage, as in the Dyadic Adjustment Scale (Spanier, 1976), the behaviour of relatives in the family home as assessed by the Camberwell Family Interview (CFI); (Vaughan and Leff, 1976), as well as measures that encompass the extended social network (Brown *et al.*, 1986; Brugha *et al.*, 1987; Henderson *et al.*, 1981). The topic will be covered more selectively later in this chapter and a detailed review of measures can also be consulted elsewhere (Brugha, 1986).

Measures of Environmental Adversity

The third and final concept is that of adversity. As pointed out already in this chapter, this construct has also proved to be surprisingly difficult to assess independently of the influence of the person being studied, and this issue will be taken up again in the next section on methodology. The topic of adversity has been at the centre of social psychiatry research for a number of years and there are many useful commentaries on the theoretical and methodological issues available elsewhere for the interested reader (Katschnig, 1986). Further conceptual difficulties have also been noted in relation to the successful delineation of measures of adversity from those of social resources (Monroe and Steiner, 1986; Brugha, 1986). To take one or two examples: a house move may be a very stressful event or it may be a very positive event that leads to an increased level of social support through the development of new personal relationships with neighbours; similarly, getting married may increase social demands and the weight of responsibility as well as providing a particularly secure form of affective social support and a reliable source of confiding. The researcher and the student examining the work of others may need to consider how carefully these kinds of ambiguities have been tackled by means of the instruments used. This topic will be given further, more detailed consideration in the discussion of life events instruments, at the end of this chapter.

METHODOLOGICAL ISSUES

In practice, the theoretical constructs identified above have been measured by means of questionnaires, structured and semi-structured interviews, independently judged ratings of data obtained by interview and the use of observational or laboratory methods. In this section, brief mention will also be made of the use of computers in social psychiatry research, both for measurement and also for the closely related tasks of data storage using complex file structures, the conduct of statistical analysis and the development of expert systems.

Although questionnaires have considerable advantages in their cost of use there are severe limitations to the kind of data that can be gathered using them. This is particularly the case where social and environmental measures are required, in contrast to the area of individual clinical assessment where dimensional measures of non-psychotic psychiatric symptoms can be obtained more easily with acceptable reliability. A particularly good example of the drawbacks of questionnaire measures arises in relation to measures of life events; this issue will also be taken up later.

Interview methods can be subdivided into those in which the investigator is satisfied with a verbatim record of the subject's response to questions (respondent-based instruments) and those in which independent judgements and ratings are preferred (investigator-based instruments). The former is obviously simpler and less demanding and is usually well suited to gathering socio-demographic data, information about present or past events and a direct measure of the subject's own opinions on a topic. Most measures of social relationships and social support fall into this category (Brugha *et al.*, 1987; Henderson *et al.*, 1981). However, there is no doubt that the most sophisticated instruments that have been developed in the field of social psychiatry are the investigator-based measures. These instruments require of the investigator that a detailed set of rating criteria be developed and used for deciding whether the information obtained during an interview can be said to represent an example of a chosen construct. For example, with the Life Events and Difficulties Scales (LEDS; Brown and Harris, 1978) the occurrence of an event is not rated during the interview but is decided upon by an independent panel of raters who are told about the event but not about the clinical state of the respondent. The panel raters are guided by a detailed set of rating rules, and formal training in their use is an essential requirement. Similarly, in the Present State Examination (PSE; Wing *et al.*, 1974) the presence of a symptom such as depressed mood cannot be positively rated simply because the respondent said 'yes', when asked whether they felt low in spirits during the past month; the interviewer is required to probe further in order to elicit information that may permit a rating to be made (during or after the interview) that accords with a set of rules to be followed at every assessment. In this sense, investigator-based methods depend on the critical examination and judgement of data gathered and are not based upon a verbatim record of the responses obtained during an interview. Other measures with similar elaborate criteria include the CFI and the HBS mentioned earlier. Not surprisingly, all of these methods have in common the need for users to undergo a special course of training.

There are relatively few instruments in the field of social psychiatry that are based on independent observations of behaviour. To some extent the CFI can be said to fall into this category. However, there is a growing body of laboratory-based work taking place now in which, for example, dyadic interactions (Hahlwag *et al.*, 1984) are recorded on videotape and subsequently rated and analysed in considerable detail.

Whilst most of the measurement techniques described so far have been principally influenced by research psychology, it is important to remember that field methods developed by sociologists and social anthropologists can also play an important role in opening up a new area of research. Patten and Press (1975) have provided a useful introduction to the topics of socio-demographic data collection, content analysis of open interviews, the use of diaries, inventories and sociometric techniques for the graphical representation of social activity. Another very useful introduction to interviewing techniques by Grad de Alarcon and Crocetti (1975) could also be consulted: apart from providing guidance on instrument standardization, reliability and validity, these workers also discuss appropriate methods for gaining the cooperation of informants, minimizing refusals, conducting and controlling interviews and the avoidance of bias.

Increasing emphasis is being given to the use of computers in measurement. Although most of the present uses of direct patient computer interviewing are concerned with assessing symptoms and cognitive functioning (Erdmann *et al.*, 1983) social psychiatrists are beginning to consider this method also. Social and epidemiological psychiatrists have for long been using computers in order to facilitate the development of case registers, which have made a considerable contribution to social psychiatry research (Gibbons *et al.*, 1983). A notable development in relation to the statistical analysis of epidemiological data is the availability of database management software that allows the storage and processing of hierarchical as well as of rectangular data sets: these usually allow the user to incorporate data error checking facilities into the system as well as structuring the data in a manner that is appropriate to the complexities of the social world (Brugha, 1986). A final area of development in computing is the use of expert systems that incorporate rules for processing data prior to statistical analysis. An early and widely used example is CATEGO-ID (Wing and Sturt, 1978), in which PSE data are processed in order to produce symptom scores, threshold levels on an eight-point scale and research diagnostic categories with equivalent ICD codes. Once implemented, expert systems have the advantage of total reliability if properly used and the potential of almost instantaneous availability at no cost over that of the initial production of the system (although it has to be said that the latter can involve considerable effort).

Because the field of social psychiatry is clearly a very wide one, the final sections of this chapter will concentrate only on those instruments that are the most highly developed and widely used and tested in two specific areas: the assessment of adversity and the assessment of social support and social networks.

Life Events Instruments

Whilst the assessment of stress by means of self-administered lists such as the Social Readjustment Rating Scale (Holmes and Rahe, 1967) has been very widely used, it is difficult to see much justification for their popularity save for their low demands on the researcher's energies. The topic has been amply discussed elsewhere (Brown and Harris, 1978), and the recent review by Katschnig (1986) provides detailed references to the numerous variations on the check-list theme that have emerged since the pioneering work of Holmes and Rahe (1967).

Katschnig (1986) has set out a system for assessing how stressful a single life event is likely to be and has proposed a taxonomy of four different levels, based on four assumptions about the stressfulness of life events. At the first level, all events are regarded as being equally stressful and the research worker is concerned with the total number reported by each subject (Rahe *et al.*, 1964; Paykel *et al.*, 1969). At the second level different weights are attached to different types or categories of life event, assuming differences in their stressfulness (Holmes and Rahe, 1967; Paykel *et al.*, 1971; Tennant and Andrews, 1976). At the third level the context and circumstances in which an event takes place are also taken into account as in the method of Brown and Harris (1978) already explained above. The LEDS panel rating method therefore works by laying down rules for assessing the stressfulness of events of the same type according to differences in the context in which they occur. Although technically demanding and time-consuming, an independent assessment of its reliability has been quite satisfactory (Tennant *et al.*, 1979). The fourth and final level adds to the other three by taking into account the subject's own (subjective) judgement of the stressfulness of the event. Whilst this would appear to be the ideal method of assessing the stressfulness of an event for any one person, it has rarely been used because of the unreliability of retrospectively reported life event data in persons with affective disturbance (Katschnig, 1986).

One of the more serious shortcomings of the check-list method may be due to the inclusion of minor events that in most cases are unlikely to have any significant effect on health (Brugha *et al.*, 1985; Rey *et al.*, 1987). Check-list methods have also suffered from the use of lengthy time periods (typically the previous year) over which reliability of recall suffers progressively. Therefore the recent development of a brief list of 12 categories of adversity that are more likely to be highly threatening (for example being fired from one's job, the serious illness or death of someone very close) may be worth considering in studies that have limited resources or in which adversity is not the sole major issue (Brugha *et al.*, 1985). Recent work by the author of this chapter, using this technique, particularly over a brief period of time (the last 3 months) has shown it to be of acceptable reliability (test–retest) and to be well corroborated by the independent report of an informant.

In spite of their considerable technical shortcomings, check-list life event inventories are almost certainly here to stay, particularly in studies that are also designed to consider additional aetiological variables. Intending users are strongly recommended to 'bite off as little as possible' by covering short recent time periods and enquiring only about events that are likely to be moderately or severely threatening. In addition, an interview rather than a questionnaire version should be used (Paykel, 1983; Oei and Zwart, 1986). However, the research worker whose central concern is with the nature of stress and its relationship to psychiatric disorder is unlikely to achieve worthwhile gains unless the full investigator-based contextual rating method is chosen.

Social Support Instruments

Social support instruments have been less widely documented and analysed and will therefore be considered in greater detail here. Table 1 shows the dimensions of social support that appear to be covered by each of a selected group of instruments. (A more detailed review can be consulted elsewhere: Brugha, 1986.) Available information on reliability is also summarized in the table.

The first detailed description of a technique for assessing social interaction in epidemiological surveys was provided by Henderson *et al.* (1978). The Social Interaction Schedule (SIS) was designed to collect information about the quantity and quality of all social contacts in the week prior to interview, as well as to obtain from the subject a nominated list of close kith and kin. Each subject was asked to nominate household members, good friends and close relatives. In order to identify attachment figures, he was then asked which of these persons was most important to him, and which of the others was considered to be of similar importance. The quantity and quality of social interaction with these persons during the previous 7 days was enquired about. Intense face to face interaction and negative and positive interactions were also quantified. Each subject was asked to state whether he had

Table 1

Source	Technique	Support areas covered	Reliability
Henderson *et al.* (1978) *Br. J. Psychiatry* **132**, 74–86	SIS Interview 76 items Time coverage: 7 days	Quality and quantity of social interaction/ Emot./Soc. ties/ Resp. Beh. v. perc.	See text
Henderson *et al.* (1981) Academic Press, Australia	ISSI Interview 52 items	Perceived availability and adequacy: attachment and social integration Soc. ties/Responsiv./ Emot.	Inter-rater: 0.7–0.8 Retest: (4 or 8 months) 0.51–0.76
Jenkins *et al.* (1981) *Soc. Sci. Med.* **15**, 195–203	SSSI Ratings based on interview	Ratings of stressfulness and supportiveness on 6 social dimensions. Tangib./Emot.	Inter-rater: 0.79–0.90
Sarason *et al.* (1983) *J. Pers. Soc. Psychol.* **44**, 127–139	SSQ-S and SSQ-N Questionnaires (S)atisfaction and (N)umber	Emot./Tangib./Soc. ties/Responsiv. 2 scales; 27 items.	Test–retest 4 weeks: 0.9–0.83 Internal (S) 0.94
Lin *et al.* (1981) *Schizophr. Bull.* **7**, 73–89	Questionnaire 4 scales 43 items	Family confidant and neighbourhood functioning Emot./ Tangib./Soc. ties/ Responsiv.	Internal Consistency varied
Holohan and Moohs (1983) *Br. J. Clin. Psychol.* **22**, 157–162	FRI and WRI Family and work Relationships Questionnaire	Family: cohesion, expressiveness, conflict Work: peer and staff support Emot./Soc. ties/ Responsiv.	Internal: 0.67–0.81
McFarlane *et al.* (1981) *Schizophr. Bull.* **7**, 90–100	SRS Questionnaire 6 areas	Help with family, finances, work, health/Emot./Soc. ties/Respons.	Test–retest 0.54–0.99

Table 1 (*continued*)

Source	Technique	Support areas covered	Reliability
Brown and Harris (1978, 1986) Tavistock, London. *Psychol. Med.* **16**, 813–831	Interview and panel rating SESS	Emot. support/ Responsiv./Beh. v. perc./Crisis support	Inter-rater: $\kappa = 0.8$
Norbeck *et al.* (1981) *Nurs. Res.* **30**, 264–269	NSSQ (Quest.) Sources and functions	Emot./Tangib./ Responsiv./Soc. ties	Retest (1 week): 0.85–0.92 Internal: 0.7–0.9
Brugha *et al.* (1987) *Soc. Psychiatry* **22**, 123–128	IMSR Interview Measure of social relationships	Emot./Tangib./Beh. v. perc./Responsiv./ Soc. ties/Social network density	Inter-rater: $\kappa = 0.7$–0.9 4-month retest: 0.6–0.8

Key:

Dimensions of social support:

Emot.	=	Emotional support
Tangib.	=	Tangible support
Respons.	=	Responsiveness of key others
Soc. ties	=	Social ties
Beh. v. perc.	=	Reported behaviour and events versus perceived (subjective) evaluation

obtained support from his principal attachment figure or from others during the previous week. These measures contributed to the assessment of the subject's primary group. The same information was obtained about social interaction with other persons who were not members of the subject's primary group. The location of members of the social network outside the household was recorded. Subjects were also asked to fill out a self-completion questionnaire, designed to tap the subject's own perception of the adequacy and availability of social interaction with members of his social network.

The SIS was found to have acceptable inter-rater reliability both by Henderson *et al.* (1978) and by Brugha *et al.* (1982). The usefulness of the SIS was confirmed by the second group of researchers, who carried out a replication in Dublin that resulted in very similar findings to those of Henderson and his colleagues (Brugha *et al.*, 1982). This can be taken as an indication of the construct validity of the instrument.

The SIS appears to have two main advantages. It provides a very detailed account of close (primary) relationships, setting no a priori limits on the number of such relationships to be considered. In contrast, most other measures, and particularly those of the self-completion type, set an upper limit on the number or range of relationships to be considered. Secondly, the SIS focuses specifically on the interactional behaviour of the subject in the week before interview; it may therefore be presumed to reflect more precisely the actual behaviour of the subject and his primary network. Most other measures either fail to specify a time period or choose a longer time period, leaving more room for respondent bias due to variations in recall ability or affective state (see Table 1).

The main disadvantage of the SIS is that it takes a trained interviewer as much as an hour to administer and, as the present author has pointed out elsewhere (Brugha, 1985), its time budget measures add little to the rest of the data gathered and produced highly skewed variables, which may pose difficulties in statistical analysis. These criticisms have resulted in the development of a modification of the SIS, the Interview Measure of Social Relationships (IMSR) (Brugha *et al.*, 1987); the reliability and to a limited extent the validity of this instrument have been assessed and found to be quite satisfactory, and its particular advantage is the relatively brief interview time of 15–20 minutes per subject. The IMSR also gathers information about the density or interrelatedness of the primary social network. A more limited questionnaire version is undergoing development.

Many workers now recommend the incorporation of measures of both the quality and quantity of personal relationships. This realization led the Canberra group to develop a second instrument, the ISSI (Duncan-Jones, 1981 a and b); because of its growing and widespread use it merits close examination. The ISSI is administered by trained lay interviewers. Unlike the earlier SIS, the ISSI uses a range of fairly non-specific time coverage questions using terms such as 'on most days', 'these days', 'usually', 'at present' and 'in an ordinary week'. Using data collected during a population survey, the authors were able to show that two separate dimensions—'attachment' and 'social integration'—were being measured. The use of confirmatory factor analysis revealed that the availability of attachment and of social integration were nearly independent of one another, but the perceived adequacy of these two areas was substantially correlated (Duncan-Jones 1981b). Other analyses showed that the internal consistency, test–retest reliability and the stability of the factor scores over time (4 months, 8 months and 12 months) were very high (Henderson *et al.*, 1981).

In order to cast further light on the validity of the instrument, 114 informants (participants) who knew subjects, who had been studied in a community survey, were also interviewed. The correlations between respondents' and informants' scores were all significant beyond the 1% level, ranging from 0.26 to 0.59 (Henderson *et al.*, 1981). Although the authors themselves regarded the correlations as acceptable, others might not find them sufficiently secure. The authors have also provided a more detailed consideration of the issue of validity (Henderson *et al.*, 1981).

There are difficulties inherent in the structure and content of the ISSI to which the authors themselves have devoted attention. One concern is whether the ISSI is an accurate measure of the social behaviour of others towards the subject, and whether it measures the subject's own view of others without being coloured by his present affective state. Supportive behaviour in itself may not be fully understood (or validly described) without considering many other factors that may be perceived only by the participants: for example, past rewards, obligations based on cultural and personal values, the duration of the relationship and the form rather than the content of interactions. These considerations indicate that both behaviour and social perceptions should be measured separately. Brown *et al.* (1986) argue that these difficulties can be surmounted by detailed questioning about actual behaviour, followed by investigator-based judgements about the provisions of close ties.

The measures of Brown *et al.* (1978) have also developed over the years as a result of the desire to augment their social account of depression. They originally used a measure of confiding and intimacy that has been adopted by several other workers (Murphy, 1982; Campbell *et al.*, 1983; Bebbington *et al.*, 1984; Dolan *et al.*, 1985; Parry and Shapiro, 1986). The person interviewed is rated as having a confidant if they have a relatively problem-free, close relationship with a sexual partner with whom they feel free to discuss any problem. Because of its emphasis on one type of personal relationship it is possible that the measure provides an unrepresentative account of the overall level of social support available to some subjects. This index also incorporated a preliminary effort at assessing crisis support. This apparently yielded negative findings, and received little attention (Brown and Harris, 1978).

A greatly expanded and more detailed procedure, the Self-evaluation and Social Support Schedule (SESS), has since been developed (O'Connor and Brown, 1984; Brown *et al.*, 1986). In its present form, the interview takes 1–2 hours to administer, and is followed by numerous 'panel' ratings based on audiotape recordings. Behavioural measures focus on the present and recent past, and self-report measures reflect the subject's feelings and attitudes. The SESS appears to emphasize very close relationships (in particular with a sexual partner), and also enquires into crisis support in relation to any life events or difficulties. It includes measures of negative and positive self-esteem. However, it is not clear whether such psychological variables can be clearly separated from other aspects of social behaviour and other cognitions. The SESS appears to be reliable between raters. Some indication of its temporal stability may be gleaned from a prospective study which showed that confiding with a very close tie predicted subsequent crisis support, though only in unmarried women (Brown *et al.*, 1986).

As with the companion measure of adversity—the LEDS—the cost in time and training incurred in using this instrument is considerable. This has not restricted the widespread use of the LEDS, developed by this group of workers, as it has considerable methodological advantages. However, comparable advantages over far less costly measures have yet to be demonstrated for the SESS. Its authors have highlighted a more general difficulty: the detailed assessment of crisis support, which forms part of the SESS, cannot be conducted prospectively. This applies to all such measures; however, it might be possible to adapt this part of the SESS to the prospective assessment of single major events, for example, sudden bereavement or the diagnosis of a fatal condition. Finally, it is not clear how the concomitant use of the LEDS and the SESS circumvents problems of overlap, for example, with marital difficulties, or the development in a close confidant of a chronic handicapping disease such as senile dementia.

There are many other questionnaire and interview-based measures, and details of a selection of these are set out in Table 1. The social support questionnaire (Sarason *et al.*, 1983) has two parts dealing with satisfaction and the number of relationships identified, termed SSQ(S) and SSQ(N), respectively (see Table 1 for further details). These have been tested on a number of different samples (Sarason *et al.*, 1983), which may be an advantage to workers who are concerned with comparability of findings.

Direct comparisons of the results of surveys and the more considered evaluation of instruments has been inhibited by the variety of techniques employed by different workers. An interesting and thought-provoking experimental evaluation of an instrument was a test of response bias carried out on the Social Relationship Scale (SRS) by McFarlane *et al.*, (1981). Nineteen post-graduate students were administered the questionnaire on two occasions: on the second occasion they were given an additional instruction to score according to what they considered good or ideal circumstances, and these responses differed significantly from those obtained from the first testing. The authors concluded that subjects would not normally use a desirable response set. The Norbeck Social Support Questionnaire (NSSQ) (Norbeck *et al.*, 1981) has also been assessed and described in some detail by its authors, who reported that no item was found to be related to a test of social desirability (Crowne and Marlowe, 1960).

The SSSI (Jenkins *et al.*, 1981) is particularly interesting in that it combines in a single measure the assessment of stress and social support, on a range of socio-economic dimensions. This approach does not permit the user to consider the effects of support and adversity separately but it does remind one that this kind of separation of function may not be all that easy to achieve even with technically more sophisticated measures such as the LEDS and the SESS. This instrument is also interview-based and has been carefully evaluated.

Although some notable progress has been made, particularly in the development of interview-based measures of social support, a great deal more work is needed on the relationship between these and other measures of psychological and social functioning. Work on measures that distinguish more clearly between participant and non-participant (observer) data is overdue, although the SESS, and in a limited way the Camberwell Family Interview, can be thought of as serving such a function. It is clear from the empirical literature that this area of research deserves further attention now and in the future (Brugha, 1988). In the meantime, the results of studies using existing methods merit careful consideration.

CONCLUSIONS

The present chapter has set out to achieve two relatively limited tasks: first, to establish some general principles for choosing or, if necessary, developing instruments for use in social psychiatry and psychiatric epidemiological research; and, second, to provide more detailed guidelines concerning two major categories of instruments in this field. Because the area is large and heterogenous and undoubtedly overlaps with matters dealt with elsewhere in this book, nothing more ambitious has been attempted. A comprehensive overview of social psychiatry instruments would fill at least one, if not several, books. In the absence of an obvious contender that serves such as function, the prudent research worker is reminded once again that what is offered here is a few pointers to existing instruments that may save time and effort by making the task of reduplicating the work of others unnecessary.

REFERENCES

Alderson, M., (1983). *An introduction to Epidemiology*, Macmillan, London.

Bebbington, P., Tennant, C., Sturt, E. and Hurry, J. (1984). The domain of life events: a comparison of two techniques of description. *Psychol. Med* **14**, 219–222.

Brewin, C. R., Wing, J. K., Mangen, S., Brugha, T. and MacCarthy, B. (1987). Principles and practice of measuring needs in the long-term mentally ill. *Psychol. Med.* **17**, 971–981.

Brown, G. and Harris, T. (1978). *The Social Origins of Depression*, Tavistock Publications, London.

Brown, G., Bhrolchain, N. and Harris, T. (1975). Social class and psychiatric disturbance among women in an urban population. *Sociology* **9**, 225–254.

Brown, G. W., Andrews, B., Harris, T., Adler, Z. and Bridge, L. (1986). Social support, self-esteem and depression. *Psychol. Med.* **16**, 813–831.

Brugha, T. S. (1985). "Dubliners". Social networks and neurosis in an Irish City. In: *Psychiatry: the State of the Art, Vol 7, Epidemiology and Community Psychiatry* (Proc. VII World Congress of Psychiatry), New York, Plenum.

Brugha, T. S. (1986). *Depressive Disorders and Personal Relationships*, MD thesis, National University of Ireland, Dublin.

Brugha, T. S. (1988). Social Support. *Current Opinion in Psychiatry*. **1** (2), 206–211.

Brugha, T. S., Conroy, R., Walsh, N., Delaney, W., O'Hanlon, J., Dondero, E., Daly, L., Hickey, N. and Bourke, G. (1982). Social networks, attachments and support in minor affective disorders: a replication. *Br. J. Psychiatry* **141**, 249–255.

Brugha, T. S., Bebbington, P., Tennant, C. and Hurry, J. (1985). The list of threatening experiences: a subset of 12 life event categories with considerable long term contextual threat. *Psychol. Med.* **15**, 189–194.

Brugha, T. S., Sturt, E., MacCarthy, B., Potter, J., Wykes, T. and Bebbington, P. E. (1987). The Interview Measure of Social Relationships: the description and evaluation of a survey instrument for assessing personal social resources. *Soc. Psychiatry* **22**, 123–128.

Campbell, E. A., Cope, S. J. and Teasdale, J. D. (1983). Social factors and affective disorders: an investigation of Brown & Harris' model. *Br. J. Psychiatry* **143**, 548–554.

Cox, J. L. (1986). *Transcultural Psychiatry*, Croom Helm, London.

Crowne, D. P. and Marlowe, D. (1960). A new scale of social desirability independent of psychpathology. *J. Consult. Psychol.* **24**, 349–354.

Dohrenwend, B. P. and Dohrenwend, B. S. (1969). *Social Status and Psychological Disorders*, Wiley, New York.

Dolan, R. J., Calloway, S. P., Fonagy, P., De Souza, V. F. A. and Wakeling, A. (1985). Life events, depression and hypothalmic–pituitary–adrenal axis function. *Br. J. Psychiatry* **147**, 429–433.

Duncan-Jones, P. (1981a). The structure of social relationships: Analysis of a survey instrument, part 1. *Soc. Psychiatry* **16**, 55–61.

Duncan-Jones, P. (1981b). The structure of social relationships: Analysis of a survey instrument, part 2. *Soc. Psychiatry* **16**, 143–149.

Erdman, H. P., Klein, M. H. and Greist, J. H. (1983). Direct patient computer interviewing. *J. Consult. Clin. Psychol.* **53**, 760–773.

Garrety, P. A. and Morris, I. (1984). A new unit for long-stay psychiatric patients: organisation, attitudes and quality of care. Psychol. Med. **14**, 183–192.

Gibbons, J., Jennings, C. and Wing, J. K. (1983). Psychiatric care in 8 register areas. Statistics for 8 psychiatric case registers in Great Britain 1976–1981. Psychiatric case register, Knowle Hospital, Fareham, Hants.

Goldthorpe, J. and Hope, K. (1974). *The Social Grading of Occupations: A New Approach and Scale*, Oxford University Press, London.

Grad de Alarcon, J. and Crocetti, A. (1975). Interviewing in psychiatric field surveys. In *Methods of Psychiatric Research* (P. Sainsbury and N. Kreitman, eds), Oxford Medical Publications, London.

Hahlwag, K., Reisner, L., Kohli, G., Vollmer, M. and Schindler, L., Revenstorf, D. (1984). Development and validity of a new system to analyse interpersonal communication: Kategoriensystem fur partnerschaftliche Interaktion. In *Marital Interaction: Analysis Modification* (K. Hahlweg and N. S. Jacobson, eds), Guilford, New York.

Henderson, S., Byrne, D. G., Duncan-Jones, P., Adcock, S., Scott, R. and Steele, G. D. (1978). Social bonds in the epidemiology of neurosis: a preliminary communication. *Br. J. Psychiatry* **132**, 463–466.

Henderson, S., Byrne, D. G. and Duncan-Jones, P. (1981). *Neurosis and the Social Environment*, Academic Press, Sydney.

Holmes, T. H. and Rahe, R. H. (1967). The Social readjustment rating scale. *J. Psychosom. Res.* **11**, 213–218.

Hurry, J. and Sturt, E. (1981). Social performance in a population sample—Relation to psychiatric symptoms. In *What is a Case—The Problem of Definition in Psychiatric Community Surveys* (J. K. Wing *et al.*, eds), Grant McIntyre, London.

Jarman, B. (1983). Identification of underprivileged areas. *Br. Med. J.* **286**, 1705–1709.

Jenkins, R., Maurs, A. H. and Belsey, E. (1981). The background, design and use of a short interview to assess social stress and support in research and clinical settings. *Soc. Sci. Med.* **15**, 195–203.

Katschnig, H. (1986). Measuring life stress—a comparison of the checklist and the panel technique. In *Life Events and Psychiatric Disorders: Controversial Issues*, Cambridge University Press, Cambridge.

McFarlane, A. H., Neale, K. A., Norman, G. R., Roy, R. G. and Streiner, D. L. (1981). Methodological issues in developing a scale to measure social support. *Schizophr. Bull.* **7**, 90–100.

Monroe, S. M. and Steiner, C. (1986). Social support and psychopathology: interrelations with pre-existing disorder, stress and personality. *J. Abnorm. Psychol.* **95**, 29–39.

Murphy, E. (1982). Social origins of depression in old age. *Br. J. Psychiatry* **141**, 135–42.

Norbeck, J. S., Lindsey, A. M. and Carrieri, V. L. (1981). The development of an instrument to measure social support. *Nurs. Res.* **30**, 264–269.

O'Connor, P. and Brown, G. W. (1984). Supportive relationships: fact or fancy? *J. Pers. Soc. Relation.* **1** 159–175.

Oei, T. I. and Zwart, F. M. (1986). The assessment of life events: self administered questionnaire versus interview. **10**, 185–190.

Parry, G. and Shapiro, D. A. (1986). Social support and life events in working class women: stress buffering or independent effects? *Arch. Gen. Psychiatry* **43**, 315–323.

Patten, M. P. and Press, J. (1975). Sociological methods in psychiatric research. In *Methods of Psychiatric Research* (P. Sainsbury and N. Kreitman, eds), Oxford University Press, Oxford.

Paykel, E. S. (1983). Methodological aspects of life events research. *J. Psychosom. Res.* **27**, 341–352.

Paykel, E. S., Myers, J. K. *et al.* (1969). Life events and depression. *Arch. of Gen. Psychiatry* **21**, 753–760.

Paykel, E. S., Prusof, B. A. and Klerman, G. L. (1971). The endogenous–neurotic continuum: rater independence and factor distributions. *J. Psychiatr. Res.* **8**, 73–90.

Platt, S. (1985). Measuring the burden of psychiatric illness on the family: an evaluation of some rating scales. *Psychol. Med.* **15**, 383–393.

Platt, S., Weymann, A., Hirsh, S. and Hewett, S. (1980). The Social Behaviour Assessment Schedule (SBAS): Rationale, contents, scoring and reliability of a new interview schedule. *Soc. Psychiatry* **15**, 455.

Rahe, R. H., Meyer, M., Smith, M., Kjaer, G. and Holmes, T. H. (1964). Social stress and illness onset. *J. Psychosom. Res.* **8**, 35–44.

Rey, J. M., Stewart, G. W., Plapz, J. M., Bashir, M. R. and Richards, I. N. (1987). Sources of unreliability of DSM III Axis IV. *Aust. NZ J. Psychiatry* **21**, 75–80.

Sarason, I. G., Levine, H. M., Basham, R. B. and Sarason, B. R. (1983). Assessing social support: the social support questionnaire. *J. Pers. Soc. Psychol.* **44**, 127–139.

Smith, C. F. (1984). Geographical approaches to mental health. In *Mental Health and the Environment*, (H. Freeman, ed.), Churchill Livingstone, Edinburgh.

Spanier, G. B. (1976). Measuring dyadic adjustment: New scales for assessing the quality of marriage and similar dyads. *J. Marriage Family* **38**, 15–28.

Sturt, E. and Wykes, T. (1987). Assessment schedules for chronic psychiatric patients. *Psychol. Med.* **17**, 485–493.

Tennant, C. and Andrews, G. (1976). A scale to measure the stress of life events. *Aust. NZ J. Psychiatry* **10**, 27–32.

Tennant, C., Smith, A., Bebbington, P. and Hurry, J. (1979). The contextual threat of life events: the concept and its reliability. *Psychol. Med.* **9**, 525–528.

Vaughan, C. F. and Leff, J. P. (1976). The measurement of expressed emotion in families of psychiatric patients. *Br. J. Soc. Clin. Psychol.* **15**, 157–165.

Webb, S. D. (1984). Rural–urban differences in mental health. In *Mental Health and the Environment*, (H. Freeman, ed.), Churchill Livingstone, Edinburgh.

Weissman, M. M. (1975). The assessment of social adjustment: A review of techniques. *Arch. Gen. Psychiatry* **32**, 357–365.

Weissman, M. M., Klerman, G. L., Prusoff, B. A., Sholomskas, M. A. and Padian, N. (1981). Depressed outpatients—results one year after treatment with drugs and/or interpersonal psychotherapy. *Arch. Gen. Psychiatry* **38**, 51–55.

Wing, L. and Gould, J. (1978). Systematic recording of behaviours and skills of retarded and psychotic children. *J. Autism Child Schizophr.* **8**, 79–97.

Wing, J. K. and Sturt, P. (1978). *The PSE-ID-CATEGO System: Supplementary Manual* (mimeo), Institute of Psychiatry, London.

Wing, J. K., Cooper, J. E. and Sartorius, N. (1974). *Measurement and Classification of Psychiatric Symptoms*, Cambridge University Press, Cambridge.

Wykes, T. (1982). A hostel ward for 'new' long-term patients: an evaluative study of a 'ward in a house'. *Psychol. Med.* Monograph suppl. no. 2. (J. K. Freeman, ed.). Cambridge University Press, Cambridge.

The Instruments of Psychiatric Research
Edited by C. Thompson

CHAPTER 12

Structured assessments of psychopathology in children and adolescents

ADRIAN ANGOLD
Departure of Psychiatry,
Duke University Medical Centre,
Durham, North Carolina, USA

INTRODUCTION

The use of structured assessments of the psychiatric status of children and adolescents has expanded enormously over the last twenty years. There are now numerous questionnaires, interviews and observational rating schedules that provide means of collecting information of interest to the psychopathologist. While this burgeoning of instrumentation represents a number of important theoretical and methodological advances, it is also a source of considerable confusion to those not intimately concerned with the niceties of methodology. In this chapter I will, therefore, concentrate on developing a strategy for selecting assessment instruments for what DSM-III/III-R (American Psychiatric Association, 1980, 1987) and ICD-9/10 (World Health Organization, 1978, 1987; Rutter *et al.*, 1975c) would call the Axis I clinical psychiatric syndromes, before presenting details of some of the most important interviews and questionnaires themselves. Further extensive discussions of many important assessment issues and evaluations of a variety of measures are to be found in recent books by Achenbach (1985), Frame and Matson (1987) and Rutter *et al.* (1988), but it should be borne in mind that the field is developing very rapidly, and that there is no substitute for discussing each individual assessment problem with someone familiar with these developments.

A STRATEGY FOR SELECTING A STRUCTURED ASSESSMENT INSTRUMENT

In presenting a strategy for selecting measures of psychopathology in young people I have focused on a series of eight questions that need to be answered in designing an assessment package. Not surprisingly, these questions relate both to scientific issues, in terms of clarifying the research problem conceptually, and practical concerns, relating to what can feasibly be done given the resources at the researchers' disposal.

Question 1: Is Pathology Really the Subject of Interest?

It is first necessary to decide whether 'pathology' as such should be the focus of attention at all. It will often be the case that behaviours, mental states or competencies within the normal range will be of interest, as, for instance in assessing the effects of environmental lead levels on IQ (Lansdown and Yule, 1986), in documenting the effects of children's temperamental traits, or studying the vicissitudes of self-esteem or the sense of self-competence. I will not discuss the assessment of self-esteem in detail here, except to note that the most widely used measures are the Piers–Harris Children's Self-concept Scale (Piers and Harris, 1969; Piers, 1977), and the Harter Perceived Competence Scale (1982). Closely related themes are also explored in the learned helplessness paradigm of Seligman and his co-workers, who have developed the Children's Attributional Style Questionnaire (CASQ; Seligman *et al.*, 1984; Seligman and Peterson, 1986).

Similarly, this chapter is not the place to focus on the details of temperament research, but informative reviews of methodological and conceptual issues in the area can be found in Rutter (1982) and Berger (1985a, pp. 6–14).

In studies of concepts such as these, effects on normal developmental processes (like the development of the self-concept in relation to factors such as parental psychopathology or adverse life events) may be the main subject of interest, and a focus on overtly pathological states may be only a secondary concern. Alternatively, the research may seek to investigate the relationship between the individual's status in a particular area of development and some sort of psychopathology (such as the relationship between self-concept and depression). Since only limited amounts of subject and researcher time are usually available, it is important to ensure that what are often very lengthy assessments of psychopathology do not use up precious resources that would be better spent on areas of more central interest.

One might also not wish to measure Axis I symptomatology because it is sometimes the case that early markers of psychiatric disturbance differ in form from the adult expression of the disorder. The most striking example relates to schizophrenia, where attentional, information processing, autonomic and social functioning deficits, which do not conform well to any current diagnostic categories, have been extensively implicated as childhood markers of vulnerability to schizophrenia (Nuechterlein, 1986), while full-blown childhood schizophrenia itself is very rare. This leads to the obvious point that any assessments that are made need to be tailored to the developmental level of the children under investigation, and that existing assessments of psychopathology may not always offer the proper tools for studying links with well-recognized adult disorders.

Projective tests have also been used in the assessment of child psychopathology, but do not directly address Axis I symptomatology. The research literature in this area also indicates that the interpretation of such tests is highly problematic, and often not very revealing, so they will not be considered further here. Reviews of the relevant literature are available in Gittelman-Klein (1978), Gittelman (1980) and French *et al.* (1983).

Question 2: What Sort of Pathology?

I wish to distinguish six broad areas of pathology that are of particular concern to developmental pathologists:

1. Psychiatric syndromes
2. Specific delays in development
3. Intellectual level
4. Impairments of psychosocial functioning
5. Problems in family functioning
6. Adverse environmental conditions

These distinctions, amongst others, are embodied in both the ICD-9/10 and DSM-III/III-R nosologies, and although there is considerable conceptual overlap between them it is important to try to clarify early on which areas are to be investigated, since the approaches best fitted to each differ in important respects.

Psychiatric syndromes refer here to material that is mostly covered by Axis I in both the ICD and DSM nosologies. This area is the central concern of this chapter, and it will be considered in detail below.

The *specific delays in development*, such as specific reading retardation, are a group of disorders which are often associated with Axis I psychiatric conditions, but which also often occur separately. These developmental delays are of particular importance from the educational point of view, and whilst the mechanisms by which they arise are unclear, age-specific population norms for attainments in these areas are available, and widely consulted. Discussions of the assessment of language delay can be found in Yule and Rutter (1987), while Gittelman (1985), French *et al.* (1983) and Schloss *et al.* (1987) provide information on a number of tests of academic performance.

Intellectual level is usually measured with a standardized IQ test, of which the best known are the Stanford–Binet (Terman and Merrill, 1973) and the Wechsler Intelligence Scale for Children—Revised (WISC–R; Wechsler, 1974). In this field, as in many others, training, skill and experience in the proper mode of administration of each test are necessities that are all too often ignored in the hurly-burly of study design and proposal writing. In planning to use these or other assessments it is necessary to be sure that sufficient staff, with suitable experience, will be available to the study, or that adequate training facilities can be provided.

Impairment of psychosocial functioning is regarded by some as being almost a *sine qua non* for the diagnosis of a psychiatric disorder, since disorders of insufficient severity to cause some problems in school or peer relationships, or the like, will often seem to be of little clinical significance. On the other hand, a child may manifest poor peer and teacher relationships that significantly interfere with his/her development, without conforming to any Axis I category. Furthermore, one might be interested in examining psychosocial impairment regardless of its causes, in which case assessments of Axis I symptomatology would be irrelevant. Until recently, there have been rather few instruments for the systematic evaluation of the social aspects of psychopathology in young people (Achenbach and Edelbrock, 1981; Boyle and Chambers, 1981; Orvaschel and Walsh, 1984), but this situation seems to be changing. DSM-III-R Axis 5 consists of a Global Assessment of Functioning scale, and a version of this scale for use with 4- to 16-year-olds, called the Children's Global Assessment Schedule (CGAS) has been developed by Shaffer and his colleagues (Shaffer et al., 1983; Bird *et al.*, 1987b). This measure seems likely to figure much more widely in research in the next five years. It is a single scale, for completion by a clinician, that provides anchoring descriptions of functioning for ten point ranges, beginning with 100–91, which describes superior functioning in all areas, and ending at 10–1, which involves the need for constant supervision, because of aggressive or self-destructive behaviour, impaired reality testing or communication, or failure to maintain personal hygiene. The severity and nature of the symptomatology that the child is manifesting and the degree of psychosocial impairment that it has resulted in are therefore assessed simultaneously. This could be a strength when direct measures of Axis I disorders are not available, but may be unhelpful when they are. The CGAS demands that the rater exercise a good deal of clinical judgement, following a complete clinical assessment of the child, but requires only minimal specific training, takes little time to complete, and has shown good test–retest stability and inter-rater reliability. A study of five second-year child psychiatry fellows who rated 19 written case vignettes twice, at an interval of 6 months, found an intraclass correlation coefficient (ICC)[1] of 0.84, representing the agreement between raters at the first rating of the vignettes and an ICC of 0.85 for agreement between the initial ratings and the re-ratings 6 months later. A group of in-patients were rated significantly worse on the CGAS than a group of out-patients, but the limited description of this part of the study makes the interpretation of this finding difficult (Shaffer *et al.*, 1983). A further study of ratings of case vignettes from Berlin (Steinhausen, 1987) found good agreement amongst four raters (ICC = 0.93), but rather poorer stability of ratings when the same cases were represented 6–8 weeks later. In this case coefficients of agreement ranged from 0.22 (not significant) for a vignette describing a child with an emotional disturbance to 0.85 for one describing an enuretic child. However, the number of raters used in this study was small, and it is not clear exactly how these stability values were arrived at.

Good inter-rater reliability was also found by Bird *et al.* (1987b), who reported an ICC of 0.83 between psychiatrists who had interviewed 91 subjects and their parents using the Diagnostic Interview Schedule for Children (DISC; see below).

Further re-ratings of 46 videotapes of these interviews by two more psychiatrists yielded ICCs of 0.87 and 0.86. These authors also found high correlations between the Child Behaviour Check-list (CBCL) Total Problem score (around 0.6) and the CBCL Social Competence Score (around 0.6 in those over age 6 years) and the CGAS. Furthermore the CGAS scores of children with DISC diagnosis were much lower (i.e. worse) than those with insufficient symptomatology to warrant a diagnosis. These findings strongly suggest that the CGAS does indeed reliably tap important aspects of the child's overall clinical state. However, it should be remembered that the CGAS was completed by clinicians who had conducted or witnessed an extensive clinical interview with the child and a parent, so that the reliability

[1] Footnote on the measurement of agreement.
The Intra-class Correlation Coefficient (ICC; Bartko and Carpenter, 1976) is a statistic based upon analysis of variance that addresses the absolute level of agreement between raters using a scale. It is superior to simple correlation coefficients for this purpose because it takes into account both the ordering of individual subjects and the absolute levels of their scores in quantifying the level of agreement. The agreement statistic now most commonly employed when categorical judgements are being made is kappa (κ) (Cohen, 1960, 1968). Kappa takes into account the level of agreement that might be expected by chance, given the base rate of the categories of interest in the population being studied. It is thus preferable to use kappa, rather than percentage agreement between raters, since the latter makes no allowance for the effects of chance agreement (see Shrout *et al.*, 1987, for a recent discussion of this topic). There are no fixed rules as to what constitutes good agreement, but ICCs or kappas above 0.6 would usually be considered satisfactory (although levels approaching unity are the goal), while levels of less than 0.4 would be considered definitely unsatisfactory.

being measured here is really that of the CGAS completed on the basis of a structured interview. How it would perform in less structured settings (such as an ordinary out-patient clinic) remains to be seen. It also seems likely that if extensive interview and questionnaire data are already available from a study, then little will be added by completing the CGAS as well. However, one might set against this fact that it can be seen as an operationalization of DSM-III-R's Axis 5, and will thus generate data of interest to those working towards the production of DSM-IV, amongst others.

Much more detailed codings of a number of areas of functioning are provided by the Social Adjustment Inventory for Children and Adolescents (SAICA; John *et al.*, 1987). This interview-based measure, which takes about 20 minutes to complete and exists in parallel forms for use with children and their parents, is probably the best available measure of social adjustment, for use in psychiatric studies.

The interview provides School functioning, Spare-time functioning, Peer interaction, Heterosexual interaction, Sibling interaction and Parental interaction subscales, which consist of items relating to activities, relationships and problems in each area. The authors state that only 4 hours of training were required for those with a higher degree and experience to achieve 95% agreement on individual and global items through co-rating interviews. The subscales mostly show moderate correlations (0.3–0.6) with the total score. Mothers' and children's reports were quite highly correlated (correlation coefficients around 0.7 for the most part), with the children tending to rate themselves less positively for the most part. The SAICA total scores were also quite highly correlated with the CBCL social competence scores ($r=0.64$ for the parental SAICA reports). There were also moderate correlations with the CGAS (0.46 and 0.52 for the parent and child report, respectively), but the two measures cover rather different material, with the SAICA being more directly focused on social functioning, so very high agreement would not be expected. Children who were suffering from a psychiatric disorder (as measured by the kiddie-SADS-E, see below) had significantly worse SAICA scores than those who were not.

All in all, the SAICA shows promise for the future; it could be used as a stand-alone instrument (given to either parents or children) or in association with measures of Axis I symptomatology to flesh out the assessment of clinical psychiatric syndromes. Its structure is especially suited for addition to other semi-structured interview assessments. A questionnaire version for group administration is also available, and normative data on over 900 English and American 8–18 year-old children are currently being collected.

Two further instruments that provide information about social functioning are the Child Behaviour Check-list and the Child and Adolescent Psychiatric Assessment, which will be discussed further below.

Problems of family functioning are of great interest to developmental pathologists, and some would see analyses at this level as being critical for understanding child psychopathology. There are a great number of assessments of family pathology, and space will not permit a detailed discussion of them here. However, discussions of a range of approaches can be found in Quinton *et al.* (1976), Rutter and Quinton (1984), Vaughan and Leff (1976), Doane (1978), Doane *et al.* (1981) and Jacob and Tennenbaum (1988).

There is overwhelming evidence that *environmental conditions*, by which I mean negative life events and chronic life difficulties, are associated with psychiatric disorder, and Axis 5 of ICD-9/10 and Axis IV of DSM-III-R address the presence and severity of psychosocial stressors.

All the problems of measurement of adult acute life events and chronic difficulties (see e.g. Katschnig, 1986 or Zimmerman, 1983 for reviews) apply to children, with the added complication that events may have different implications and meanings for children than they do for adults (Johnson, 1986). A comparative review of a number of check-list measures of life stress in childhood and adolescence is provided by Johnson (1986) while Goodyer *et al.* (1985), Monck and Dobbs (1985) and Sandberg *et al.* (1987) have developed measures of life events and chronic life difficulties that attempt to deal with the problem of independence of life stresses and psychiatric disorder.

Question 3: What Model of Psychopathology?

Assuming that psychopathology is indeed to be the central focus of the research, then the question of what theoretical model of psychopathology is to be employed. Broadly speaking there are two main traditions to choose from:

1. The continuous–empirical tradition
2. The categorical–diagnostic tradition

In essence the decision is whether or not to make Axis I diagnoses. The continuous–empirical tradition (see e.g. Achenbach and Edelbrock, 1978) has tended to focus scores on continuous scales and to define psychopathology in terms of quantitative deviation from empirically determined population means. Scales conceived in this tradition can offer symptom counts, overall disturbance scores, various types of subscale scores and sometimes cluster-analytically derived diagnostic groupings.

Measures of this sort are typically questionnaires for completion by teachers, parents or the children themselves. Extensive population norms may be available, and a real strength of such measures is that an individual child's performance can be referenced to such norms. However, such measures usually cannot provide Axis I diagnoses, and are indeed often based on a model of psychiatric disorder that is at some variance to the current DSM and ICD nosologies. On the other hand, there is evidence of considerable overlap between the diagnostic concepts of these two traditions (Edelbrock and Costello, 1988b), and combinations of the two approaches may prove superior to an exclusive reliance on only one.

The categorical–diagnostic tradition proceeds by the delineation of clinical disorders in a descriptive sense, and the diagnostic process thus consists of determining whether a child conforms to a particular description or not. Two related types of 'diagnosis-fitting' process are used, which I will call the heuristic and the algorithmic methods. In the former (as espoused in ICD-9) the clinician is called upon to decide which single diagnostic description best fits the child. The second form, best exemplified by DSM-III/III-R, demands that symptoms be evaluated and counted, and that when a certain number of symptoms of a disorder are present, the diagnosis is allotted. Thus in the child psychiatric field, multiple diagnoses will often prove to be applicable to a single individual.

The relatively complex nature of the symptom judgements required for making such diagnoses, which often require the evaluation of quantitative and qualitative deviation from normality, duration and frequency of occurrence, usually mean that interviews are required for making Axis I diagnoses. There has been a powerful swing towards categorical diagnostic evaluations over the last decade or so, which has brought with it a flush of new interviews. In most cases these are a good deal more time-consuming than the continuous–empirical instruments, and often necessitate the use of highly trained interviewers. Assessments of this sort will therefore almost always prove more expensive than continuous–empirical counterparts.

Question 4: What Sources of Information?

Until recently it was customary to place most weight on adult reports of children's behaviour and psychiatric problems (e.g. Rutter *et al.*, 1970). However, it has emerged that adults are not very good informants about some aspects of their children's mental states. In general, parents often seem to have only limited knowledge of their children's internal mental states, and to report less in the way of depressive and anxiety symptoms than their children would report. In effect parents seem to be relatively insensitive to their children's internalizing symptoms (Edelbrock *et al.*, 1985; Angold *et al.*, 1987). On the other hand adults seem to be the better informants about many externalizing or conduct disorder items, such as fighting or disobedience (Edelbrock *et al.*, 1985). The best adult informant for these items will be the one who has most contact with the child in the setting of interest. Thus teachers are good informants about school behaviour and performance, while parents are more informative about home life.

Very high levels of agreement between informants cannot be expected (Weissman *et al.*, 1987; Angold *et al.*, 1987), with the result that some workers submit all the diagnostic material to one or more raters, who then produce an overall 'best estimate' diagnosis (see e.g. Weissman *et al.*, 1984). This procedure at least produces a single diagnosis for each child, but the weighting of the information from different sources is left to the individual best estimator, with the result that some of the advantages of using a structured assessment are lost in the unstructured best-estimating process.

Much more work needs to be done on methods of combining information from different informants, but a start has been made towards formalizing this process (Reich and Earls, 1987), and it is probable that further methodological advances will be forthcoming in this area in the near future (see also Hoier and Kerr, 1988, for further discussion of the use of extrafamilial sources of information).

Question 5: Broad-band or Narrow-band Assessment?

Broad-band measures are those that produce an overall rating of psychiatric disturbance or cover a broad range of specific diagnostic categories. Many broad-band measures contain subscales that provide scores or diagnoses in specific symptom subareas. With continuous measures, these subscales have often been derived from factor or cluster analyses of normal and/or psychiatrically disturbed populations, while with categorical diagnostic measures the subscales will usually be operationalizations of one of the standard nosological systems (DSM-III/R, or its congeners, or ICD-9/10). Broad-band measures are obviously useful for studies that are not aimed at investigating a specific pathology, or where diagnostic heterogeneity is to be expected, as, for example, in studies of the children of psychiatrically disturbed parents, or studies of the psychiatric sequelae of adverse life events (see e.g. Beardslee *et al.*, 1983; Goodyer *et al.*, 1985).

Narrow-band measures will be appropriate when individual psychiatric disorders are the focus of interest (as in studies of the aetiology of depression). The assessment of autism and the related pervasive developmental disorders is an example of a special area where very highly focused narrow-band assessment is required. An introduction to the assessment of autism can be found in Rutter and Schopler (1988). These authors recommend, for specific diagnostic purposes, a combination of a detailed standardized parental interview specifically designed to elicit the key features of autism (e.g. Wing and Gould, 1978, or Le Couteur *et al.*, 1988), and a standardized observation system, such as the Childhood Autism Rating Scale (Schopler *et al.*, 1986) or the Autism Diagnostic Observation Schedule (Lord *et al.*, 1988).

Of course, mixtures of narrow- and broad-band measures may be indicated, and may offer a useful compromise when assessment resources are scarce. For instance, in a study primarily of anxiety disorders, one might employ a relatively time-consuming structured interview to evaluate anxiety, but use a simple parental report scale to provide broad coverage of a range of other symptoms.

Question 6: How Will the Information Be Collected?

There are four basic choices in answer to this question:

1. By self-report questionnaire
2. By interview
3. By observation
4. By testing

Each of these options has advantages and disadvantages, and often a combination of techniques will be necessary.

Self-report questionnaires are usually relatively quick and easy to complete, and may be suitable for group administration, which means that very large numbers of subjects can be processed in settings where they congregate, such as schools. For some of the available questionnaires quite extensive normative data are available, so that the results of any new study can be compared with those of the normative studies, which is often helpful for interpretive purposes.

Unaided self-completion of a questionnaire obviously requires a reasonable level of literacy on the part of a subject, and this may be a particular problem with young subjects. It can, however, be overcome by having someone read the questions out.

On the other hand, the form of these questionnaires means that they usually do not produce categorical diagnoses according to the DSM or ICD nosologies. They also rely upon the subject's understanding of the question being asked, and do not allow any room for explanation or clarification. Since there is no opportunity for cross-questioning or detailed exploration of the nature of the symptoms reported, it seems likely that sometimes non-pathological material will be reported in answer to questions aimed at eliciting psychopathology (Angold, 1988), while some people with high thresholds for reporting may fail to acknowledge material that a clinician would regard as being highly significant. However, in spite of this, the most widely used self-reports have usually been repeatedly shown to distinguish clinically disordered subjects from non-disordered subjects, so for many purposes they may be quite satisfactory.

Interviews represent the standard method of making Axis I phenomenological diagnoses, since they represent an operationalization of ordinary clinical practice. Direct interviews usually take longer than questionnaires, and often require clinical skills from the interviewer. Interviewers will also need to have completed a specific training course in the use of the interview. All of those drawbacks will often be offset, however, by the fact that an interview may be the only available way to collect some sorts of detailed information, since subjects will tolerate relatively long interviews much better than very long questionnaires (Edelbrock and Costello, 1988a). Furthermore, most interviews adopt a screen/skip structure to speed administration and to avoid seemingly endless series of tedious negatives. For instance, detailed questions about depressive symptoms may only be asked if screening questions about depressed mood are answered in the affirmative. If depressed mood proves to be absent, then the interviewer skips to the next part of the interview. This sort of flexibility allows very extensive areas of symptomatology to be covered efficiently, in a way that is really not feasible with questionnaires.

Another major source of information is direct *observation*. A number of the semi-structured interview schedules contain codings for observations of mental status. There is also enormous scope for making observations of school behaviour, family life and peer interactions. However, the development of coding schemes is a highly technical affair, and direct observations will always be very labour intensive, and therefore expensive. Any observational study will need expert consultation from someone well versed in these issues (see Bakeman and Gottman, 1987; Gettinger and Kratochwill, 1987; Sackett, 1987; Reid *et al.*, 1988) for a discussion of many of the major points).

I have already commented upon the place of formal *testing* in the assessment of IQ and the specific developmental delays (see also Berger, 1985b), and Tupper (1986), Teeter (1986) and Stoddart and Knights (1986) review a variety of neuropsychological test batteries for children, and so I will not consider this area further here.

Question 7: What Sort of Interview?

If the decision to use an interview is made, then it will be necessary to decide what sort of interview will be most appropriate. There are two basic types of structured interview, which are nowadays usually called 'fully structured' (or 'highly structured' or just 'structured') and 'semi-structured' (some authors use other terms; see e.g. Richardson *et al.*, 1965). This distinction is important in that it encapsulates rather different approaches to the collection of information. In the fully structured interview, the interviewer directs a series of questions to the interviewee, which should be delivered verbatim. Such interviews have the advantage that the variability due to differences in the phrasing of questions is reduced, and, so long as the interview is properly conducted, one knows exactly what has been asked of each subject. If such interviews are to work well, the questions need to be very carefully phrased to be suitable for use with children of varying ages, but once good questions have been prepared the interviewers need relatively little training, and do not need to be clinically experienced (Edelbrock and Costello, 1988a). The disadvantage here is that, in general, one has simply to accept the interviewee's assessment of whether a symptom is present or not, and each interviewee may be using a scale of symptom severity different from that employed in clinical practice, or simply misunderstanding the intention of the questions (see Breslau *et al.*, 1987 for an example). When instructions to ask unspecified clarifying questions, when in doubt about the validity of the answer to a previous question, are included in the rubric of the interview, then the opportunity for variations in interview content become greater, with a consequent loss of some of the advantages of the highly structured format.

Semi-structured interviews employ a rather different approach to standardizing information collection; the interviewer is expected to pursue questioning until he or she has determined whether or not a particular symptom or behaviour is present, according to a pre-specified glossary definition. Quite detailed questions will often be provided on the interview schedule, but the interviewer is expected to use whatever questioning seems necessary to come to a fine decision as to the presence or absence of symptoms. Thus, the semi-structured interview can be seen as a 'questionnaire' directed to the interviewer about the subject, while the fully structured interview is aimed directly at the subject. Not surprisingly, therefore, semi-structured interviews usually call for more highly clinically qualified (and therefore more expensive) interviewers, and greater amounts of specific interview training, before the interviewer is ready to begin fieldwork. The advantage of this approach lies in the fact that complex judgements may be explored more fully, and the final coding may be more confidently seen as reflecting clinical severity judgements. On the other hand, if careful attention is not paid to interviewer standardization, interviewers will gradually diverge in their interviewing styles, so that rather different information will be collected by each one. Thus continuous monitoring of interviewer performance is really required if semi-structured interviews are to be used.

One problem with many of the interviews to be reviewed below is that they are tied to a single nosological system, usually DSM-III or DSM-III-R. This means that only a subset of the symptoms that might be considered relevant to a particular diagnosis will be included, since those items that are not required for making a DSM diagnosis will be missed out. Items can always be added, but there will be no information about the reliability of the new items unless it is provided by the investigator who is using the instrument.

Question 8: What Time-frame Should Be Covered?

The answer to this question will greatly affect the range of instruments available. For instance, there are few measures that are designed to generate lifetime diagnoses of the sort that are required for most family-genetic studies. At the other end of the spectrum, if an instrument to measure change is required, then its time-frame should be relatively short. Sometimes two different measures may be required; for instance, a diagnostic interview that covers the preceding year may be used to establish the presence or absence of depression during that period, while a questionnaire covering the previous 2 weeks is used as a measure of current mood, prior to some intervention.

RATING SCALES AND CHECK-LISTS

I will review here only a small group of the available rating scales and check-lists for child psychopathology (further useful information is available in Barkley, 1988). These will usually be those that have been most widely used or researched, or which offer features that are otherwise not widely available. With respect to the broad-based questionnaires, those that are available probably fulfil most needs for a questionnaire of this sort as far as parent and teacher reports are concerned, but child self-reports have been much less adequately investigated. This situation is beginning to change, with the appearance of a child-completed version of the Child Behaviour Check-list.

Child Behaviour Check-list (CBCL)

The CBCL is a 138-item scale for use with 4–16-year-olds (although normative data on 2–3-year-olds have recently appeared (Achenbach *et al.*, 1987a)). It is available in forms for completion by parents, teachers and children themselves (Achenbach, 1966; Achenbach, 1978; Achenbach and Edelbrock, 1979; Edelbrock and Achenbach, 1980; Achenbach and Edelbrock, 1981; Achenbach *et al.*, 1987b), and assesses both a wide range of pathological behaviours (118 items) and the child's social competence (20 items in the parent version). It is probably the currently most widely used instrument of its kind. The teacher's report form does not contain some items, such as nightmares, that teachers cannot be expected to know about. These are replaced by questions about school behaviour. Each item refers to the preceding 6 months and is scored on a 0–1–2 scale (0 = not true; 1 = somewhat or sometimes true; 2 = very true or often true). It takes 15–30 minutes to complete.

The social competence scale provides information about spare-time activities, social life and school life, and from this age- and sex-specific profile scores can then be derived. One-week test–retest stability for the social competence scale was in excess of 0.99 (ICC) in a study of 72 mothers of non-referred children (Achenbach and Edelbrock, 1981) while 3-month stability was 0.927. Inter-interviewer reliability, computed from CBCLs obtained by three interviewers on 241 triads of children, was 0.927. However, somewhat lower test–retest stability was reported from a study of 104 Dutch children (ICC = 0.77) with interviews conducted 3–4 weeks apart (Verhulst *et al.*, 1985a).

The test–retest stability for the behaviour problems scales was similarly gratifying, with values of 0.95 and 0.75 being reported from the American and Dutch studies, respectively, for the parent-completed version. A test–retest study of teacher reports on 22 children completed 3–4 weeks apart resulted in an intra-class correlation coefficient of 0.84 (Verhulst *et al.*, 1985a).

High levels of inter-parent agreement have also been obtained, with ICCs on the behaviour problem scale and social competence scale being 0.97 and 0.98, respectively, in the US sample and 0.70 and 0.69 from the Dutch sample.

Large population surveys from the US (N=1,442) and Holland (N=2439) have provided valuable normative data on the frequencies of individual items in the general population, and these are broadly similar in these two countries (Achenbach and Edelbrock, 1981; Verhulst *et al.*, 1985a and b; Achenbach *et al.*, 1987c and d). CBCLs filled out by the parents of children being seen in child mental health settings were factor-analysed to yield separate problem profiles for girls and boys in age groups 4–5, 6–11 and 12–16 years (Achenbach, 1978; Achenbach and Edelbrock, 1979; Edelbrock and Achenbach, 1980; Achenbach and Edelbrock, 1981). Two higher-order factors, which Achenbach and Edelbrock labelled 'internalizing' and 'externalizing', emerged while eight to nine somewhat varying lower-order factors ranging from delinquency to schizoid behaviour appeared for each of the age and sex groups. It should be noted that the test–retest stabilities and levels of inter-parental agreement on the individual factor scores are sometimes much lower than those reported above for total scores.

The CBCL has been shown to be predictive of scores on other well-established continuous measures of psychopathology (Barkley, 1988) and also to predict psychiatric disorders as measured by both highly structured (Costello *et al.*, 1985) and semi-structured (Verhulst *et al.*, 1985b) interviews with parents and, in the latter case, the children themselves.

In summary, the wide item coverage of the CBCL, its availability in parent, teacher and child forms, its easy administration, good standardization and widespread use, make it a very attractive instrument for many purposes. However, as a screening instrument for two-stage studies, it is probably unnecessarily long, and its performance in this area (Verhulst *et al.*, 1985a; Bird *et al.*, 1987a) does not suggest that it is better than a much shorter and more quickly completed instrument like the Rutter A and B scales (Boyle and Jones, 1985). The parent version and the teacher report form share with the Rutter scales the property of predicting disorder better in combination than when used separately.

Conners Rating Scales (CRS)

The very widely used Conners Parent and Teacher Rating Scales each exist in at least three forms: Original (93 and 39 items, respectively (Conners, 1969, 1973)); Revised (49 and 28 items, respectively (Goyette *et al.*, 1978)); and Abbreviated (ten items in each case (Goyette *et al.*, 1978)). Each item is rated on a four-point (0–3) scale ('not at all', 'just a little', 'pretty much', 'very much') (Conners, 1985).

All of these scales are weighted towards the conduct disorders and hyperactivity, and the Revised and Abbreviated forms are only suitable for assessing externalizing spectrum disorders. The various forms require between 3 and 15 minutes for completion. The original form is intended for use with 6–14 year-olds, while the Revised and Abbreviated versions are designed for use with 3–17 year-olds.

Overall test–retest stabilities have usually been satisfactory, ranging from around 0.7 to 0.9 over a 1-month interval, but with a good deal of variation across the factor scores (Conners, 1973; O'Connor *et al.*, 1980). Higher test–retest stabilities have been found for the teacher Revised scale over 1 week (0.97 for the total score).

To make matters still more complicated, several forms of the Abbreviated scales exist, although Conners recommends the use of that reported in Goyette *et al.* (1978). The Iowa Conners Teacher Rating Scale (Loney and Milich, 1981; Milich *et al.*, 1980) is a ten-item scale consisting of supposedly pure hyperactivity and aggressivity items.

Inter-teacher agreements for the original teacher scale have been very different for different factors, ranging from 0.09 to 0.89 (Trites *et al.*, 1981; Trites *et al.*, 1982). The lower levels of agreement have been over factors reflecting emotional or internalizing problems. Agreement between parents and teachers has been reported as around 0.3–0.4.

Inter-rater reliabilities for the factors of the parent Revised scale ranged from 0.46 to 0.57 (product–moment correlations), while inter-parent agreement was between 0.55 and 0.71 (Mash and Johnston, 1983).

Very substantial normative data from a number of countries exist for the original teacher form of the questionnaire for children aged 4–12, but the factor structures reported by these different groups are variable, which makes generalization difficult.

On the other hand, only limited normative data are available for the Original parent form, while Goyette *et al.* (1978) provide data on 570 3–7 year-old children on whom Revised parent evaluations were collected.

A mass of evidence supports the ability of these scales, in their various forms, to distinguish hyperactive and conduct disordered children from normal children and those with other psychiatric disturbances. They correlate with other measures of conduct disorder and hyperactivity and observational measures of classroom behaviour (see Barkley, 1988 for references). There is also evidence that they are sensitive to treatment effects in hyperactivity. In this latter respect, it should be noted that there is a marked practice effect with repeated administrations of the questionnaires (Ullman *et al.*, 1985), and Conners suggests that the scale should be administered at least twice before assessing treatment effects.

Behaviour Problem Check-list (BPC)

The Behaviour Problem Check-list is the third of the triad of widely disseminated and extensively investigated broad-band instruments. It exists in Original (Quay and Peterson, 1975; Quay, 1977) and Revised (Quay, 1983; Quay and Peterson, 1983, 1984; Aman *et al.*, 1983; Aman and Werry, 1984) forms, but in this case the revision resulted in a lengthening from 55 to 89 items. This revision was undertaken to expand coverage of hyperactivity and psychotic behaviour and to improve the psychometric properties of some of the shorter subscales. This Revised version is the one that should now be used, since the original is no longer supported by its authors.

Each behaviour is rated by a parent or teacher or other adult in close contact with the child on a 0–1–2 scale ('not a problem', 'mild problem', 'serious problem'). It takes 15–20 minutes to complete, and is designed for use with 5–15-year-olds.

The original version had good test–retest stability (0.7–0.9 for the factor scores), although inter-informant variability has been greater (Barkley, 1988). Very extensive evidence supports the BPC's use as a measure of psychopathology, and particularly externalizing disorders. It has also been found to be responsive to treatment effects following psychotherapy and stimulant medication (see Barkley, 1988 for references).

Evidence is emerging that the Revised scale has adequate test–retest stability (coefficients 0.49–0.83 for the subscales) and shows reasonable inter-teacher and inter-parent agreement (0.52–0.85 and 0.55–0.93, respectively), and it differentiates clinic and normal children (Aman and Werry, 1984). The factor structure seems similar in US and New Zealand samples (Aman *et al.*, 1983), and there are now said to be four 'major' scales of the RBPC measuring Conduct disorder, Socialized aggression, Attention problems, Immaturity and Anxiety–Withdrawal, while two 'minor' scales measure Psychotic behaviour and Motor excess.

The RBPC does not seem to have any really significant advantages over the Revised Conners scale if conduct disorder or hyperactivity are the areas of interest, and much more psychometric information is available for the Conners at this stage, but if psychotic behaviour is to be measured then it may be useful (although perhaps an interview is more appropriate for the adequate assessment of psychosis). However, if emotional disorders are a real focus of interest then the CBCL seems to be indicated, since neither the Conners nor the RBPC really cover this area very well. The additional length of the CBCL is the price that has to be paid for broader coverage.

If an instrument is to be used for screening purposes and only crude delineation of the type of pathology is required then the Rutter A (2) (parent) and Rutter B (2) (teacher) (Rutter, 1967; Rutter *et al.*, 1970) scales still have a place in the assessment armamentarium for children in middle childhood or adolescence. The parent version consists of 18 items in three different formats, while the teacher version consists of 26 items in a 0–1–2 response format ('doesn't apply', 'applies somewhat', 'certainly applies'). Population data on large samples are available (Rutter *et al.*, 1970; Rutter *et al.*, 1975a and b; Rutter *et al.*, 1976) and test–retest reliability is adequate, with a product–moment correlation of 0.74 over a 2-month interview for 83 maternal ratings. Inter-parent agreement is reasonable (r=0.64 for 35 parent pairs) (Rutter *et al.*, 1970; Zimmerman-Tansella *et al.*, 1978). The scale discriminates between neurotic and antisocial disorders, and predicts the presence of psychiatric disorder (as measured by interview). However, as its author points out, these scales probably under-identify disorder (and particularly emotional disorder), especially in adolescents (Rutter *et al.*, 1976).

When emotional disorders are the central focus of interest and there is no need to collect information about conduct problems, there is rather a dearth of well-standardized instruments. However, there are a variety of scales for depression and anxiety, usually based on adult models. Notable features in this area are that these scales have often been more recently developed, and that they provide child self-report forms. Indeed, it would seem unwise at this stage to conduct studies of emotional or internalizing disorders without including some child self-report measures.

Scales to measure childhood and adolescent depression have recently been the subject of at least two recent reviews (Costello, 1986; Costello and Angold, 1988), and so only two instruments will be briefly mentioned here.

Children's Depression Inventory (CDI)

The Children's Depression Inventory (Kovaks, 1983) is the best-known depression scale. This 27-item self-report questionnaire for 7–17 year-olds presents three statements describing each symptom at three different levels of intensity from 'not a problem' to 'severe', and covers a time-frame of the previous 2 weeks, taking 10–20 minutes to complete. This format seems to demand a greater effort of memory than is required by most of the other questionnaires in this area, and this might be a problem for younger children. The CDI covers quite a broad range of depressive symptoms, although not all of those included in the DSM or ICD definitions of depression. Satisfactory test–retest stability over 9 weeks of 0.84 (product–moment correlation) has been reported. However, there are conflicting findings over the CDI's ability to distinguish between clinically referred and normal children, and between depressed and non-depressed referred children (Costello and Angold, 1988).

Mood and Feelings Questionnaire (MFQ)

The Mood and Feelings Questionnaire (Angold *et al.*, 1988) is a new 32-item questionnaire that covers all the symptoms of depression mentioned in ICD-10 and DSM-III and DSM-III-R and employs a simple 0–1–2 ('true'; 'sometimes', 'not true') response scale. It exists in both parent and child report versions, and the child version has been found to have good test–retest stability, in a study of 20 adolescent psychiatric in-patients (Spearman coefficient = 0.81). However, as has been noted with other scales and interviews, there is a fall in scores between the first and second administration. It has been found to discriminate between psychiatrically referred and non-referred children, and to distinguish between children with high depression scores according to the Diagnostic Interview Schedule for Children (Angold *et al.*, 1988).

Revised Children's Manifest Anxiety Scale (RCMAS)

The Revised Children's Manifest Anxiety Scale (Reynolds and Paget, 1981, 1983; Reynolds, 1982) is a 37-item yes/no self-rating scale, which yields three narrow-band anxiety factors (physiological, worry/oversensitivity and concentration), and a total anxiety factor. It exists only in a child-report form. It has been found to correlate moderately with other measures of childhood anxiety, and the worry/oversensitivity scale has proved sensitive to the presence of DSM-III anxiety disorders (Mattison and Bagnato, 1987; Mattison *et al.*, 1988).

When childhood fears (rather than anxiety disorders *per se*) are the subject of interest, then the 80-item Fear Survey Schedule for Children (Scherer and

Nakamura, 1968) or the 81-item Louisville Fear Survey Schedule are available (Miller *et al.*, 1971, 1972). Further reviews of scales for childhood anxiety can be found in Johnson and Melamed (1979), Barrios *et al.* (1981) and Frances and Ollendick (1987).

DIAGNOSTIC INTERVIEWS

The literature on diagnostic interviews is distinguished from that on questionnaire measures by its much more meagre attention to psychometric issues. This is partly due to the more recent emergence of the structured interview as a generally accepted form of assessment, and this is particularly true of the face to face interview with the child (Edelbrock and Costello, 1988a). A second reason is that, since the interviews are usually quite time-consuming, large methodological studies are expensive and require considerable facilities. The interviews considered here are those that are leaders in their fields or that show important promise for the future. Further discussion of these and some other instruments can be found in a recent review by Edelbrock and Costello (1988), while Young *et al.* (1987) review the present state of research on structured interviews. Gutterman *et al.* (1987), p. 624) also provide a useful comparative table showing the DSM-III categories covered by a number of the interviews discussed here. The highly structured interviews were developed primarily with the needs of epidemiological research in mind, while the semi-structured interviews were usually initially intended for clinical research. However, there is no evidence that the highly structured interviews are unsatisfactory for use in clinical settings, or that the semi-structured interviews cannot be used in epidemiological studies. Indeed, at least two of the semi-structured interviews (K-SADS and CAPA) exist in forms that are intended for epidemiological studies.

Fully structured interviews

Diagnostic Interview Schedule for Children (DISC)

There can be no doubt that the DISC is the most extensively methodologically evaluated of all the interviews to be discussed here (Costello *et al.*, 1984; Edelbrock *et al.*, 1985, 1986). A great deal of time was spent in the design and testing of the individual questions and the organization of the interview and its skip structures. It exists in forms for completion with the parent and child and forms to generate DSM-III and DSM-III-R diagnoses, and contains ratings of 264 items in the child version and 302 items in the parent version, covering a broad range of child psychiatric disorders for children aged 6–18 years. It can also be scored to produce 27 scale scores, and various computer diagnostic algorithms for scoring the results of the interview are available

(Cohen *et al.*, 1987b). Lay (non-clinical) interviewers require only 2–3 days of training, and the interview with the child takes about 40–60 minutes to complete, while the parent version requires about 60–70 minutes. Most items are 0–1–2 ('no or never', 'somewhat, sometimes or a little', 'yes, often or a lot'), and cover a time-frame of the previous year, but information about onset and duration is also obtained for many items.

Inter-rater reliability on scoring videotapes has been found to be very high (r=0.94–1.0 for the symptom scores). Test–retest stability examined by re-interviewing 242 parent–child pairs at a median interval of 9 days, with different interviewers conducting the two interviews, was 0.90 (ICC) for the parent interview total score and between 0.44 and 0.86 for the other 26 symptom clusters. In fact, stability was satisfactory for all but the obsessive-compulsive, schizoid-psychotic and manic scales. A rather different picture emerged from the child reports, where, broadly speaking, the stabilities with children under 10 were disappointing, leading the authors of the DISC to suggest that stability was only really sufficiently high for the reporting of fears (Edelbrock *et al.*, 1985). On the other hand, the stability scores for the over 10s were mostly satisfactory, with ICCs mostly in the 0.6–0.8 range. However, this was not true of reports of affective, obsessive-compulsive or schizoid/psychotic symptoms in the 10–13-year-olds, or manic symptoms at any age, where the ICCs were mostly in the 0.2–0.5 range. A more recent study by Breslau (1987) has found that both parents and children seem to be misunderstanding the intent of the questions about obsessive-compulsive and psychotic phenomena, with the result that they over-report their presence. When the interview was rescored by a clinician in the light of notes taken during the interview that included the interviewees' responses to being asked for examples of the supposed symptoms, it was found that many of the positive reports could be reclassified as being negative. However, at the time of writing, no version of the DISC incorporating the changes suggested by Breslau to deal with this problem is available.

A further important finding from the DISC reliability study was that children reported substantially fewer, and less severe, symptoms in the second interview than they had in the first, such that the mean total symptom score for the second interview was 23% lower than for the first interview. A drop of only 5% was found for the parental reports.

The DISC successfully discriminates between psychiatric and paediatric referrals, and its scale scores correlate with equivalent profile scores on the CBCL (Costello *et al.*, 1984; Edelbrock *et al.*, 1985).

Thus the DISC provides wide coverage of the psychopathology of childhood, and in most areas provides questioning that leads to high test–retest stability, except with younger children. It has been subjected to more stringent psychometric testing than any of the other interviews reviewed here, and it would be unwise to assume that any of them would perform any better in these respects.

Diagnostic Interview for Children and Adolescents (DICA)

The DICA (Herjanic and Campbell, 1977; Herjanic and Reich, 1982) is a highly structured interview for use with children aged 6 years and above. It exists in forms for administration to parents or children and takes about 40–45 minutes to complete. Only a short period of interviewer training is necessary, and interviewers do not need to have had clinical experience. It provides coverage of 18 DSM-III diagnoses through questioning about 900 items in a branching structure (in a 'no', 'sometimes', 'yes' format), and can also be scored to yield ICD-9 diagnoses (Reich *et al.*, 1981). The DICA-P (parent version) also includes a section covering the child's developmental and medical history. It can also be scored to generate a variety of scale scores, and current and past diagnoses can be made.

A small study of inter-rater reliability (ten raters with two taped interviews) found an average agreement on symptoms of 95% (Herjanic and Reich, 1982). Test–retest stability over a 1–7-day period, using different interviewers for the two interviews with 27 psychiatric in-patients, aged 7–17 years, found very good levels of agreement for the six specific diagnostic categories examined (kappas ranging from 0.76 to 1.0). This study also found that the mean number of diagnoses per child fell from 3.6 at the first interview to 2.3 at the second (Welner *et al.*, 1987). This drop may have been due to individuals becoming less anxious as they settled into the ward environment, but it is also reminiscent of the findings with the DISC (Edelbrock *et al.*, 1985), where most of the children were out-patients. Agreement between DICA diagnoses and the hospital discharge diagnosis was rather poor in the Welner *et al.* (1987) study, but considering that the DICA was producing multiple diagnoses, whereas the clinicians were using a diagnostic hierarchy, and probably reporting only what they regarded as being the main diagnosis, this is not surprising, and cannot really be taken as evidence of invalidity as far as the DICA is concerned. The DICA has been found to discriminate between paediatric and psychiatric clinic referrals (Herjanic and Campbell, 1977), although the methods of analysis used in this study make it hard to tell just how the parent and child interviews performed as a whole. A comparison of 42 children each having a parent with a panic disorder and 42 children from families where neither parent had a psychiatric disorder found much higher rates of disorder (especially emotional disorder) in the children of the disordered probands.

The very promising test–retest stability results achieved with the DICA to date suggest that it is worthy of further investigation; it also has the advantage of being scorable for ICD-9 diagnoses, but at this stage it is probably fair to say that the DISC is the market leader as far as highly structured interviews for children are concerned.

Semi-structured Diagnostic Interviews

Schedule for Affective Disorders and Schizophrenia for School-age Children (Kiddie-SADS, K-SADS)

The K-SADS (Puig-Antich and Chambers, 1978) is probably the most widely used semi-structured diagnostic interview. It covers a broad range of child psychiatric diagnoses, but its content is heavily weighted towards depression. It was designed for use with children aged 6–17, and is now available in forms for generating current (K-SADS-P; NB in this case the 'P' is for Present and not Parent as in most other interviews) and lifetime (K-SADS-E (Orvaschel *et al.*, 1982a); where the 'E' stands for Epidemiological), and DSM-III and DSM-III-R diagnoses. It is intended for administration by clinically sophisticated interviewers, who are familiar with the use of research diagnostic criteria, and who have also received extensive interview-specific training. However, the K-SADS-P has been used with lay interviewers (Hodges *et al.*, 1987). It requires 60 minutes or more for completion.

The first 15 minutes of the interview is spent in unstructured conversation designed to establish rapport, elicit the history of the present condition, and form a general impression of the child's problems. More structured specific symptom areas are then covered, although the questioning is still supposed to be flexible and guided by clinical acumen. Many of the 273 items in the K-SADS-P are rated on six-point intensity scales that have symptom-specific anchoring definitions. These definitions include various combinations of intensity, duration, frequency, environmental responsiveness, psychosocial impairment and observation in their formulations of symptom severity. In the Epidemiologic version codings are made for the current episode and the last week on an X–1–2 scale ('not applicable/no information', 'No', 'Yes'). At the end of the interview with the child the interviewer completes 11 observational ratings.

The K-SADS differs from most interviews in directing that the parent should be interviewed first and then the child should be seen by the same interviewer, who is then expected to resolve any discrepancies between the child's reports and those of the parent. The interviewer then completes a single record representing his or her conflation of the two interviews. This procedure obviously requires considerable clinical judgement, and is subject to the criticism that the process of combining the information is quite uncontrolled, and it is impossible to recover the specific information that was obtained from each interviewee. This method also seems likely to bias the results of the interview in favour of the parental reports (Angold *et al.*,

1987), and some workers have preferred to score the interviews with the parent and the child separately (see e.g. Weissman *et al.*, 1987). When this is done the usual high level of parent–child disagreement appears.

A preliminary study of inter-rater reliability using an early draft of the K-SADS-P has been reported as finding a mean ICC for the depressive syndrome score of 0.86 for the interview with the parent and 0.89 for the child, but no other details are given (Chambers *et al.*, 1985). The test–retest stability of the K-SADS-P over a 2–3-day period has been examined using three rater pairs and 52 subjects aged 6–17 years (Chambers *et al.*, 1985). Individual symptoms were mostly moderately stable (average ICC = 0.55, ranging from 0.09 to 0.89). The 12 summary scores were not surprisingly more stable than the individual items (average ICC = 0.68, ranging from 0.41 to 0.81), while the categorical diagnoses showed rather variable reliability (κ = 0.24–0.70). Rather unexpectedly, the highest level of specific diagnostic agreement was for non-major depressive disorders (κ = 0.70) while agreement for major depressive disorder was only 0.54 (κ). The kappa coefficient for agreement over Conduct disorder was 0.63, while that for Anxiety disorder was frankly low, at only 0.24. It seems probable that attempts to subtype these rather global categories further would have led to still lower levels of diagnostic agreement.

The K-SADS-E has been found to pick up disorders that were diagnosed 6–24 months earlier using the K-SADS-P (Orvaschel *et al.*, 1982a).

Little further attention has been paid to the psychometric properties of the K-SADS, although two recent studies have indicated that it produces diagnoses similar to those produced by the CAS and the DISC (Hodges *et al.*, 1987; Cohen *et al.*, 1987a). However, one might argue that given the flimsy psychometric evidence attaching to these comparators it is hard to be sure exactly what this means.

Interview Schedule for Children (ISC)

The Interview Schedule for Children (Kovacs, 1983) is structurally similar to the K-SADS-P. Parents and children are interviewed separately, but the final diagnosis is arrived at in a group conference, after all the diagnostic information has been collected. The central core of the interview is strongly weighted towards depression, but a number of add-on sections are now available, and it is the only interview reviewed here to include some personality disorder diagnoses (borderline, compulsive, histrionic and schizotypal). It also exists in a follow-up version. Extensive clinical experience and interview-specific training is required of interviewers using the ISC. Many of these features are reflections of the specific studies for which it was designed, and it has not been much used outside the domain of its originator (Kovacs *et al.*, 1984a and b). There are no published studies of the ISC's psychometric properties, although Edelbrock and Costello (1988b) report good inter-rater reliability for co-ratings of live interviews (ICCs ranging from 0.64 to 1.0), from an unpublished study.

Child Assessment Schedule (CAS)

The Child Assessment Schedule (Hodges *et al.*, 1981, 1982a and b) is a semi-structured interview for children aged 7–12, divided into 11 content areas. It has recently undergone a series of modifications and now generates DSM-III diagnoses of quite a wide range of the most commonly occurring childhood disorders, and several scale scores can also be calculated. However, a number of conditions, such as eating disorders, psychotic symptomatology and substance abuse disorders, are not fully covered, although screening questions about them are present. A number of items that do not correspond to DSM-III criteria, but which are of clinical interest, are also included. The CAS now exists in child, adolescent and parent report forms (Hodges *et al.*, 1987), and takes about 45–75 minutes to complete. Although originally developed for use by experienced clinicians (Hodges *et al.*, 1982a), the CAS has now been used by lay interviewers in a study reported by its originator (Hodges *et al.*, 1987). The first part of the CAS (which essentially corresponds to the originally developed interview) consists of approximately 75 questions about the various content areas, which are scored on a five-point scale ('yes', 'no', 'ambiguous', 'not applicable', 'no response'). This is followed by questioning about the onset and duration of positive symptoms. Finally, there are 53 observational items for rating intra-interview behaviour.

Inter-rater reliability assessed from independent ratings of videotapes of child interviews by four raters averaged 0.90 for the total score and was greater than 0.70 for 12 of the 20 content areas or symptom complexes covered by the interview. The reliability of the DSM-III diagnoses generated by the CAS has not been reported to date. Diagnostic concordance with the K-SAS-P, administered by lay interviewers, was found to be moderate in a study of 30 clinically-referred children (kappas between 0.36 and 0.75). CAS scores have been found to discriminate between inpatient, outpatient and normal groups, and to correlate with scores on the Child Behavior Checklist and Spielberger's (1973) State-Trait Anxiety Inventory for Children (Hodges *et al.*, 1982a, b; Verhulst, Berden & Sanders-Woudstra, 1985b).

Child and Adolescent Psychiatric Assessment (CAPA)

The Child and Adolescent Psychiatric Assessment (Angold *et al.*, 1987) is a new semi-structured interview developed at the MRC Child Psychiatry Unit in London, building upon the Isle of Wight Interviews (Rutter and Graham, 1968; Graham and Rutter, 1968), and advances in the K-SADS and the

Present State Examination (Wing, 1974). It is suitable for use with 8–16 year-olds and exists in parent and child and clinical and epidemiological forms. It covers a wide range of diagnoses, and is the only available instrument that generates DSM-III, DSM-IIIR and ICD-10 diagnoses, as well as providing ratings of items of psychiatric interest not specifically mentioned in any of these nosologies, and detailed assessment of psychosocial impairment in a number of functional areas. Ratings of symptom intensity (on a 0–1–2–3 scale: 'absent', 'possibly present', 'definitely present', 'severe'), frequency, duration and onset are made for about 250 items. The basic time-frame of the CAPA is the preceding 3 months, and if symptoms are present during this period then their date of onset is determined. The interview usually takes 45–120 minutes to complete.

Like the K-SADS, the CAPA begins with a relatively unstructured initial section to promote the establishment of rapport and to gain an overview of likely problem areas. Systematic questioning is then pursued, with detailed probes being provided in a two-tier structure, with some being essentially compulsory, unless the information has already been obtained in the course of the interview, while others are provided for clarification if this is necessary. Questioning is directed towards determining whether symptoms as defined in an extensive glossary are present. A particular feature of the CAPA glossary is an attempt to produce more rigorous and formally coherent definitions of symptom intensity than have been available until now. Substantial training is required to produce sufficient familiarity with both the glossary and the interview schedule itself. However, interviewers do not have to be clinically experienced, although training proceeds more rapidly if they are.

The final section of the CAPA is a 65-item intra-interview observational schedule, again backed by an extensive glossary.

To date no psychometric data on the CAPA are available, but it has proved acceptable in practice, and reliability studies are currently under way.

CONCLUSIONS

There is no single best strategy for rating psychiatric disturbance in children, but a range of different approaches are available, and the quality of the psychometric evaluation of individual instruments is improving. All of the rating scales, questionnaires and interviews discussed in this chapter have both strengths and weaknesses, and how these balance out in the face of the needs of each individual assessment problem will determine which ones to pick. It is usually a good idea to try out one or two of the more likely choices, to see how they operate in practice, and to get a feel for the sort of information that they provide (although this can be difficult with semi-structured interviews). In the end, the appropriateness of item coverage, personal preference for a particular style of assessment, and resource availability, will often be the main deciding factors, and a realistic evaluation of these in relation to the eight questions outlined in the first part of this chapter will usually result in a workable assessment package.

REFERENCES

Achenbach, T. M. (1966). The classification of children's psychiatric symptoms: A factor-analytic study. *Psychol. monographs* **80**, (7, whole no. 165).

Achenbach, T. M. (1978). The child behaviour profile: I. Boys aged 6–11. *J. Consult. Clin. Psychol.* **46**, 478–488.

Achenbach, T. M. (1985). *Assessment and Taxonomy of Child and Adolescent Psychopathology*, Sage, London.

Achenbach, T. M. and Edelbrock, C. S. (1978). The classification of child psychopathology: A review and analysis of empirical efforts. *Psychol. Rev.* **85**, 1275–1301.

Achenbach, T. M. and Edelbrock, C. S. (1979). The child behaviour profile: II. Boys aged 12–16 and girls aged 6–11 and 12–16. *J. Consult. Clin. Psychol.* **47**, 223–233.

Achenbach, T. M. and Edelbrock, C. S. (1981). Behavioral problems and competencies reported by parents of normal and disturbed children aged four through sixteen. *Monographs Soc. Res. Child Devel.* **46** (whole no. 1).

Achenbach, T. M., Edelbrock, C. S. and Howell (1987a). *J. Abnorm. Child Psychol.* **15**, 629–650.

Achenbach, T. M., McConaughy and Howell (1987b). *Psychol. Bull.* **101**, 213–232.

Achenbach, T. M., Verhulst, F. C., Baron, G. D. and Akkerhuis, G. W. (1987c). Epidemiological comparisons of American and Dutch children: I. Behavioral/emotional problems and competencies reported by parents for ages 4 to 16. *J. Am. Acad. Child Adol. Psychiatry* **26**, 317–325.

Achenbach, T. M., Verhulst, F. C., Edelbrock, C., Baron, G. D. and Akkerhuis, G. W. (1987d). Epidemiological comparisons of American and Dutch children: II. Behavioral/emotional problems reported by teachers for ages 6 to 11. *J. Am. Acad. Child Adol. Psychiatry* **26**, 326–332.

Aman, M. G. and Werry, J. S. (1984). The revised behavior problem checklist in clinic attenders and non-attenders; Age and sex effects. *J. Clin. Child Psychol.* **13**, 3–237.

Aman, M. G., Werry, J. S., Fitzpatrick, J., Lowe, M. and Waters, J. (1983). Factor structure and norms for the revised behavior problem checklist in New Zealand children. *Aust. NZ J. Psychiatry* **17**, 354–360.

American Psychiatric Association (1980). *Diagnostic and Statistical Manual*, 3rd edn, American Psychiatric Association, Washington, DC.

American Psychiatric Association (1987). *Diagnostic and Statistical Manual*, 3rd ed (Revised), American Psychiatric Association, Washington, DC.

Angold, A. (1988). Childhood and adolescent depression: I. Epidemiological and aetiological aspects. *Br. J. Psychiatry* **152**, 601–617.

Angold, A., Weissman, M. M., John, K., Merikangas, K. R., Prusoff, B. A., Wickramaratne, P. and Gammon, G. D. (1987). Parent and child reports of depressive symptoms. *J. Child Psychol. Psychiatry* **28**, 901–915.

Angold, A., Costello, E. J., Pickles, A., Winder, F. and Silver, D. (1988). The development of a questionnaire for use in epidemiological studies of depression in children and adolescents (submitted for publication).

Bakeman, R. and Gottman, J. M. (1987). Applying observational methods: A systematic view. In *Handbook of Infant Development* J. D. Osofsky, Wiley, Chichester, pp. 818–851.

Barkley, R. A. (1988). Child behavior rating scales and checklists. In *Assessment and Diagnosis in Child Psychopathology* (M. Rutter, A. H. Tuma and I. S. Lann, eds), Guilford, New York, pp. 113–155.

Barrios, B. A., Hartmann, D. P. and Shigetomi, C. (1981). Fears and anxieties in children. In *Behavioral Assessment of Childhood Disorders* (E. D. Mash and L. G. Terdal, eds), Guilford, New York.

Bartko, J. and Carpenter, W. T. (1976). On the methods and theory of reliability. *J. Nerv. Ment. Dis.* **163**, 307–317.

Beardslee, W. R., Bemporad, J., Keller, M. B. and Klerman, G. L. (1983). Children of parents with major affective disorder: A review. *Am. J. Psychiatry* **140**, 825–832.

Berger, M. (1985a). Temperament and individual differences. In *Child and Adolescent Psychiatry: Modern Approaches* (M. Rutter and L. Hersov, eds), Blackwell, London, pp. 3–16.

Berger, M. (1985b). Psychological assessment and testing. In *Child and Adolescent Psychiatry: Modern Approaches* (M. Rutter and L. Hersov, eds), Blackwell, London, pp. 264–279.

Bird, H. R., Canino, G., Gould, M. S., Ribera, J., Rubio-Stipec, M., Woodbury, M., Huertas-Goldman, S. and Sesman, M. (1987a). Use of the Child Behavior Checklist as a screening instrument for epidemiological research in child psychiatry: Results of a pilot study. *J. Am. Acad. Child Adol. Psychiatry* **26**, 207–213.

Bird, H. R., Canino, G., Rubio-Stipec, M. and Ribera, J. C. (1987b). Further measures of the psychometric properties of the children's global assessment scale. *Arch. Gen. Psychiatry* **44**, 821–824.

Boyle, M. H. and Chambers, L. W. (1981). Indices of social well-being applicable to children: A review. *Soc. Sci. Med.* **15**, 161–171.

Boyle, M. H. and Jones, S. C. (1985). Selecting measures of emotional and behavioural disorders of childhood for use in general populations. *J. Child Psychol. Psychiatry* **26**, 137–159.

Breslau, N. (1987). Inquiring about the bizarre: False positives in Diagnostic Interview Schedule for Children (DISC) ascertainment of obsessions, compulsions, and psychotic symptoms. *J. Am. Acad. Child Adol. Psychiatry* **26**, 639–644.

Chambers, W. J., Puig-Antich, J., Hirsch, M., Paez, P., Ambrosini, P. J., Tabrizi, M. A. and Davies, M. (1985). The assessment of affective disorders in children and adolescents by sem-structured interview: Test–retest reliability of the schedule for affective disorders and schizophrenia for school-age children, present episode version. *Arch. Gen. Psychiatry* **42**, 696–702.

Cohen, J. (1960). A coefficient of agreement for nominal scales. *Educ. Psychol. Measurement* **20**, 37–46.

Cohen, J. (1968). Weighted kappa: Nominal scale agreement with provision for scaled disagreement or partial credit. *Psychol. Bull.* **70**, 213–220.

Cohen, P., O'Connor, P., Lewis, S., Velez, C. N. and Malachowski, B. (1987a). Comparison of DISC and K-SADS-P interviews of an epidemiological sample of children. *J. Am. Acad. Child Adol. Psychiatry* **26**, 662–667.

Cohen, P., Velez, C. N., Kohn, M., Schwab-Stone, M. and Johnson, J. (1987b). Child psychiatric diagnosis by computer algorithm: Theoretical issues and empirical tests. *J. Am. Acad. Child Adol. Psychiatry* **26**, 631–638.

Conners, C. K. (1969). A teacher rating scale for use in drug studies with children. *Am. J. Psychiatry* **126**, 884–888.

Conners, C. K. (1973). Rating scales for use in drug studies with children. *Psychopharmacol. Bull.* Special issue: *Pharmacotherapy with Children,* 24–84.

Conners, C. K. (1985). *The Conners Rating Scales: Instruments for the Assessment of Childhood Psychopathology,* unpublished manuscript, Washington, DC.

Costello, A. J. (1986). Assessment and Diagnosis of Affective Disorders in Children. *J. Child Psychol. Psychiatry* **27**, 565–574.

Costello, E. J. and Angold, A. (1988). Scales to assess child and adolescent depression; Checklists, Screen and Nets. *J. Am. Acad. Child and Adol. Psychiatry* (in press).

Costello, A. J., Edelbrock, C. S., Dulcan, M. K., Kalas, R. and Klaric, S. H. (1984). *Development and Testing of the NIMH Diagnostic Interview Schedule for Children in a Clinic Population: Final Report* (contract no. RFP-DB-81-0027) Center for Epidemiologic Studies–NIMH, Rockville, MD.

Costello, E. J., Edelbrock, C. S. and Costello, A. J. (1985). Validity of the NIMH Diagnostic Interview Schedule for Children: A comparison between psychiatric and pediatric referrals. *J. Abnorm. Child Psychol.* **13**, 579–595.

Cronbach, L. J. (1970). *Essentials of Test Validation*, Harper & Row, New York.

Doane, J. A. (1978). Family interaction and communication deviance in disturbed and normal families: A review of research. *Family Process.* **17**, 357–376.

Doane, J. A., West, K. L., Goldstein, M. J., Rodnick, E. H. and Jones, J. E. (1981). Parental communication deviance and affective style: Predictors of subsequent schizophrenia spectrum disorders in vulnerable adolescents. *Arch. Gen. Psychiatry* **38**.

Edelbrock, C. and Achenbach, T. M. (1980). A typology of child behavior profile patterns: Distribution and correlates for disturbed children aged 6–16. *J. Abnorm. Child Psychol.* **8**, 441–470.

Edelbrock, C. and Costello, A. J. (1988a). Structured psychiatric interviews for children. In *Assessment and Diagnosis in Child Psychopathology (*M. Rutter, A. H. Tuma and I. S. Lann, eds), Guilford Press, New York.

Edelbrock, C. and Costello, A. J. (1988b). Convergence between statistically derived behaviour problem syndromes and child psychiatric diagnoses. *J. Abnorm. Child Psychol.* **16**, 219–231.

Edelbrock, C. S., Costello, A. J., Dulcan, M. K. and Kalas, R. (1985). Age differences in the reliability of the psychiatric interview of the child. *Child Development*, **56**, 265–275.

Edelbrock, C., Costello, A. J., Dulcan, M. K., Conover, M. C. and Kalas, R. (1986). Parent–child agreement on child psychiatric symptoms assessed via structured interview. *J. Child Psychol. Psychiatry* **27**, 181–190.

Frame, C. L. and Matson, J. L. (1987). *Handbook of Assessment in Childhood Psychopathology*, Plenum, New York.

Frances, G. and Ollendick, T. H. (1987). Anxiety disorders. In *Handbook of Assessment in Child Psychopathology* (C. L. Frame and J. L. Matson, eds), Plenum, New York.

French, J., Graves, P. A. and Levitt, E. E. (1983). Objective and projective testing of children. In *Handbook of Clinical Child Psychology* (E. Walker and M. Roberts eds), Wiley, New York.

Gettinger, M. and Kratochwill, T. R. (1987). Behavioral assessment. In *Handbook of Assessment in Childhood Psychopathology* (C. L. Frame and J. L. Matson eds), Plenum, New York.

Gittelman, R. (1980). The role of psychological tests for differential diagnosis in child psychiatry. *J. Am. Acad. Child Psychiatry* **19**, 413–438.

Gittelman, R. (1985). The use of psychological tests in clinical practice with children. In *The Clinical Guide to Child Psychiatry* (D. Shaffer, A. A. Erhardt, and L. L. Greenhill, eds), Free Press, New York, pp. 447–474.

Gittelman-Klein, R. (1978). Validity of projective tests for psychodiagnosis in children. In *Critical Issues in Psychiatric Diagnosis* (R. L. Spitzer and D. F. Klein, eds), Raven, New York.

Goodyer, I., Kolvin, I. and Gatzanis, S. (1985). Recent undesirable life events and psychiatric disorder in childhood and adolescence. *Br. J. Psychiatry* **147**, 517–523.

Goyette, C. H., Conners, C. K. and Ulrich, R. F. (1978). Normative data on the revised Conners parent and teacher rating scales. *J. Abnorm. Child Psychol.* **6**, 221–236.

Graham, P. and Rutter, M. (1968). The reliability and validity of the psychiatry assessment of the child: II. Interview with the parent. *Br. J. Psychiatry* 581–592.

Gutterman, E. M., O'Brien, J. D. and Young, J. G. (1987). Structured diagnostic interviews for children and adolescents: Current status and future directions. *J. Am. Acad. Child Adol. Psychiatry* **26**, 621–630.

Harter, S. (1982). The perceived competence scale for children. *Child Development* **53**, 87–97.

Herjanic, B. and Campbell, W. (1977). Differentiating psychiatrically disturbed children on the basis of a structured interview. *J. Abnorm. Child Psychol.* **5**, 127–134.

Herjanic, B. and Reich, W. (1982). Development of a structured psychiatric interview for children: Agreement between child and parent on individual symptoms. *J. Abnorm. Child Psychol.* **10**, 307–324.

Herjanic, B., Herjanic, M., Brown, F. and Wheatt, T. (1975). Are children reliable reporters? *J. Abnorm. Child Psychol.* **3**, 41–48.

Hodges, K., Klein, J., Fitch, P., McKnew, D. and Cytryn, L. (1981). The Child Assessment Schedule. *Catalog Selected Documents Psychol.* **11**, 56.

Hodges, K., Kline, J., Stern, L., Cytryn, L. and McKnew, D. (1982a). The development of a child assessment interview for research and clinical use. *J. Abnorm. Child Psychol.* **10**, 173–189.

Hodges, K., McKnew, D., Burbach, D. J. and Roebuck, L. (1987). Diagnostic concordance between the Child Assessment Schedule (CAS) and the Schedule for Affective Disorders and Schizophrenia for School-age Children (K-SADS) in an outpatient sample using lay interviewers. *J. Am. Acad. Child Adol. Psychiatry* **26**, 654–661.

Hodges, K., McKnew, D., Cytryn, L., Stern, L. and Kline, J. (1982b). The Child Assessment Schedule (CAS) diagnostic interview: A report on reliability and validity. *J. Am. Acad. Child Psychiatry* **21**, 468–473.

Hoier, T. S. and Kerr, M. M. (1988). Extrafamilial information sources in the study of childhood depression. *J. Am. Acad. Child Adol. Psychiatry* **27**, 21–33.

Jacob, T. and Tennenbaum, D. L. (1988). Family assessment methods. In *Assessment and Diagnosis in Child Psychopathology* (M. Rutter, A. H. Tuma and I. S. Lann, eds), Guilford Press, New York.

John, K., Gammon, G. D., Prusoff, B. A. and Warner, V. (1987). The social adjustment inventory for children and adolescents (SAICA): Testing a new semi-structured interview. *J. Am. Acad. Child Adol. Psychiatry* **26**, 898–911.

Johnson, J. H. (1986). *Life Events as Stressors in Childhood and Sdolescence*, Sage, London.

Johnson, S. B. and Melamed, B. G. (1979). The assessment and treatment of children's fears. In *Advances in Clinical Psychology*, Vol. 2. (B. B. Lahey and A. E. Kazdin, eds), Plenum, New York.

Katschnig, H. (1986). Measuring life stress—a comparison of the checklist and the panel technique. In *Life Events and Psychiatric Disorders: Controversial Issues* (H. Katschnig, ed.), Cambridge University Press, London.

Kovacs, M. (1983). The children's depression inventory: A self-rated depression scale for school-aged youngsters, unpublished manuscript.

Kovacs, M., Feinberg, T. L., Crouse-Novak, M. L., Paulauskas, S. L. and Finkelstein, R. (1984a). Depressive disorders in childhood. *Arch. Gen. Psychiatry* **41**, 229–237.

Kovacs, M., Feinberg, T. L., Crouse-Novak, M., Paulauskas, S. L., Pollock, M. and Finkelstein, R. (1984b). Depressive disorders in childhood II: A longitudinal study of the risk for a subsequent major depression. *Arch. Gen. Psychiatry* **41**, 643–649.

Lansdown, R. and Yule, W. (eds) (1986). *The Lead Debate: The Environment, Toxicology and Child Health*, Croom Helm, London.

Le Couteur, A., Rutter, M., Lord, C., Rios, P., Robertson, S., Holdgrafer, M. and McLennan, J. (1988). Autism Diagnostic Interview: A standardized investigator-based instrument. *J. Autism Dev. Dis.* (in press).

Loney, J. and Milich, R. S. (1981). Hyperactivity, inattention, and aggression in clinical practice. In *Advances in Behavioral Pediatrics,* Vol. 2 (M. Wolraich and D. K. Routh, eds), JAI Press, Greenwich, CT.

Lord, K., Rutter, M., Goode, S., Heemsbergen, J., Jordan, H., Mawhood, L. and Schopler, E. (1988). Autism diagnostic observation schedule. A standardized observation of social and communicative behavior. *J. Autism Dev. Dis.* (in press).

Mash, E. J. and Johnston, C. (1983). Parental perceptions of child behavior problems, parenting, self esteem, and mothers' reported stress in younger and older hyperactive and normal children. *J. Consult. Clin. Psychol.* **51**, 69–99.

Mattison, R. E. and Bagnato, S. J. (1987). Empirical measurement of overanxious disorder in boys 8 to 12 years old. *J. Am. Acad. Child Adol. Psychiatry* **26**, 536–540.

Mattison, R. E., Bagnato, S. J. and Brubaker, B. H. (1988). Diagnostic utility of the revised children's manifest anxiety scale in children with DSM-III anxiety disorders. *J. Anxiety Dis.* **2**, 147–155.

Milich, R., Roberts, M. A., Loney, J. and Caputo, J. (1980). Differentiating practice effects and statistical regression on the Conners Hyperkinesis Index. *J. Abnorm. Child Psychol.* **8**, 549–552.

Miller, L. C., Barrett, C. L., Hampe, E. and Noble, H. (1971). Factor structure of childhood fears. *J. Consult. Clin. Psychol.* **39**, 264–268.

Miller, L. C., Barrett, C. L., Hampe, E. and Noble, H. (1972). Revised anxiety scale for the Louisville Behavior Checklist. *Psychol. Rep.* **29**, 503–511.

Monck, E. and Dobbs, R. (1985). Measuring life events in an adolescent population: Methodological issues and related findings. *Psychol. Med.* **15**, 841–850.

Nuechterlein, K. H. (1986). Childhood precursors of adult schizophrenia. *J. Child Psychol. Psychiatry* **27**, 133–144.

O'Connor, M., Foch, T., Sherry, R. and Plomin, R. (1980). A twin study of specific behavioral problems of socialization as viewed by parents. *J. Abnorm. Child Psychol.* **8**, 189–199.

Orvaschel, H. and Walsh, G. (1984). The assessment of adaptive functioning in children: a review of existing measures suitable for epidemiological and clinical services research (DHHS Pub. No. (ADM) 84–1343) Washington, DC, US Government Printing Office.

Orvaschel, H., Puig-Antich, J., Chambers, M. D., Tabrizi, M. A. and Johnson, R.

(1982a) Retrospective assessment of prepubertal major depression with the Kiddie-SADS-E. *J. Am. Acad. Child Psychiatry* **4**, 392–297.

Orvaschel, H., Thompson, W. D., Belanger, A., Prusoff, B. A. and Kidd, K. K. (1982b). Comparison of the Family History Method to Direct Interview. *J. Affect. Dis.* **4**, 49–59.

Piers, E. (1977). *The Piers–Harris Children's Self-Concept Test: Research Monograph No. 1*, Counselor Recordings and Tests, Nashville.

Piers, E. and Harris, D. (1969). *The Piers–Harris Children's Self-Concept Scale*, Counselor Recordings and Tests, Nashville.

Puig-Antich, J. and Chambers, W. (1978). The schedule for affective disorders and schizophrenia for school-aged children, unpublished interview schedule, New York State Psychiatric Institute.

Quay, H. C. (1977). Measuring dimensions of deviant behavior: The Behavior Problem Checklist. *J. Abnorm. Child Psychol.* **5**, 277–287.

Quay, H. C. (1983). A dimensional approach to behavior disorder: The Revised Behavior Problem Checklist. *School Psychol. Rev.* **12**, 244–249.

Quay, H. C. and Peterson, D. R. (1975). *Manual for the Behavior Problem Checklist*, unpublished manuscript, University of Miami.

Quay, H. C. and Peterson, D. R. (1983). Interim manual for the Revised Behavior Problem Checklist, unpublished manuscript, University of Miami.

Quay, H. C. and Peterson, D. R. (1984). Appendix I to the interim manual for the Revised Behavior Problem Checklist, unpublished manuscript, University of Miami.

Quinton, D., Rutter, M. and Rowlands, O. (1976). An evaluation of an assessment interview of marriage, *Psychol. Med.* **14**, 107–124.

Reich, W. and Earls, F. (1987). Rules for making psychiatric diagnoses in children on the basis of multiple sources of information: Preliminary strategies. *J. Abnorm. Child Psychol.* **15**, 601–616.

Reich, W., Herjanic, B., Welner, Z. and Gandhy, P. R. (1981). Development of a structured psychiatric interview for children: Agreement on diagnosis comparing child and parent interviews. *J. Abnorm. Child Psychol.* **10**, 325–336.

Reid, J. B., Patterson, G. R., Baldwin, D. V. and Dishion, T. J. (1988). Observations in the assessment of childhood disorders. In *Assessment and Diagnosis in Child Psychopathology* (M. Rutter, A. H. Tuma and I. S. Lann, eds), Guilford Press, New York.

Reynolds, C. R. (1982). Convergent and divergent validity of the Revised Children's Manifest Anxiety Scale. *Educ. Psychol. Measurement* **42**, 1205–1212.

Reynolds, C. R. and Paget, K. D. (1981). Factor analysis of the Revised Children's Manifest Anxiety Scale for blacks, whites, males and females with a national normative sample. *J. Clin. Consult. Psychol.* **49**, 352–359.

Reynolds, C. R. and Paget, K. D. (1983). National normative and reliability data for the Revised Children's Manifest Anxiety Scale. *School Psychol. Rev.* **12**, 324–336.

Richardson, S. A., Dohrenwend, B. S. and Klein, D. (1965). *Interviewing: Its Form and Function*, Basic Books, New York.

Rutter, M. (1967). A children's behaviour questionnaire for completion by teachers: Preliminary findings. *J. Child Psychol. Psychiatry* **8**, 1–11.

Rutter, M. (1982). Temperament: concepts, issues and problems. In *Temperamental Differences in Infants and Young Children* (R. Porter and G. M. Collins, eds), Pitman, London.

Rutter, M. and Graham, P. (1968). The reliability and validity of the psychiatric assessment of the child: I. Interview with the parent. *Br. J. Psychiatry* 563–579.

Rutter, M. and Quinton, D. (1984). Parental psychiatric disorder: Effects on children. *Psychol. Med.* **14**, 853–880.

Rutter, M. and Schopler, E. (1988). Autism and pervasive developmental disorders. In *Assessment and Diagnosis in Child Psychopathology* (M. Rutter, A. H. Tuma and I. S. Lann, eds), Guilford Press, New York, pp. 408–434.

Rutter, M., Tizard, J. and Whitmore, K. (1970). *Education, Health and Behavior*, Longman, London.

Rutter, M., Cox, A., Tupling, C., Berger, M. and Yule, W. (1975a). Attainment and adjustment in two geographical areas I. The prevalence of psychiatric disorder. *Br. J. Psychiatry* **126**, 493–509.

Rutter, M., Yule, B., Quinton, D., Rowlands, O., Yule, W. and Berger, M. (1975b). Attainment and adjustment in two geographical areas II: Some factors accounting for area differences. *Br. J. Psychiatry* **126**, 520–533.

Rutter, M., Shaffer, D. and Sturge, C. (1975c). *A Guide to a Multi-axial Classification Scheme for Psychiatric Disorders in Childhood and Adolescence*, Frowde, London.

Rutter, M., Graham, P., Chadwick, O. F. D. and Yule, W. (1976). Adolescent turmoil: Fact or fiction? *J. Child Psychol. Psychiatry* **17**, 35–56.

Sackett, G. P. (1987). Analysis of sequential social interaction data: Some issues, recent developments, and a causal inference model. In *Handbook of Infant Development* (J. D. Osofsky, ed.), Wiley, Chichester, pp. 855–878.

Sandberg, S., Rutter, M., Giles, S. and Owen, A. (1987). The Children's Life Events and Long-term Experiences Assessment, unpublished manuscript, MRC Child Psychiatry Unit, London.

Scherer, M. W. and Nakamura, C. Y. (1968). A Fear Survey Schedule for Children (FSSC): A factor analytic comparison with manifest anxiety (CMAS). *Behav. Res. Ther.* **6**, 173–182.

Schopler, E., Reichler, R. J. and Renner, B. R. (1986). *The Childhood Autism Rating Scale (Cars) for Diagnostic Screening and Classification of Autism*, Irvington, New York.

Seligman, M. E. P. and Peterson, C. (1986). A learned helplessness perspective on childhood depression: Theory and research. In *Depression in Young People: Clinical and Developmental Perspectives* (M. Rutter, C. E. Izard and P. B. Read, eds), Guilford Press, New York, pp. 223–249.

Seligman, M. E. P., Peterson, C., Kaslow, N. J., Tanenbaum, R. L., Alloy, L. B. and Abramson, L. Y. (1984). Explanatory style and depressive symptoms among school children. *J. Abnorm. Psychol.* **93**, 235–238.

Shaffer, D., Gould, M. S., Brasic, J., Ambrosini, P., Fisher, P., Bird, H. and Aluwahlia, S. (1983). A children's global assessment scale (CGAS). *Arch. Gen. Psychiatry* **40**, 1228–1231.

Shrout, P. E., Spitzer, R. L. and Fleiss, J. L. (1987). Quantification of agreement in psychiatric diagnosis revisited. *Arch. Gen. Psychiatry* **44**, 172–177.

Spielberger, C. D. (1973). *Manual for the State–Trait Anxiety Inventory for Children* Consulting Psychologists Press, Palo Alto, CA.

Steinhausen, H. C. (1987). Global assessment of child psychopathology. *J. Am. Acad. Child Adol. Psychiatry* **26**, 203–206.

Stoddart, C. and Knights, R. M. (1986). Neuropsychological assessment of children: Alternative approaches. In *Child Neuropsychology*, Vol. 2, Clinical Practice (J. E. Obrzut and G. W. Hynd, eds), Academic Press, London.

Teeter, P. A. (1986). Standard neuropsychological batteries for children. In *Child Neuropsychology*, Vol. 2, Clinical Practice (J. E. Obrzut and G. W. Hynd, eds), Academic Press, London.

Terman, L. M. and Merrill, M. A. (1973). *The Stanford–Binet Intelligence Scale*, Houghton Mifflin, Boston.

Trites, R. L., Blouin, A. G., Ferguson, H. B. and Lynch, G. W. (1981). The Conners Teacher Rating Scale: An epidemiological inter-rater reliability and follow-up investigation. In *Psychosocial Aspects of Drug Treatment for Hyperactivity* (K. Gadow and J. Loney, eds), Westview Press, Boulder, CO.

Trites, R. L., Blouin, A. G. and Laprade, K. (1982). Factor analysis of the Conners Teacher Rating Scaler based on a large normative sample. *J. Consult. Clin. Psychol.* **50**, 615–623.

Tupper, D. E. (1986). Neuropsychological screening and soft signs. In *Child Neuropsychology*, Vol. 2, Clinical Practice (J. E. Obrzut and G. W. Hynd, eds), Academic Press, London.

Ullman, R. K., Sleator, E. K. and Sprague, R. L. (1985). A change of mind: Conners Abbreviated Rating Scales reconsidered. *J. Abnorm. Child Psychol.* **13**, 553–566.

Vaughn, C. E. and Leff, J. P. (1976). The measurement of Expressed Emotion in the families of psychiatric patients. *Br. J. Soc. Clin. Psychol.* **15**, 157–165.

Verhulst, F. C., Akkerhuis, G. W. and Althaus, M. (1985a). Mental health in Dutch children: (I) a cross-cultural comparison. *Acta Psychiatr. Scand. Supple. 323,* 1–108.

Verhulst, F. C., Berden, G. F. M. G. and Sanders-Woudstra, J. A. R. (1985b). Mental health in Dutch children: (II) the prevalence of psychiatric disorder and relationship between measures. *Acta Psychiatr. Scand. Suppl. 324,* 1–45.

Wechsler, D. (1974). *Wechsler Intelligence Scale for Children—Revised (WISC-R),* Psychological Corporation, New York.

Weissman, M. M., Prusoff, B. A., Gammon, G. D., Merikangas, R., Leckman, J. F. and Kidd, K. K. (1984). Psychopathology in the children (ages 6–18) of depressed and normal parents. *J. Am. Acad. Child Psychiatry* **231**, 78–84.

Weissman, M. M., Wickramaratne, P., Warner, V., John, K., Prusoff, B. A., Merikangas, K. R. and Gammon, G. D. (1987). Assessing psychiatric disorders in children; discrepancies between mothers' and children's reports. *Arch. Gen. Psychiatry* **44**, 747–753.

Welner, Z., Reich, W., Herjanic, B., Jung, K. G. and Amado, H. (1987). Reliability, validity, and parent–child agreement studies of the Diagnostic Interview for Children and Adolescents (DICA). *J. Am. Acad. Child Adol. Psychiatry* **26**, 649–653.

Wing, J. K. (1974). *Measurement and Classification of Psychiatric Symptoms,* Oxford University Press, Oxford.

Wing, L. and Gould, J. (1978). Systematic recording of behaviors and skills of retarded and psychotic children. *J. Autism Child. Schizophr.* **8**, 79–97.

World Health Organization (1978). *Mental Disorders: Glossary and Guide to Their Classification in Accordance with the Ninth Revision of the International Classification of Diseases*, World Health Organization, Geneva.

World Health Organization (1987). *Tenth Revision of the International Classification of Diseases Chapter V (F): Mental, Behavioural and Developmental Disorders. Clinical Descriptions and Diagnostic Guidelines—1986 Draft for Field Trials*, World Health Organization, Geneva.

Young, J. G. O'Brien, J. D., Gutterman, E. M. and Cohen, P. (1987). Research on the clinical interview. *J. Am. Acad. Child Adol. Psychiatry* **26**, 613–620.

Yule, W. and Rutter, M. (eds) (1987). *Language Development and Disorders*, Blackwell, Oxford.

Zimmerman, M. (1983). Methodological issues in the assessment of life events: A review of issues and research. *Clin. Psychol. Rev.* **3**, 339–370.

Zimmerman-Tansella, C., Minghetti, S., Tacconi, A. and Tansella, M. (1978). The

Children's Behaviour Questionnaire for completion by teachers in an Italian sample. Preliminary results. *J. Child Psychol. Psychiatry* **19**, 167–173.

The Instruments of Psychiatric Research
Edited by C. Thompson

CHAPTER 13

Rating scales in old age psychiatry

J. R. M. Copeland[1] and K. C. M. Wilson[2]
[1]*Department of Psychiatry and Institute of Human Ageing, University of Liverpool, Liverpool, UK*

[2]*Royal Liverpool and Mossley Hill Hospitals, University of Liverpool, Liverpool, UK*

INTRODUCTION

Some of the Needs

The needs which rating scales are expected to fulfil in old age psychiatry differ little from those in other age groups.

For most studies, a simple, but accurate, description of the illness is the first requirement. This may be at the symptom, syndrome or differential diagnostic level. The importance of a reliable diagnosis both for aetiological investigations and the management of patients has been firmly established. Although diagnosis is only one stage in the description or formulation of an illness, which should include social and psychological factors, it is for many investigators the beginning of their study. Interviews are now available for assessing diagnosis in elderly people in a reliable manner and some validity date are also available. For most studies, but particularly for epidemiological studies comparing illness levels between populations, some authors would argue the importance of a computerized diagnosis, and these are also now becoming available (see below).

The limitations of cross-sectional studies have led increasingly to longitudinal designs. These bring the difficulty of measuring change over time. Many scales developed for hospital-based patients are too insensitive for recording change in community samples. Theoretically at least, the symptoms required for determining diagnosis may not be those which show most change as the condition advances. In practice, however, these theoretical objections may not be very apparent and many scales can be used for both purposes.

The identification and definition of 'cases' are crucial to most epidemiological studies. It cannot be emphasized sufficiently strongly (Copeland, 1981) that cases are concepts, not objects, and therefore only exist in so far as they are defined, and must be defined appropriately for each study. Thus the concept and definition of a case will vary from study to study. This will create difficulties when trying to extrapolate the findings of one study to another. Of particular interest is the recognition of 'early cases'. Clearly if therapeutic benefits for dementia are to be maximized, recognition of the illness must occur before substantial permanent brain damage has taken place. Perhaps biological markers will one day indicate the stages of a psychiatric illness, but even these could pose similar difficulties of interpretation in the early stages of illness. Answers to some of these problems could emerge from current longitudinal studies, but so far it has been difficult to isolate prognostic features.

If diagnosis is to be of help to planners of services, some concept of severity will be important. Severity has been difficult to formulate because it is not unidimensional. It is possible to obtain reasonable inter-rater agreement on, say, a five-point scale of severity left undefined, but as such a scale uses a number of different parameters it is difficult to interpret. Investigators have to decide what aspects of severity are important, and then develop individual scales for measuring these. Is it to be degrees of suicidal risk, the abruptness and intensity of the symptoms at the onset of an illness, or increasing danger of death, that are important for the study? A method of staging the progression of an illness may be an acceptable alternative. This would be helpful in a slow but progressive condition such as dementia. Stages would be related to disability and handicap at each stage, and also draw attention to deviations from the established course of the illness which might indicate different aetiological subgroups.

If the planner of services wishes to know into which facility to admit a patient, then ratings of the degree and impact on daily living of physical handicap, mobility, incontinence, feeding and hygiene, etc. will be required. Here the relationship between baseline ability and the effects of the illness will help to determine their amenability to rehabilitation.

It may be as important to understand why certain people successfully survive unpleasant life events as to understand why others succumb. The study and measurement of life events has progressed steadily over the last decade, but the measurement of coping strategies in the elderly has not gained consistent attention, and the assessment of personality factors has lagged behind the small advances made by psychiatry of other age groups.

Some of the Problems

We have already hinted that one of the difficulties with rating phenomena in the behavioural sciences is that of rating concepts rather than objects. Since the rating of objects itself involves perception and not all persons perceive similarly, difficulties can arise even here. The additional problem with concepts is that they deal with the individual's interpretation of events, so that the individual is already armed with an idiosyncratic view when he or she attempts to record what is perceived. The important thing, as we have said, is to remember that concepts are not objects, and that a concept is only useful in so far as it successfully fulfils its purpose. The other side of this is that concepts are not fixed, and will vary according to the purpose for which they are to be used. All this makes the creation of rating scales of behaviour particularly hazardous when they seek to interpret, rather than measure, what is observed.

A rating scale that may work well in one setting or for one purpose may not be suitable for another. The question is whether there can be a minimum or core concept of, say, depression or 'caseness', which will be useful for a range of applications, which most investigators will recognize or agree with and to which they can add additional features of particular interest to their own studies. The indications are that this may be the case up to a point, and that ideas such as 'depressive mood' or 'syndrome case' levels for diagnosis, for examples, may form a useful set of basic ideas which can be defined and measured and then elaborated to provide for the individual purpose. When using such measures developed by others, the investigator must be prepared to compromise on his or her own ideas in the interests of a wider communication. There is thus the problem that, although on the one hand it is desirable for workers to use similar methods so that the results of studies can be compared, on the other there is a limit to the degree of compromise that is acceptable before the particular measures become no longer appropriate. Perhaps some of the reasons why so much research remains unintelligible to the planners of services may be because the measures used have deviated too far from the purposes of the study or there has been a failure to appreciate that the core 'minimum concept' requires elaboration before it can be applied to a practical situation.

The rating of behaviour concerned with ageing has yet a further problem; what constitutes normal ageing is still largely unknown. At what point are phenomena to be regarded as deviant or abnormal? It is probably better not to build in assumptions, but rather to rate what is found and, if necessary, to make a second rating of abnormality, and even a third to indicate whether, for example, loss of appetite is due to psychiatric or physical illness. This at least allows second thoughts on the data, and reinterpretation if necessary.

Most rating scales deal only with psychiatric morbidity and associated problems. As we have observed, they do not attempt to rate what is sometimes called 'positive living'. Such assets may be important when trying to understand the ability to cope with physical, mental and social problems in old age. It would also be useful to have some measure of successful ageing, but this is not easy to develop. Some years ago, the gradual withdrawal from active participation in life and reconciliation to limited objectives consistent with physical and mental decline was seen as successful ageing. However, as it is not at all certain how much such decline is actually due to ageing and how much to neglect or disuse, such views may be premature. Is increasing fatigue due to the poor recovery of ageing muscles, or to lack of exercise and increasing unfitness which can be reversed? Does the brain becomes less active from loss of cortical tissue, or lack of use as society makes fewer demands upon the aged?

Much that determines morbidity may have to do with individual lifestyle and personal goals which are difficult to measure. Elderly people appear over-optimistic when asked to judge their general health, or perhaps do not recognize chronic disability as a problem of health, but rather a problem of ageing, so that when asked to assess their health they rate it optimistically against the absence of acute illness. Young investigators must remember when dealing with elderly people that there may be at least one, and probably two, generations gap between them and their subjects. Cultural differences make it difficult to extrapolate from one generation to another. If an elderly person living in a physically squalid environment says that he feels happy, is that a denial of the physical squalor or an ability to be happy in spite of it, bred of years of having to put up with similar conditions which the investigator might find intolerable, but which the subject has long since learned to ignore? It may also have to do with expectations. Older generations brought up before the welfare state, often in childhood poverty, may feel their expectations to have been wildly superseded for the better, ending their days in their own council house, even though the roof is leaking.

On the whole, elderly people are much easier to interview than younger people; they have more time, are more likely to be found at home, and are often eager for company. Even so, their behaviour may seem paradoxical. They do not, on the whole, like to be patronized and although they may tolerate it kindly at the time may again refuse to be re-interviewed. It is particularly dangerous for young investigators to become emotionally involved with their subjects, and bring gifts which may be construed as charity and cause embarrassment and even anger.

Investigators must beware of accepting the common stereotypes of the elderly often provided by well-meaning health and social workers who see only the most severely physically and mentally ill, or socially deprived. Community subjects are different and are often as active and motivated as younger people. Scales and interviews developed for hospital samples may therefore not be appropriate in the community. Asking a relative about a subject's incontinence and whether or not he loses his way home may be particularly embarrassing when faced with a retired accountant, who is president of his local golf club, or the ex-builder's labourer who is the local darts champion.

Another danger is to assume too easily that when older persons do not behave like younger persons it is due to morbidity. One third of elderly people say that they do not feel depressive mood when many other symptoms point inevitably to the presence of a depressive illness. This is unlike the experience with younger age groups. It is tempting to talk about the elderly person's 'denial' of depressive mood because younger age groups appear to experience this symptom with depressive illness. It is just possible that older persons are not so much denying depression as not understanding the term, or even expressing depressive mood in a different manner, such as 'feeling cold or empty inside'. Again, these are likely to be due to cultural differences between generations. They can seriously influence case selection when using rating scales developed for younger age groups which have not been standardized for elderly people, or may lead to health and social workers failing to recognize illness.

A practical problem which must be tackled by psychologists is the distress and anger often displayed by elderly persons who fail to perform well on psychological tests. This may lead to premature termination of the interview, or a refusal to participate in the future, as well as influence other interview responses. It may be a feature of rating scales undertaken in the community on relatively well people, who may feel insulted by the low level of skill which the investigator appears to expect of them, a particular problem with subjects in the early stages of dementia. New techniques have to be developed to overcome this problem.

Changes of environment sometimes produce symptoms such as disorientation. Whether they do so in those who are not at least partially intellectually impaired is not certain. The relative isolation and deprivation of information that occurs in some institutions may also affect scores which depend upon a knowledge of current events. Whether such deprivation has a long-term effect on intellectual function, and how much of it is reversible, is also uncertain.

Some general problems that exist in all assessments are exaggerated in the assessment of the elderly person. One source of error is simply the carelessness of the raters. Hall (1974) has shown that the reliability of nurses' ratings falls when the ward staffing level is low. Many professional and other workers have varying experience and strong personal attitudes and prejudices about older people which may affect their ratings. These problems point to the importance of training the raters in the procedures.

Much is sometimes made of the limited span of interest and increased fatiguability of elderly people which is said to necessitate shorter interviews and less complicated scales. Like so many of the misconceptions about older age, they are probably based on severely ill hospital populations, and may not apply to community samples. Elderly people living in the community can, on the whole, tolerate long interviews as well as younger persons. Some may be less knowledgeable about the need for such investigations, and therefore less tolerant or refuse to be re-interviewed at a later date.

Nevertheless, subjects do grow weary of multiple assessments. Rating scales and interviews tend to be developed for a specific purpose such as the measurement or identification of depressive mood or illness. At the same time it is necessary to exclude other syndromes, and to relate the findings to social needs, handicap, coping abilities, and so on, but the thoroughness with which each of these needs to be accomplished in order to provide a definite answer precludes any number of them being used in practice. The investigator must carefully select only those which are essential to the purpose, or any patient will become too fatigued and terminate the interview or, perhaps worse, accept the interview grudgingly and then refuse to be followed up at a later date. It would often be useful to have two versions of a scale: one to provide an in-depth study and a much shorter version to provide background information and tentative hypotheses for related studies.

Certainly, for large surveys as much information as possible must be collected at one interview because of the considerable cost. The move has therefore been towards multi-purpose assessments which can establish a reliable diagnosis and at the same time a range of background information which may be used to suggest further, more focused studies on a smaller scale.

ASSESSMENTS, INTERVIEWS AND SCALES

Many of the existing interviews and scales have been developed for specific problems or for use by particular professional workers and may not have general applicability. Many also have little evidence of reliability and validity testing.

Organic States Including Dementia

Some Problems and Requirements of Assessment

There is a danger in using simple scales to assess mental states. Much agreement on diagnosis can be reached using mental state data alone, but few would disagree that historical data are of great importance, especially for subdividing diagnosis into subcategories. Simple scales measuring only one aspect of mental state are sometimes mistaken by the unwary for diagnostic scales. They do not furnish a differential psychiatric diagnosis. The most they do is assess a psychiatric syndrome. In this instance, an organic syndrome may, of course, be associated not only with an organic illness but also with serious forms of depression, even schizophrenia. Such syndromes often co-exist. For example, high scores on the Mini Mental State (Folstein *et al.*, 1975) may be incorrectly used as evidence of *organic illness*, even of dementia, and lead to the over-diagnosis of one or the other. Such assessments do have important but limited application. Recently, attempts have been made to develop more comprehensive interviews which rely either on an intuitive differential diagnosis by the psychiatric interviewer, or may be used by a trained non-psychiatrist when the differential diagnosis is made by a computer.

Scales such as the Mini Mental State, although they may not diagnose dementia specifically, have been used extensively for screening populations in a two-stage design, whereby those subjects nominated by scores on the screening interview are re-interviewed by psychiatrists. However, such screening methods are not very efficient, because they make no attempt to exclude depression and other illnesses at the screening stage, and gather little general mental state information. They have the merit of being quick and easy to apply, with little training. However, in community samples, where the major consumption of time is in travelling to the home of the subject and making repeat visits to find them at home, a few minutes extra interview time is of little practical importance.

Attempts to describe stages in the organic illness, related to disability, handicap and the need for certain services, have been made by Reisberg *et al.* (1982a). However, the need for certain services and management may be determined by specific behavioural problems unrelated to the stages of illness.

It is important to be able to distinguish the recent onset of an organic illness from a long-standing chronic state of low intelligence, as may follow head injury or stroke, from congenital conditions of mental impairment, and chronic psychiatric states such as schizophrenia. Although a history can often be obtained from a relative, surviving relatives may be unaware of the early background of the patient, or the patient may be living alone. Attempts have been made to develop psychological tests which would identify such conditions—the National Adult Reading Test is one example.

Specific tests designed to detect early memory and cognitive impairment are required to provide good confirmation of the diagnosis of dementia. Psychological tests ought to provide better information in the early stages than clinical observations. The distribution of cognitive deficits and other mental impairment could be related to different forms of dementing illness. Differential patterns of impairment assessed over time might help to identify subcategories of dementia. A number of test batteries have been developed, notably those by Kendrick *et al.*(1979), the Halstead–Reitan Battery (Reitan, 1955) and the Luria–Nebraska Neuropsychological Battery (Golden *et al.*,

1979). The length of these tests has limited their clinical and research use. Attempts are now being made to produce user-friendly computer tests.

Scales for the assessment of changes in mental state and behaviour over time are of interest for longitudinal studies and the evaluation of therapy. One of the first, the Sandoz scale, is still in use.

Some scales which rely on the subject's reply for their rating and on the accumulation of scores as symptoms increase in number with severity, may appear to improve if the subject's condition deteriorates to the point where items cannot be rated and have to be omitted. Similarly, in some illnesses, outstanding symptoms may overshadow others, so that the number of symptoms appears to decline. These pose particular problems for the estimation of severity in the later stages of dementia unless other devices are introduced.

The More Popular Assessments

The Blessed Dementia Rating Scale (BDRS; Blessed *et al.*, 1968) is still widely used for assessing the severity of previously diagnosed dementia. It has some 50 items, taking about 30 minutes to administer. Items of cognition make up the Memory and Information Tests (MIT) and items of behaviour the Dementia Rating Scale (DRS; Kay, 1977). Blessed *et al.* used their dementia scale to demonstrate a highly significant correlation between mean brain cortical plaque counts and scores for dementia, and performance on psychological tests. Their findings suggested that psychological and pathological indices were closely related to one another, although the correlation declined sharply in clinically severe sufferers. They were able to conclude that pathological differences between normal subjects and those with mild, moderate and severe dementia were quantitative. Few other scales have had this degree of neuropathological validation, although this state of affairs is now changing rapidly. Lloyd (1970) used the scale in a pilot study and found it to have good test–retest reliability. Hodkinson (1972), in a large multicentre study on hospital in-patients, identified the ten most useful questions for differentiating between normal and abnormal cognitive functioning. Dysphasic patients were excluded from the study. He claimed that this shorter version, 'the Mental Test Score', gave comparable results to the full Blessed scale, for the identification of cognitive impairment. However, he acknowledged that the coarser gradations of the abbreviated form may not perform as well in the recognition of serial changes, important in the diagnosis of confusional states. Quershi and Hodkinson (1974) attempted to validate the Mental Test Score further by comparing it to the Roth–Hopkins test 'Roth and Hopkins, 1953) and a modified version of the Tooting Bec questionnaire. High correlations between all three tests were found, but the shorter test achieved greatest compliance. Thompson and Blessed (1987) found the scale to be useful as a simple test of mental impairment in functionally and mildly organically ill psychogeriatric patients attending a day hospital. Little *et al.* (1987) followed up 181 elderly patients living at home, using the short Mental Test Score, the Inglis Paired Associate Learning Test (Inglis, 1959) and the Psychogeriatric Assessment Schedule devised by Bergmann (unpublished) to find that the Mental Test Score was the most useful of the three for screening for organic disorder and for predicting change over a 2-year period.

The Blessed scale was also used by Perry *et al.* (1978) to demonstrate a satisfactory correlation between the deficiency of brain choline acetyltransferase in Alzheimer's disease, and scale scores during life. Most of the studies comparing the Blessed scale with brain neuropathology have concentrated on dementias of the Alzheimer type. The scale has not been developed to discriminate between this disorder and multi-infarct dementia. However, where a single score is required as an indication of the severity of already diagnosed dementia, the Blessed scale can be recommended with confidence, and the shortened version may well serve as a useful rapid screening device for organic disorder, i.e. possible dementia, for clinical use.

The Mini Mental State Examination (MMSE) has been used extensively in the USA, where it was chosen as the sole cognitive component for the Diagnostic Interview Schedule (Robins *et al.*, 1981). Whereas the Blessed scale concentrates on memory and orientation, the MMSE attempts to assess a wider range of types of deficits, which may be found in Alzheimer's disease and associated dementias. The test consists of two parts: verbal and performance. Four verbal subtests have a maximum score of 21 points and evaluate orientation in time, memory and attention. Two performance subtests have a maximum score of 9 points, and involve the naming of objects, execution of written or spoken orders, writing, and copying a complex polygon. In the original studies by Folstein *et al.* (1975) the scale was tested on two series of patients. The first was a group of 69 elderly persons suffering from affective disorders alone, affective disorders with cognitive impairment, dementia, and a group of normal subjects. The second group consisted of 137 elderly consecutive admissions to hospital suffering from a variety of psychiatric illnesses. Serial tests were undertaken to demonstrate change over time, and the ability to separate cases of dementia from other conditions. Concurrent validity tested against the WAIS subtest, and inter-rater reliability and test–retest reliability at 24 hours and 28 days, were found to be satisfactory. The scale takes between 5 and 10 minutes to administer.

Nelson *et al.* (1986) reviewed the 11 validation studies on the MMSE comprising data on 859 subjects. Most of these studies correlated scores with clinical descriptions using DSM-III diagnoses and various radiological investigations. The authors drew attention to the lack of validative work carried out in community and non-hospital populations. Dick *et al.* (1984), using the scale in the context of neurological and neurosurgical admissions, found that race and socio-economic status significantly affected the scores.

Tsai and Tsuang (1979) have reported positive correlations between the Mini Mental State Score and CT scans indicating cortical atrophy.

With a cut-off score between 23 and 24 on the MMSE, most non-dementing elderly subjects rarely score below 24. Anthony *et al.* (1982) found that 87% of their sample of patients with clinical dementia scored below 23 points, and similar findings were reported by Roth *et al.* (1986).

The CAMDEX (see below) incorporates the MMSE as an integral part of its schedule. The GMS–AGECAT package (see below), although not including it, suggests its use alongside these interviews in order to preserve comparability with the American studies.

Other Scales for the Assessment of Organic States

Although the search has always been for the shortest possible scale which will yield satisfactory results, it is doubtful whether scales shorter than those described above can be of much practical use. Most clinicians would probably claim that moderate to severe dementias can be distinguished by answers to as few as five questions, but the illness is usually obvious to the investigator at this stage, and an informant's account, however brief, leaves little doubt about the diagnosis. Short scales have not been shown to be useful in the identification of early or mild cases of dementia, an area fraught with difficulty because mild cognitive disturbance can result from many different causes. The view that only subjects with early dementia are likely to be cogniti' ely affected by depression, unfamiliar surroundings, etc., is an interesting one but not yet proven. Many of the early scales relied heavily on memory impairment, for example the Mental Status Questionnaire (Kahn *et al.*, 1960), and the not dissimilar Short Portable Mental Status Questionnaire developed by Pfeiffer (1975), consisting of ten questions concerned with orientation, remote and recent memory, but also evaluating attention and concentration by the serial subtraction of 3s. Pfeiffer was able to show a good test–retest reliability for his scores and postulate that normal adults would fail only one item, but 28% of his community sample failed two items. As usual in these scales, level of education and social class had a confounding influence on the scores. Later Fillenbaum (1980) found a sensitivity of 0.98 and a specificity of 0.55 for organic brain syndrome when using a cutting score of more than two items. Three items were found to be responsible for over 90% of the discrimination between normal individuals and those with organic brain syndrome. They are the now familiar ones: full date of birth; current day of the week; and name of the previous President of the United States.

The Alzheimer Disease Assessment Scale (ADAS) has been developed recently by Mohs *et al.* (1983) and Rosen *et al.* (1984). It consists of items for assessing both the cognitive and non-cognitive deficits usually associated with Alzheimer's disease which has been confirmed neuropathologically. The cognitive and memory tests account for some 60% of the items, which cover memory, disorientation, dyspraxia and dysphasia, and also attempt to rate depression and other affective states. Inter-rater reliability and success at rating change 12 months later were regarded as satisfactory. Its validity was tested against the Dementia Rating Scale, the Memory Information Test (part of the Blessed Dementia Scale) and the Sandoz Clinical Assessment Geriatric Scale.

The ADAS represents a compromise between the brief rating scales mentioned above and a more thorough assessment of individual impairments by separate specific tests. The 45 minutes or so which are required for its administration is not dissimilar from that required for the comprehensive diagnostic assessments to be described later. Investigators, however, may find it descriptively useful when mapping changes in cognitive and other deficits over time. The graded severity of the items may hamper inter-rater reliability, as they appear to depend on relatively subjective observations, although overall inter-rater reliability is claimed to be high.

The Staff Assessment of Confusion Scale (Slater and Lipman, 1977) is worth mentioning because it is one of the few scales which has been standardized in community residential settings, and could serve as a simple case-finding procedure, preliminary to a larger investigation. 457 residents in 11 homes were rated to determine their levels of mental confusion. Validity was tested against the ratings of the head of each home, and on a number of other scales.

There are few scales specifically designed for psychopharmacological research with elderly persons. The Sandoz Clinical Assessment Geriatric Scale (SCAG) was devised with this primary purpose, and the authors claim that it is a valid and reliable instrument for assessing psychopathology in older people (Shader *et al.*, 1974). It differs from some of the other interviews discussed above by requiring a trained observer to make the ratings on the basis of extensive observations of the patient. A shorter, self-assessment scale, has been designed, but has limitations in its applicability to demented patients (Yesavage *et al.*, 1981). The original scale was used in the assessment of Hydergine as a treatment for dementia (Lowe and Weil, 1982). Rosen *et al.* (1984) criticized the scale for its lack of justification of item selection, and its poor inter-rater reliability. It is doubtful whether psychopharmacological research requires specific scales.

It is also worth mentioning the scale developed by Hasegawa (1983), which although not used extensively outside Japan has formed the basis of a number of epidemiological studies of dementia and organic states in that country.

The Differentiation Between Senile Dementia of the Alzheimer Type and Multi-infarct Dementia

The distinction between Alzheimer's and multi-infarct dementia is important because investigators have regarded these disorders as having differing aetiologies. Recently, some authors have challenged this view and it is certainly true that mixed forms exist. Meanwhile, Hachinski's ischaemic score is the most popular method of attempting to make the distinction. The scale itself is based on clinical features described by Slater and Roth, in Mayer-Gross *et al.* (1969). It consists of 13 ratings producing a weighted score. The ratings concern such items as abrupt onset, stepwise deterioration, fluctuating course, nocturnal confusion, etc. In the original articles these were left undefined but a useful description can be found in Wade and Hachinski (1987), and Roth (1981) gives some further helpful suggestions for improving the definitions of terms. In the original studies (Hachinski *et al.*, 1975) 24 patients of comparable age, blood pressure and degree of dementia were classified by the ischaemic score based on clinical features, into multi-infarct and primary degenerative dementia. Regional cerebral blood-flow was measured by the intra-carotid xenon-133 method. There was no correlation between degree of dementia and cerebral blood flow in the primary degenerative group, but an inverse relationship was demonstrated in the multi-infarct group, determined by the Hachinski score. Thus, some validation of the score was obtained. The authors found that the ischaemic score was bimodal in distribution, differentiating multi-infarct dementia from Alzheimer-type with no overlap. Further studies have confirmed that the dementing population tends to separate into groups, scoring less than 4 and greater than 7 (Harrison *et al.*, 1979). In the group scoring more than 7, further evidence of multiple infarction can usually be obtained by special investigation such as EEG, computed tomography scan or positron emission tomography (Harrison *et al.*, 1979; Loeb and Gandolfo, 1983; Frackowiak *et al.*, 1980). The authors stress that the scores do not represent a linear scale of severity and that those achieving maximum scores do not necessarily have a more advanced illness than those achieving lower scores. Rosen *et al.* (1979), examining 14 elderly demented patients brought to autopsy, found that scores ranging from 2 to 5 were obtained in those with Alzheimer-type dementia, whereas those with multi-infarct dementia and a combination of the two diagnoses had scores ranging from 7 to 14. Rosen *et al.* modified the scale and eliminated items such as 'fluctuating course' and 'nocturnal confusion', which they did not find contributed to the diagnostic differentiation, and they omitted 'relative preservation of personality' because such data were not available in their study. One of the problems of the Hachinski scale is the overall lack of precise definitions and rating instructions for each of the items and the lack of a structured examination for making the ratings.

Attempts have now been made to standardize appropriate questions and answers, and both Copeland *et al.* in that part of the GMS–AGECAT package called the History and Aetiology Schedule, and Roth *et al.* in the CAMDEX, have incorporated such questions in their interviews. Data have not yet been published to show whether or not such standardization leads to improved reliability. Although validated samples are relatively small, it is probably safe to assume that scores below 4 effectively eliminate the presence of multi-infarct dementia.

Hovaguimian and his colleagues in Geneva (personal communication) have recently been developing a clinical interview for the differential diagnosis of dementia between Alzheimer's disease and multi-infarct types, and are adapting it for computer use.

The Clinical Staging of Dementia

To be able to stage dementia in terms of severity, or at least the advancement of the disease, would be exceedingly useful. Reisberg *et al.* (1982) have developed the Global Deterioration Scale (GDS) and the Brief Cognitive Rating Scale (BCRS). The GDS grades dementia on seven levels, mainly by disabilities of memory. This is a somewhat narrow approach which might be considered to limit its usefulness for research. The scale appears to have been developed on clinical grounds, and then tested against more established measures. It is now popular in the USA. There is no standardized method provided for acquiring the necessary information to allot subjects to the scale levels, although some of the information must be derived from psychological tests, from Mental State examination, from family members or health and social workers. Clearly, the amount of information available will vary from subject to subject and from study to study, as there is no insistence on a minimum or maximum amount. Thus, for research there may be difficulties with reliability. The seven staged clinical descriptions relate to the spectrum of clinical presentation between normality and severe Alzheimer's disease. The five axes contributing to these clinical profiles have each been graded into seven degrees of severity. The scale is described by Reisberg *et al.* (1982a, 1982b, 1983, 1984).

Fifty consecutive out-patients were studied and grouped by the stage of dementia according to GDS definitions. A number of tests were carried out on the population, including Mental Status questionnaire scores, WAIS subtests and the GUILD test battery. The global clinical parameters measured have also been found to relate to behavioural aspects and neuroradiology (De Leon *et al.*, 1979, 1980, 1983a, b and c). The prognostic success of the stages of dementia as measured by the scale have been examined in the community, and found to be of value over a 27-month period (Reisberg *et al.*, 1983).

The scale would appear to require a clinician to assemble the information and to decide which Reisberg stage best describes the individual patient. Stage 3 out of 7 is considered by Reisberg and his co-workers to be the lowest level of impairment indicating the probable development of dementia, provided that other causes of organic brain syndrome have been excluded. Apart from the excessive dependence upon memory, the scale descriptions appear to have good face validity and relate closely to clinical observation. However, the lack of reliability arising from the variable amount of data available on individual patients and between studies is likely to make the scale less useful for longitudinal research aimed at mapping change over time. Some degree of standardization and more specific instructions on how to allot subjects to levels would greatly increase the value of the scale for research, as no other method of clinical staging seems to have been developed.

Gurland *et al.* (1983) described the use of the CARE interview (see below). The scales of pervasive dementia and pervasive depression derived from scores on items in this interview do provide an alternative method of staging dementia for those requiring a comprehensive assessment not only of psychiatric disorder but also physical and social problems, social disability and need.

Another interview which may be useful for staging dementia is the GBS scale developed by Gottfries *et al.* (1982) (see below). This scale assesses a number of parameters each on seven points of severity, which could be used for the staging of the disorder. The scale is designed to be used by trained nurses and psychologists as well as psychiatrists.

Psychological Tests for Organic Disorders

Psychological tests should have several important functions in the assessment of elderly people for research. They ought to be useful as an aid to diagnosis, for screening and to assess areas of cognitive and other psychological functioning which might help to discriminate between different forms of dementia on cross-sectional studies, and by their differential patterning over time serve to be useful for both diagnosis and prognosis. Another use for psychological tests would be the assessment of pre-morbid cognitive level. It can be said immediately that few of these functions are at present being satisfied by current tests. Cowan *et al.* (1975) and others were unable to show that psychological tests were superior to clinical judgement in diagnosing elderly psychiatric inpatients. When controlling for severity of initial illness, she was able to demonstrate change over time using psychological tests, which others had found difficult. These changes, however, seemed to be less sensitive than clinical judgement. Ron *et al.* (1979) has found psychological tests to be useful in the diagnosis of dementia.

One of the best documented and validated test batteries is that devised by Kendrick. Kendrick *et al.* (1965) developed a sophisticated learning and memory test—the Synonym Learning Test (SLT)—based on a technique pioneered by Shapiro and Nelson (1955), and later modified by Walton and Black (1957). Kendrick also introduced the Digit Copying Test (DCT) of motor speed, which is likely to be impaired in depression. However, the SLT proved to be stressful, both for the examinee and the examiner, resulting in a high drop-out rate for the examinee (Gibson and Kendrick, 1976; Kendrick *et al.*, 1978, 1979). It has now been replaced by the Object Learning Test (OLT), which has proved to have better compliance. The concurrent validity of the tests has been studied and shown to differentiate clearly between dementing and non-dementing subjects (Gibson, 1979; Kendrick *et al.*, 1979). The construct validity of the tests has been studied by factor analysis (Gibson, 1979). Normal and depressed patients were found to be similar in terms of the factors identified, but demented patients differed in that the factors were non-definable. All three scores, the OLT, the SLT and the DCT, were found to correlate with cortical brain atrophy, the Evans ratio and planimetry as determined by CT scan. Jacoby and Levy (1980a and b) and Naguib and Levy (1982) have studied the predictive value of the DCT in senile dementia and found that the scores were associated with increased likelihood of death within 30 months. The Kendrick battery has been found to function less well with chronically institutionalized subjects (Gibson *et al.*, 1980). It is recommended, therefore, that it should not be used on patients who have been in hospital for longer than 3 weeks. Kendrick claims that his cognitive tests can be used to screen for the presence of dementia, but are not designed to distinguish between its various forms. He also claims they are useful for differential diagnosis from other conditions, particularly for distinguishing between dementing, pseudo-dementing, depressive and normal modes of response (Kendrick, 1985). Both the OLT and the DCT appear to be reliable and can be shown to have concurrent, content and construct validity. Undoubtedly, the Kendrick tests are the best validated and most reliable available for work with the elderly. They have been developed on moderate to severe cases of dementia in hospital samples, and no claim at present is made for the detection of early cases. The initial impression from our own studies is that the tests in their present form are unlikely to diagnose early cases but this might be overcome by modifying cut-off points.

Recently, some claim has been made for the WAIS (Crookes, 1974) for the diagnosis of early cases of dementia. In other studies it has been shown that by comparing the verbal and performance subtests a deterioration index can be computed. Ron *et al.* (1979) demonstrated that in demented patients performance tests were substantially more affected than verbal tests. This was not the case in patients suffering from depressive pseudo-dementia.

Crookes found that for dementia in both sexes the highest score was the vocabulary score and the lowest were those for block design and digit symbol.

The Halstead–Reitan battery (Reitan, 1955) is popular in the USA. However, it is not specifically designed for the elderly and takes several hours to administer. Similar problems also attend the Luria–Nebraska Neuropsychological Battery (Golden *et al.*, 1979). Kendrick compared these batteries with his own much shorter tests, and found high correlation rates, indicating that as much information could be gained from the short test as from the long battery (Drinkwater, 1981). He concluded that such complicated batteries were not efficient methods for assessing the elderly. The Alzheimer Disease Assessment Scale by Rosen *et al.* (1984) already discussed above might be mentioned here, and the Extended Dementia Scale of Hersch (1979), which is again short, but mainly for use with more severely ill populations. Huppert and Tym (1986) considered the level of item difficulty in this scale inappropriate for the well-preserved or only mildly impaired elderly.

The level of pre-morbid intelligence has important implications for the differential diagnosis of dementia. Bergmann *et al*, (1971), in following up the subjects studied by Kay *et al.* (1964), found that a proportion of those who had been diagnosed as suffering from dementia had failed to progress, and probably represented long-standing cases of low intelligence or mental handicap. Such subjects would be recognized most easily from an informant's interview, but if such were not available a psychological test serving the same function would be useful. The National Adult Reading Test (NART) (Nelson, 1982) attempts this assessment. Nelson based the test on the observation that reading ability was comparatively well preserved in dementia. The test requires the subject to read a list of 50 irregularly spelt words, and the number of errors in pronunciation is recorded. The words have graded difficulty, and previous knowledge of the word is necessary to know the correct pronunciation, which cannot be inferred by the English spelling. In 1975, Nelson and McKenna showed that reading ability and intelligence quotient on the WAIS correlated highly in 129 non-demented subjects aged between 20 and 70 years. No significant effect of age or social class was found. In 1978, Nelson and O'Connell showed that there were no differences in patients with and without pre-senile dementia, on the basis of which they claimed that the error score was resistant to pre-senile dementia. They themselves offer no data for elderly people, nor do they appear as yet to have done any stringent longitudinal studies. However, Binks and Davies (1984) have applied the NART to community samples of elderly people, validated against psychiatric diagnosis and computer diagnostic levels. Tentative findings indicated that the mentally impaired sample made significantly more errors. They therefore conclude that it is likely that the NART is dementia-sensitive, although possibly to a much lesser extent than other tests, such as the Mill Hill Vocabulary Test. More extensive testing is required. It is likely that the NART will be affected by dementia severe enough to affect most intellectual function, but may be particularly applicable in the early stages. This scale could make an important contribution to diagnosis.

A number of other tests have been introduced, but require more extensive trials. The Selective Reminding Test developed by Buschke (1973) relies mainly on verbal memory tasks requiring the immediate and delayed recall of a list of 12 words. Subscores are aimed to assess whether defects arise in encoding, or in the storage or retrieval of information. This test has been successfully used in the USA for measuring the improvement in memory function following trials of oral physostigmine (Beller *et al.*, 1985).

The difficulty with many psychological tests is their face validity. The latter is important for gaining the patient's cooperation and sometimes that of the examiner. The everyday relevance can be questioned of tests which examine artificial skills such as remembering word lists. To overcome this difficulty, a number of tests have been developed which are said to resemble the simple tasks of daily living. One of these is the Misplaced Objects Test (MOT) (Crooke *et al.*, 1979). These authors claim good reliability and good patient tolerance for this test, in which the patient places and replaces common objects on the ground floor plan of a house. However, Searle (1984) found that the MOT correlated highly with other mental tests in community samples, adding little further information. Similar tests by the same group are the Facial Recognition and Name–Face Association tests, using photographic material (Ferris *et al.*, 1980), the Shopping List Test (McCarthy *et al.*, 1981) and the Telephone Number Task (Crooke *et al.*, 1980). Again it could be asked how much relevance, placing objects on the two-dimensional ground plan of a house, has to mislaying spectacles in a real home. However, the semblance of a game may make such tests more acceptable to the subject. More sophisticated tests such as those by Tinkleberg *et al.* (1984), consisting of a computerized test of divided attention, are interesting, but require further development. Nevertheless, computer-assisted tests as a whole have found increasing acceptance among elderly people. Carr *et al.* (1982) warn that computer testing does not necessarily produce the same answers as conventional testing. Subjects may read the screen correctly, but make verbal responses when motor responses are required, or accidentally press the wrong button. Forced-choice responses may overwhelm the subject in indecision. The interest in the development of computer tests is now considerable among research groups in Britain and the USA. It is, however, likely that these tests will be suited to institution-based subjects. The development of portable computers for home assessments for epidemiological surveys may require different techniques if they are to be acceptable to well and mildly ill subjects.

Depressive States

Most epidemiological studies show that about one-third of elderly persons, who otherwise have substantial symptoms of depressive illness, do not admit to depressive mood. They may present with somatic symptoms, feelings of emptiness or deadness inside, loneliness, or complaints of memory loss. Conventional methods for assessing depression may therefore not suffice for older adults. Zung and Green (1973) suggested using a classification criterion of 40 for his scale, which correctly identified 88% of depressives, but wrongly classified 44% of non-depressives. He acknowledged that the scale had a relatively poor specificity when used in elderly populations (Zung, 1975). In particular, it appears to miss depressives who are presenting in the guise of somatic illness (Raft *et al.*, 1977), and its use has been further criticized in the elderly by Carroll *et al.* (1973) and Weiss *et al.* (1986). Gallagher *et al.* (1983) examined the congruence between conventional cut-off scores on the Beck Depression Inventory and selected diagnostic criteria in a sample of 102 elders seeking psychological treatment. Only around 17% were misclassified by conventional BDI cut-off scores. As usual, minor depressive disorders were less clearly identified than major depressive disorders or non-depressed states. The Hamilton Rating Scale (1960) could be similarly criticized.

Brink *et al.* (1982), having reviewed problems in the use of psychometric tests to identify depression in older populations, then present their own Geriatric Depression Scale (GDS) consisting of 100 items covering seven common manifestations of depression in later life, somatic concern, lowered affect, cognitive impairment, feelings of discrimination, impaired motivation, lack of future orientation and impaired self-esteem. When compared with the results of both the Zung and Hamilton scales on the same patients, the GDS was just superior to the others in differentiating between the control and target samples. Reasonable evidence for reliability and validity is presented in both the 1982 paper and that by Yesavage *et al.* (1983). Although the authors present the GDS as a self-rating scale, it can be completed by an interviewer questioning the subject. Recently Bird *et al.* (1987) have reported their self-rating scale SELFCARE (D), which they claim to be an acceptable and economic screening test for depression in a primary care population of elderly subjects. It was compared with independent psychiatric assessment in 75 patients attending general practitioners. Specificity was 98%, sensitivity 77%, and positive predictive value 96% in a sample with prevalence at 41.3% and kappa values of agreement of 0.77. A number of studies are now using this scale in the UK and the USA so that further information on its performance is likely to be available before long.

The Identification of Illness for Case-Finding Studies

Kay *et al.* (1985) in Hobart found that the MMSE performed satisfactorily for the identification of moderate and severe dementia in a population sample. It was brief to administer and required little training. Against DSM-III criteria, the sensitivity was 100% and the specificity 86% using the 30-item version and a cutting point of 23/24. However, for mild dementia it was much less satisfactory; sensitivity was only 59% and specificity 93%. They concluded that it is only satisfactory for detecting probable cases of moderate or severe dementia. However, most screening instruments will discriminate satisfactorily at this level. Henderson (1986) wonders whether a single question to an informant would not distinguish equally well. Its performance in the National Institute of Mental Health (USA) catchment area study has raised some doubts about its screening ability for large samples. As the MMSE is not a diagnostic scale and would therefore pick up organic states simulated by other conditions, the six month prevalence rate of 3.4% for severe cognitive impairment is low compared with other studies (Weissman *et al.*, 1985).

The Survey Psychiatric Assessment Schedule (SPAS) (Bond *et al.*, 1980) is derived from the Geriatric Mental State (see below) and adapted to be given as a questionnaire by trained non-professional staff of the consumer research type. It covers three broad diagnostic areas: organic; schizophrenic, paranoid and affective disorders; and the psychoneuroses. Its reliability was tested by a 'split half' design. It appeared to perform satisfactorily for identifying organic disorders but less so for functional disorders and co-morbid states. It has been used for surveying large samples rapidly to obtain crude prevalence figures.

There are a number of brief screening methods for organic disorders, other than the MMSE and the SPAS. Most will identify subjects with organic symptoms but will not distinguish between those of organic or functional aetiology. Recently McWilliam *et al.* (1988) have developed the community version of the Geriatric Mental State (see below) as a screening interview using an Organic/Depression Index and the computer diagnosis AGECAT to nominate cases and provide a differential diagnosis for all subjects interviewed. Interviewers should be trained and the interview takes some 15–20 minutes on subjects who are not ill (about two-thirds of the population) and up to 30 minutes on ill subjects. Once again it is stressed that in community surveys where subjects are examined at home, it is the time of travel which is costly, rather than the actual interview time. McWilliam *et al.* (1988), using a 'split half' design on a random community sample of 1070 subjects, report high sensitivity and specificity of 100% and 92% respectively for organic disorders, and 88% and 83% for cases of depression. The positive predictive value for organic cases in the community is reported as 46% and that for depressive disorders 43%. As the positive predictive value is dependent on prevalence it is always low in community samples. The nomination of cases can be undertaken on the spot. Some further validity data on the outcome of cases nominated are now becoming available.

Interviews Aimed at Differential Diagnosis

Many of the scales already mentioned assess individual aspects of mental state but cannot alone be used for the differential diagnosis of psychiatric syndromes. Also, it is no longer feasible for psychiatrists to be used for the identification of cases in epidemiological field studies, nor in many geographical areas will they be available to examine cases nominated by a screening device. In any case, it has been argued that clinical methods of diagnosis are no longer sufficiently reliable for comparative studies of prevalence and incidence. In 1976 Copeland *et al.* and Gurland *et al.* described the Geriatric Mental State and how it was derived partly from the Present State Examination (Wing *et al.*, 1974) and the Mental Status Schedule (Spitzer *et al.*, 1964) with the addition of many new items covering organic and other states. Since then, the interview has been modified as a result of field studies. By an analysis of data sets a community version has been developed (GMSA), and an informant interview added, the History and Aetiology Schedule (HAS). This latter deals in detail with type of onset of the illness, its early course, past and family history of mental and physical illness, history of alcohol and drug abuse, head trauma, previous occupational level, educational attainment, and standard items for calculating the Hachinski score (Hachinski *et al.*, 1975). A Social Status Schedule has been developed for assessing the need and provision of health and social services, and a Physical Status Schedule. Satisfactory reliability studies have now been undertaken, including those by Henderson *et al.* (1983) and Hooijer *et al.* (to be submitted). Good levels of inter-rater reliability have been shown, and satisfactory levels of test–retest reliability. The reliability of individual items of frequent occurrence has also been shown to be satisfactory. A comprehensive computerized diagnostic system, AGECAT, can now be applied to the data from the GMS–AGECAT package. In stages I and II, data from the GMS provide levels of confidence of diagnosis for each subject on eight syndromes—organic states, schizophrenia, mania, depression (psychotic and neurotic types), hypochondriasis, obsessional, phobic and anxious states—thus identifying co-morbid states, and emerge with a principal diagnosis, an alternative diagnosis if appropriate, organic and depression scores and an organic/depression index for the on-spot recognition of cases (see above). Symptom profiles allow comparison of different clinical pictures and a recording of change in symptom levels over time. The third stage of AGECAT takes data from the informant interview (HAS) and provides a breakdown of organic states into acute, subacute and chronic, those drug, alcohol or trauma related, and provides tentative diagnoses of multi-infarct and Alzheimer-type dementia. AGECAT diagnosis has been tested against psychiatrists' diagnoses in a number of studies in Britain and Australia (n = 1118) and has been shown to have good agreement with DSM-III diagnoses. The overall agreement with psychiatrists' diagnoses for organic states and dementia reaches kappa values of 0.80 and above for organic disorders and 0.76 and above for depression (Copeland *et al.*, 1986, 1988). In 1986 Copeland *et al.* reported the first study of the outcome of AGECAT diagnosis; further outcome studies and studies involving CAT and neuropathological studies are to be reported. Psychological tests have also been undertaken as part of the studies, but have not been included as an integral part of the interviews because of the difficulties of finding culture-free tests. The use of the GMSA as a screening interview for case identification has been discussed above. Copeland *et al.* (1986) discuss what is meant by the term 'case' in the context of their studies. A manual is available but the authors recommend a short training course. GMSA takes some 20 minutes to give on average, and the HAS a similar time. Interviewers do not need to be medically qualified. The interviews have been translated by need into some 14 languages other than English and are at present being used in large studies in Europe, Latin America and Asia. The authors claim that this method provides a reliable procedure by which prevalence and incidence studies can be undertaken and compared between different populations at reasonable cost. A much shorter "B" version is now available for dementia studies.

A recent assessment procedure for dementia has been reported by Roth *et al.* (1986): the CAMDEX interview. This interview is also a standardized method of interviewing consisting of structured questions concerned with information on current physical and mental state, personal and family history, and the onset and course of the illness. It includes an interview with a relative or care-giver. Items for the calculation of the Hachinski ischaemic score, the Blessed dementia score and the MMSE are included. A substantial part of the interview, however, is given to psychological testing which attempts to assess a range of functioning such as orientation, language, memory, praxis, attention, perception, calculation and abstract thinking. The whole interview is said to require some 60 minutes with the patient and 20 further minutes for the informant interview. The authors report very high inter-rater reliability rates where r = 0.99 for the patient's interview, 0.97 for the cognitive part of the examination and 0.90 for the informant's interview. This was assessed on 40 subjects. In a sample of 97 subjects, consisting of 17 normal persons, 49 with dementia, 14 with clouding of consciousness and 12 depressed subjects, the cognitive score was found to have a sensitivity of 92% and a specificity of 96% for identifying organic disorder from normal and depressive states. But this must be compared with the figures of 94% sensitivity and 85% specificity for the MMSE, which is much shorter to administer. The principal purpose of the CAMDEX interview is said to be for making a differential diagnosis, but this work has so far not been reported. No standardized computer diagnosis has been developed, although the information is available for DSM-III diagnoses to be applied by the interviewer. The application of the interview has so far been reported only on small samples and it is likely that the large psychological component will make it difficult to use the interview outside the cultural setting for which it was developed.

Assessments of Daily Living

The Performance test of Activities of Daily Living (PADL) (Kuriansky *et al.*, 1976) was first developed for the US/UK Cross-national Project in order to assess the ability to perform simple everyday tasks in hospital-based elderly subjects, particularly those unable to complete formal interviews. It continues to be used in a variety of ongoing studies. It has the advantage of face validity since it uses common objects to assess 16 activities thought to be of value for predicting the need for services. Each activity is broken down into basic movements and rated independently. Good inter-rater reliability has been recorded and scores have been shown to correlate significantly with patient's current health and outcome. Two and a half days of training are required.

Rating Scales Designed for Nurses and Other Workers

The Nurses' Observation Scale for In-patient Evaluation (NOSIE) (Honigfield and Klett, 1965) was developed as a behaviour rating scale sufficiently sensitive to measure therapeutic change in the schizophrenic patient. It draws on the skill of nursing personnel to make unobtrusive observations of patient behaviour. Although not designed for use with the older subject this scale has been widely used in all age groups and could be of use in non-demented institutionalized patients.

Although the Physical and Mental Impairment of Evaluation Scale (PAMIE), unlike the NOSIE, was developed especially for an older population, it has only been standardized on males. It was designed to quantify behavioural problems in the functionally ill and would appear to have little application to dementia.

Wilkinson and Graham-White (1980) report good reliability and validity studies for a scale designed to assess orientation, behaviour and physical capacity in the elderly mentally ill, the Psycho-geriatric Dependency Rating Scale (PGDRS). The scale is brief and reliability is satisfactory if the scale is completed by a group of nurses working together, but can be reduced if ward staffing levels are low. Concurrent validity was tested by using the scale to predict the allocation of individuals to different patient groups according to service requirement and then comparing the result with actual practice. Prognostic ability was tested against outcome over 18 months in community-based subjects and those in residential care. This could prove a useful scale, especially applicable to dementing illness, but particular attention should be given to reliability.

The GBS scale (Gottfries *et al.*, 1982) was developed for use by nurses, psychologists and psychiatrists. Designed mainly for the assessment of dementia and to demonstrate treatment changes over time, it addresses motor, intellectual and emotional functions together with common dementia symptoms. The authors claim that it can be used to assess the severity of dementia on a number of subtests with reasonable accuracy but is not for determining diagnosis. Changing patterns of subscores, progressing from memory impairment through emotional to motor disorder, have been shown to accompany the progress of the illness (Brane and Gottfries, 1985; Brane, 1986). The scale has also been used successfully to demonstrate the effects of treatment (Karlsson *et al.*, 1985). In addition it may offer a useful method for staging dementia.

Comprehensive Interviews

A number of interviews have been developed to assess a wide range of disability, both physical and mental, as well as social problems and the need for health and social services. One example is the Older Americans Resources and Services multidimensional assessment questionnaire (OARS; Fillenbaum and Smeyer, 1981). This interview was developed for an evaluative programme of resource allocation. Of the two parts, A consists of an assessment of social and economic status, mental and physical health and activities of daily living, each scored on a six-point scale. Part B tackles the assessment for services, the rating of current usage, category of provider and currently perceived need for 24 services generically defined. Two days are required to train interviewers. The authors claim to be able to assess the effect of service provision, over time. The OARS was used by Blazer and Williams *et al.* (1980) in their community studies. Because it relies on global mental health ratings rather than the rating of precise psychopathology, it has probably now been superseded by newer methods.

In 1982 Lawton *et al.* developed the Philadelphia Geriatric Center multilevel assessment instrument. Information is gathered in seven domains: physical health, activities of daily living, cognitive function, time use, personal adjustment, social interaction (including psychiatric symptoms) and perceived environment. Some demographic information is also sought, and the results processed to provide scores on four areas: behavioural competence, psychological well-being, perceived quality of life and environmental quality. Individual components can be used without reference to the interview as a whole, but training is recommended.

Of the available methods for the clinical assessment of behaviour, the Stockton Geriatric Rating Scale (Meer and Baker, 1966) has gained some measure of acceptance in the UK. The scale is the product of factor analyses of items originally selected according to the clinical experience of the authors. Satisfactory evidence is produced for the internal consistency, inter-rater reliability and validity of the scale. Four stable factors emerged: physical disability, apathy, communication failure and socially irritating behaviour. Validity was tested against three separate follow-up studies. The SGRS has recently been incorporated in the CAPE (see below). Dequeker (1974) found a version of the SGRS of value for measuring the results of rehabilitation. It had also been used to assess the help required by patients in different hospital departments and wards, and has been employed for longitudinal surveys.

One of the most popular interviews in Britain for the clinical assessment of the cognitive and behavioural disability of elderly subjects for both service use and service-oriented research is the Clifton Assessment Procedures for the Elderly (CAPE; Pattie and Gilleard, 1975, 1976, 1978, 1979). As well as assessing cognitive function, the scales are concerned with problems of bathing, dressing, incontinence, mobility and personal appearance. Containing a shortened version of the Stockton scale, the CAPE was originally devised as a brief measure of psychological functioning for a chronic psychiatric patient group. A satisfactory level of concurrent and predictive validity has now been shown against the criteria of psychiatric diagnosis and outcome. Further validation on acute and non-acute hospital samples has revealed the ability to discriminate between patient groups, and some predictive validity within groups. In addition, the CAPE has recently been validated against the outcome of day hospital and day centre care (Bell and Gilleard, 1986). A shortened version of the scale based on the information/orientation and the physical disability subscales has also been validated (Pattie, 1981). A recent article has highlighted problems of inter-rater reliability in the scoring of the psychomotor (maze) subtest (McPherson *et al.*, 1986). The CAPE in its present form is intended for a group of moderately ill subjects. It is not suitable for field surveys with large proportions of normal people for whom questions about incontinence might be distressing. A nurse may take up to 1 hour to complete and interpret the scale.

The Comprehensive Assessment and Referral Evaluation (CARE) (Gurland *et al.*, 1983, 1977) is designed to 'reliably elicit, record, grade and classify' information on the psychiatric, physical, nutritional, economic and social problems of the older person. Having been constructed specifically for the studies of the US/UK cross-national project, it contains the Geriatric Mental State, and therefore the computer diagnosis AGECAT can be applied to it. It was designed for use in the community with both patients and non-patients, and can be administered by different types of staff, provided they are trained in the method. A variety of scales has been developed, including one for assessing degrees of dependency. For those not wishing to use the computer diagnosis, an algorithm is provided for diagnosing pervasive depression and dementia. The original interview took on average about 1½ hours to complete, but shorter versions are now available. Reliability and validity studies have been undertaken and are described by the authors. For those research workers requiring a full description of their subjects, especially for studies evaluating the provision of services, this interview offers a full and well-tried method.

We have attempted to review the best and most useful scales which are now available for assessing elderly psychiatric patients and non-patients and to comment on others which are available. Inevitably the choice is personal and no doubt some excellent recent scales with, as yet, little documentation, will have been omitted. Similarly, the choice reflects an Anglo-Saxon bias and well-developed scales and interviews published in languages other than English may have been overlooked. The scene is changing rapidly and will soon be overtaken by computer-based interviews as computers become smaller and more powerful and sufficiently well behaved to accompany interviewers into the field.

REFERENCES

Anthony, J. C., Le Resche, L. and Niaz, U. (1982). Limits of the Mini-Mental State as a screening test for dementia and delirium among hospital patients. *Psychol. Med.* **12**, 397–408.

Bell, J. S. and Gilleard, C. J. (1986). Psychometric day centre outcome. *Br. J. Clin. Psychol.* **25**, 195–200.

Beller, S. A., Overall, J. E. and Swann, A. (1985). Efficacy of oral physostigmine in treatment of primary degenerative dementia. *Psychopharmacology* **87**, 147–151.

Bergmann, K., Kay, D. W. K., Foster, E. M., McKechnie, A. A. and Roth, M. (1971). A follow up study of randomly selected community residents to assess the effects of chronic brain syndrome and cerebrovascular disease. *Proceedings of the Fifth Congress of Psychiatry*, Part II, pp. 856–865.

Binks, M. G. and Davies, A. D. M. (1984). The contribution of the national adult reading text to the detection of dementia amongst community dwelling old people. Paper delivered at the British Society of Gerontology, Leeds.

Bird, A. S., MacDonald, A. J. D., Mann, A. H. and Philpot, M. P. (1987). Preliminary experience with the Selfcare (D); a self rating depression questionnaire for use in elderly, non-institutionalised subjects. *Int. J. Geriatric Psychiatry* **2**, 31–38.

Blazer, D. and Williams, C. D. (1980). Epidemiology of dysphoria and depression in an elderly population. *Am. J. Psychiatry* **137**, 439–444.

Blessed, G., Tomlinson, B. E. and Roth, M. (1968). The association between qualitat-

ive measures of dementia and senile change in the cerebral grey matter of elderly subjects. *Br. J. Psychiatry* **114**, 797–811.
Bond, J., Brookes, P., Carstaires, V. and Giles, L. (1980). The reliability of a Survey Psychiatric Assessment Schedule for the Elderly. *Br. J. Psychiatry* **137**, 148–162.
Brane, G. (1986). Normal ageing and dementia disorders, coping and crisis in the family. *Prog. Neuropsychopharmacol. Biol. Psychiatry* **10**, 287–295.
Brane, G. and Gottfries, C. G. (1985). *Treatment with monoamine drugs in Alzheimer's disease and senile dementia; aspects on aetiology, pathogenesis, diagnosis and treatment*, Editions de l'universite de Bruxelles.
Brink, T. L., Yesavage, J. A., Lum, O., Heersema, P. H., Adey, M. and Rose, T. L. (1982). Screening tests for geriatric depression. *Clin. Gerontol.* **1**, 37–43.
Buschke, H. (1973). Selective reminding for analyses of memory and learning. *J. Verbal Learn. Verbal Behav.* **12**, 543–550.
Carr, A. C., Wilson, S. L., Ghosh, A., Ancill, R. J. and Woods, R. T. (1982). Automated testing of geriatric patients using a microcomputer based system. *Int. J. Man–Machine Studies* **17**, 297–300.
Carroll, B. J., Fielding, J. M. and Blashki, T. G. (1973). Depression rating scales, a critical review. *Arch. Gen. Psychiatry* **28**, 361–366.
Copeland, J. R. M. (1981). *Mental illness amongst the elderly in London; contribution to epidemiology and prevention of mental illness in old age* (G. Magnussen and J. Neilson, eds), J. Buch Nordisk Samrad for Eldreaktivitet, Denmark.
Copeland, J. R. M., Kelleher, M. J., Duckworth, G. and Smith, A. (1976). Reliability of psychiatric assessment in older patients. *Int. J. Ag Hum. Dev.* **7**, 313–322.
Copeland, J. R. M., Dewey, M. E. and Griffiths-Jones, H. M. (1986). A standardised assessment of the mental state and diagnoses in the elderly; GMS and AGECAT. *Psychol. Med.* **16**, 89–99.
Copeland, J. R. M., Dewey, M. E., Henderson, A. S., Kay, D. W. K., Neal, C. D., Harrison, M. A. M., McWilliam, C., Forshaw, D. and Shiwach, R. (1988). The Geriatric Mental State (GMS) used in the Community. Replication studies of the computerised diagnoses of AGECAT. *Psychol. Med.* (in press).
Cowan, D. W., Wright, P. M., De Gourlay, A. J., Smith, A., Barron, G., De Gruchy, J., Copeland, J. R. M., Kelleher, M. J. and Kellett, J. M. (1975). A comparative psychometric assessment of psychogeriatric and geriatric patients. *Br. J. Psychiatry* **127**, 33–41.
Crooke, T., Ferris, S. and McCarthy, M. (1979). The Misplaced Objects Task, a brief test for memory dysfunction in the aged. *J. Am. Geriatric Soc.* **27**, 284–287.
Crooke, T., Ferris, S., McCarthy, M. and Rae, D. (1980). Utility of digit recall tasks for assessing memory in the aged. *J. Consult. Clin. Psychol.* **48**, 228–233.
Crookes, J. (1974). Indices of early dementia on the WAIS. *Psychol. Rep.* **136**, 109–119.
De Leon, M. J., Ferris, S. H., Blau, I. *et al.* (1979). Correlations between CT changes and behavioural deficits in senile dementia. *Lancet* **ii**, 859.
De Leon, M. J., Ferris, S. H. and George, A. E. (1980). Computed tomography evaluations of brain behaviour relationships in senile dementia of the Alzheimer's type. Neurobiol. Aging **1**, 69–79.
De Leon, M. J., George, A. E. and Ferris, S. J. (1983a). Regional Correlation of PET and CT in senile dementia of the Alzheimer's type. *Am. J. Neuroradiol.* **4**, 553–556.
De Leon, M. J., Ferris, S. H. and George, A. E. (1983b). Computed tomography and positron emission tomography evaluations of normal Ageing and Alzheimers disease. *J. Cereb. Blood Flow Metab.* **3**, 391–394.

De Leon, M. J., Ferris, S. H. and George, A. E. (1983c). Positron emission tomography studies of ageing and Alzheimer's disease. *Am. J. Neuroradiol.* **4**, 568–571.

Dequeker, J. (1974). Mediische Nevalidatie (Medical Rehabilitation) Acco, Leuven. Quoted by J. J. Van der Plaas in *Functional Assessment* (D. W. K. Kay and G. D. Burrows, eds), *Handbook of Studies on Psychiatry and Old Age*, Elsevier, Amsterdam.

Dick, J. P R. *et al.* (1984). Mini Mental State Examination in neurological patients. *J. Neurol Neurosurg. Psychol.* **47**, 496–498.

Drinkwater, J. (1981). The Kendrick Battery and other neuropsychological assessments in known cases of brain damage. Paper read at the Kendrick Battery Workshop, University of Hull.

Ferris, S. H., Crook, T., Clark, E., McCarthy, M. and Rae, D. (1980). Facial recognition memory deficits in normal ageing and senile dementia, *J. Gerontol.* **35**, 707–714.

Fillenbaum, G. G. (1980). Comparison of two brief tests of organic brain impairment. The MSQ and the short portable MSQ. *J. Am. Geriatric Soc.* **28**, 381–384.

Fillenbaum, G. G. and Smeyer, M. A. (1981). The development, validity and reliability of the OARS multidimensional functional assessment questionnaire. *J. Gerontol.* **36**, 428–434.

Folstein, M. F., Folstein, S. E. and McHugh, P. R. (1975). Mini mental State; a practical method for grading the cognitive state of patients for the clinician. *J. Psychiatr. Res.* **12**, 189–198.

Frackowiak, R. S., Lenzi, G. L., Jones, T. and Heather, J. D. (1980). Quantitative measurement of regional cerebral blood flow and oxygen metabolism in man, using 150 and positron emission tomography: theory, procedure and normal values. *J. Comput. Assist. Tomography* **4**, 727–736.

Gallagher, D., Brackenridge, J., Steinmetz, J. and Thompson, L. (1983). The Beck Depression Inventory and Research Diagnostic Criteria, congruence in an older population. *J. Consult. Clin. Psychol.* **51**, 945–646.

Gibson, A. J. (1979). Institutionalisation. Its effect on the cognitive status of long stay psychiatric patients who are elderly, unpublished doctoral dissertation, University of Hull Library.

Gibson, A. J. and Kendrick, D. C. (1976). The development of a visual learning test to replace the SLT in the Kendrick Battery. *Bull. Br. Psych. Soc.* **29**, 200–201.

Gibson, A. J., Moyes, I. C. A. and Kendrick, D. C. (1980). Cognitive assessment of the elderly long stay patient. *Br. J. Psychiatry* **137**, 537–557.

Golden, C., Hammeke, T. A. and Purish, A. D. (1979). *Luria–Nebraska Neuropsychological Test Battery Manual*, Western Psychological services, Los Angeles.

Gottfries, C. G., Brane, G., Gullberg, B. and Steen, G. (1982). A new rating scale for dementia syndromes. *Arch. Gerontol. Geriatrics* **1**, 311–330.

Gurland, B. J., Copeland, J. R. M., Sharpe, L., Kelleher, M. J., Kuriansky, J. B. and Simon, R. J. (1977). Assessment of the older person in the community. *Int. J. Aging Hum. Dev.* **8**, 1–8.

Gurland, B. J., Fleiss, J. L., Goldberg, K., Sharpe, L., Copeland, J. R. M., Kelleher, M. J. and Kellett, J. M. (1976). A semi-structured clinical interview for the assessment of diagnosis and mental state in the elderly. The Geriatric Mental State Schedule 2, A factor analysis. *Psychol. Med.* **6**, 451–459.

Gurland, B. J., Copeland, J. R. M., Kelleher, M. J., Kuriansky, J., Sharpe, L. and Dean, L. (1983). *The Mind and Mood of Ageing, the Mental Health Problems of the Community Elderly in New York and London*, Haworth Press, New York/ Croom Helm, London.

Hachinski, V. C., Illiff, L. D., Zihka, E., Du Boulay, G. H., McCallister, V. L., Marshall, J., Russell, R. W. R. and Symon, L. (1975). Cerebral Blood flow in Dementia. *Arch. Neurol.* **32**, 632–637.

Hall, P. (1974). Differential diagnosis and treatment of depression in the elderly. *Gerontol. Clin.* **16**, 126–136.

Hamilton, M. (1960). A rating scale for depression *J. Neurol. Neurosurg. Psychiat.*, **23,** 56.

Harrison, M. J. G., Thomas, D. J., Du Boulay, G. H. and Marshall, J. (1979). Multi infarct dementia. *J. Neurol. Sci.* **40**, 97–103.

Hasegawa, K. (1983). The clinical assessment of dementia in the aged; a dementia screening scale for psychogeriatric patients. In *Ageing in the Eighties and Beyond* (M. Bergener *et al.*, eds), Springer, New York, pp. 207–218.

Henderson, A. S. (1986). The epidemiology of Alzheimer's disease. *Br. Med. Bull.* **42**, 3–10.

Henderson, A. S., Duncan-Jones, P. and Finlay Jones, R. A. (1983). The reliability of the GMS community survey version. *Acta Psychiatr. Scand.* **67**, 281–289.

Hersch, E. L. (1979). Development and application of the extended scale of dementia. *J. Am. Gerontol. Soc.* **27**, 348–354.

Hodkinson, H. M. (1972). Evaluation of a Mental Test score for assessment of mental impairment in the elderly. *Age Ageing*, **1**, 233–238.

Honigfield G. and Klett, C. J. (1965). The Nurses Observation Scale for inpatient evaluation. *J. Clin. Psychol.* **21**, 65–71.

Hooijer, C., Jonker, C., Reivey, M.E., Van Tilburg, E. Copeland, J. R. M. (1989). A standardised interview for the elderly (GMS). Five issues of reliability using a Dutch language version. Submitted to *Psychol Med.*

Huppert, F. A. and Tym, E. (1986). Clinical and neuropsychological assessment of dementia. Br. Med. Bull. **42**, 11–18.

Inglis, J. (1959). A paired associate learning test for use with elderly psychiatric patients. *J. Ment. Sci.* **105**, 440–448.

Jacoby, R. J. and Levy, R. (1980a). Computed tomography in the elderly. 2, Senile dementia, diagnoses and functional impairement. *Br. J. Psychiatry* **136**, 259–269.

Jacoby, R., J. and Levy, R. (1980b). Computed tomography in the elderly. 3, Affective disorder. *Br. J. Psychiatry* **136**, 270–275.

Kahn, R. L., Goldfarb, A., Pollack, M. and Gerber, I. E. (1960). The relationship of mental and physical status in institutionalised aged persons. *Am. J. Psychiatry* **117**, 120–124.

Karlsson, I., Widerlov, E., Melin, E. V., Nyth, A. L., Brane, G. A. M., Rehfeld, R. E., Bissette, G. and Nemeroff, C. B. (1985). Changes in CSF neuropeptides and environmental stimulation in dementia. *Nord. Psykiatr. Tidsskr.* **39**, 76–81.

Kay, D. W. K. (1977). The epidemiology and identification of brain deficit in the elderly. In *Cognitive and Emotional Disturbances in the Elderly* (C. Esdorfer and R. O. Friedel, eds), Year Book Medical Publishers, Chicago.

Kay, D. W. K., Baemish, R. and Roth, M. (1964). Old age mental disorders in Newcastle upon Tyne. Part 1, A study of the prevalence. *Br. J. Psychiatry* **110**, 146–158.

Kay, D. W. K., Henderson, A. S., Scott, R., Wilson, J., Rickwood, D. Grayson, D. A. (1985). Dementia and depression amongst the elderly living in the Hobart Community; the effect of the diagnostic criteria on prevalence rates. *Psychol. Med.* **15**, 771–778.

Kendrick, D. C. (1985). *The Kendrick Cognitive Tests for the Elderly*, Nelson, Windsor.

Kendrick, D. C., Parboosingh, R. C. and Post, F. (1965). A synonym learning test for the use with elderly psychiatric patients. *Br. J. Soc. Clin. Psychol.* **4**, 63–71.

Kendrick, D. C., Gibson, A. J. and Moyes, I. C. A. (1978). The Kendrick Battery Mark II. *Bull. Br. Psych. Soc.* **31**, 177–178.

Kendrick, D. C., Gibson, A. J. and Moyes, C. A. (1979). The revised Kendrick Battery; clinical studies. *Br. J. Soc. Clin. Psychol.* **18**, 329–339.

Kuriansky, J. B., Gurland, B. J., Fleiss, J. L. and Cowan, D. W. (1976). The assessment of self care capacity in geriatric psychiatric patients by objective and subjective methods. *J. Clin. Psychol.* **32**, 95–102.

Lawton, M. P., *et al.* (1982). A research and service orientated multi-level assessment instrument. *J. Gerontol.* **37**, 91–99.

Little, A., Hemsley, D., Bergmann, K., Volans, J. and Levy, R. (1987). Comparison of the sensitivity of three instruments for the detection of cognitive decline in elderly living at home. *Br. J. Psychiatry* **150**, 808–814.

Lloyd, C. M. (1970). Royal College of Physicians study of mental disease in the elderly. Report of the findings of a pilot study in London. Royal College of Physicians, London.

Loeb, C. and Gandolfo, C. (1983). Diagnostic evaluation of degenerative and vascular dementia. *Stroke* **14**, 399–401.

Lowe, D. M. and Weil, C. (1982). Hydergine in senile mental impairment. *Gerontology* **28**, 54–74.

McCarthy, M., Ferris, S. H., Clark, E. and Crook, T. (1981). Acquisition and retention of categorised material in normal ageing and senile dementia. *Exp. Aging Res.* **7**, 127–135.

McPherson, F. M., Gamsu, C. V., Cockram, L. L. and Gromley, A. J. (1986). Interscorer agreement in scoring errors on the PM (Maze) test of the CAPE. *Br. J. Clin. Psychol.* **25**, 225–226.

McWilliam, C., Copeland, J. R. M., Dewey, M. E. and Wood, N. (1988). The Geriatric Mental State Examination as a case finding instrument in the community. *Br. J. Psychiatry* **151**, 205–208.

Meer, B. and Baker, J. A. (1966). The Stockton Geriatric Rating Scale. *J. Gerontol.* **21**, 392–403.

Mayer-Gross, W., Slater, E. and Roth, M. (1969). *Clinical Psychiatry*, 3rd edn, Bailliere Tindall, London.

Mohs, R. C., Rosen, W. G. and Davies, K. L. (1983). The Alzheimer's disease assessment scale: an instrument for assessing treatment efficacy. *Psychopharmacol. Bull.* **19**, 448–449.

Naguib, M. and Levy, R. (1982). Prediction of outcome of senile dementia—A computed tomography study. *Br. J. Psychiatry* **140**, 263–267.

Nelson, H. E. (1982). *National Adult Reading Test (NART) for the assessment of premorbid intelligence in patients with dementia; test manual*, NFER, Windsor.

Nelson, H. E. and McKenna, P. (1975). The use of current reading ability in the assessment of dementia. *Br. J. Clin. Psychol.* **14**, 256–267.

Nelson, H. E. and O'Connell, A. (1978). Dementia, the estimated premorbid intelligence level using the new adult reading test. *Cortex* **14**, 234–244.

Nelson, A. Fogal, B. S. and Faust, D. (1986). Bedside cognitive screening instruments: A critical assessment. *J. Nerv. Ment. Dis.* **174**, 73–83.

Pattie, A. H. (1981). A survey version of the Clifton Assessment Procedures for the elderly. *Br. J. Clin. Psychol.* **20**, 173–178.

Pattie, A. H. and Gilleard, C. J. (1975). A brief psychogeriatric assessment schedule validation against psychiatric diagnoses and discharge from hospital. *Br. J. Psychiatry* **127**, 489–493.

Pattie, A. H. and Gilleard, C. J. (1976). The Clifton Assessment Schedule; further validation of a psychogeriatric assessment Schedule. *Br. J. Psychiatry* **129**, 68–72.

Pattie, A. H. and Gilleard, C. J. (1978). The two year predictive validity of the Clifton Assessment Schedule and the shortened Stockton Geriatric Rating Scale. *Br. J. Psychiatry* **133**, 457–460.

Pattie, A. H. and Gilleard, C. J. (1979). Psychological assessment and care of the elderly. *Soc. Work Today* **10**, 46.

Perry, E. K., Tomlinson, B. E., Blessed, G., Bergmann, K., Gibson, P. H. and Perry, R. H. (1978). Correlation of cholinergic abnormalities with senile plaques and mental test scores in senile dementia. *Br. Med. J.* **2**, 1457–1459.

Pfeiffer, E. (1975). A Short Portable Mental Status Questionnaire for the assessment of organic brain deficit in elderly patients. *J. Am. Geriatric Soc.* **23**, 433–441.

Quershi, K. N. and Hodkinson, H. M. (1974). Evaluation of a ten question mental test in the institutionalised elderly. *Age Ageing* **3**, 152–157.

Raft, D., Spencer, R. F., Toomey, T. and Brogan, D. (1977). Depression in medical outpatients; the use of the Zung scale. *Dis. Nerv. System* **38**, 999–1004.

Reisberg, B., Ferris, S. H., De Leon, M. J., *et al.* (1982a). The global deterioration scale, an instrument for the assessment of primary degenerative dementia (PDD). *Am. J. Psychiatry* **139**, 1136–1139.

Reisberg, B., Ferris, S. H. and Crook, T. (1982b). Signs, symptoms and course of age associated cognitive decline. In *Alzheimer's disease. A report of Progress in Research* (S. Corkin, K. L. Davis and J. H. Growden, eds), Raven Press, New York, pp. 177–181.

Reisberg, B., Shulman, E., Ferris, S. H., *et al.* (1983). Clinical assessment of age associated cognitive decline and primary degenerative dementia prognostic concomitants. *Psychopharmacol. Bull.* **19**, 734–739.

Reisberg, B., Ferris, S., Anand, R., *et al.* (1984). Clinical Assessment of cognition in the aged. In *Biology and Treatment of the Elderly* (C. A. Shamoin, ed.), American Psychiatric Press, Washington, DC, pp. 17–37.

Reitan, R. M. (1955). Investigation of the validity of Halstead's measures of biological intelligence. *Arch. Neurol. Psychiatry* **73**, 28–35.

Robins, I. N., Helzer, J. E., Croughan, J. and Ratcliffe, K. S. (1981). National Institute of Mental Health, Diagnostic Interview Schedule. *Arch. Gen. Psychiatry* **38**, 381–389.

Ron, M. A., Toone, B. K., Garralda, M. E. and Lishman, W. A. (1979). Diagnostic accuracy in pre senile dementia. *Br. J. Psychiatry* **134**, 161–168.

Rosen, W. G., Terry, R. D., Fuld, P. A., Katzman, R. and Peck, A. (1979). Pathological verification of ischaemic score in differention of dementias. *Ann. Neurol.* **7**, 486–488.

Rosen, W. G., Mohs, R. C. and Davis, K. L. (1984). A new rating scale for Alzheimer's disease. *Am. J. Psychiatry* **141**, 1356–1364.

Roth, M. (1986). Differential diagnoses of psychiatric disorders in old age. *Hosp. Pract.* **15**, 111–125.

Roth, M. (1981). The diagnosis of dementia in late and middle life. In *The Epidemiology of Dementia* (J. A. Mortimer and L. M. Shuman, eds), Oxford University Press, New York, pp. 24–61.

Roth, M. and Hopkins, B. (1953). Psychological test performance in patients over sixty. 1. Senile psychosis and affective disorders of old age. *J. Ment. Sci.* **99**, 439–450.

Roth, M., Tym, E., Mountjoy, C. Q., Hupport, F. A., Hendrie, H., Verma, S., Goddard, R. (1986) CAMDEX. A standardized instrument for the diagnosis of mental disorder of the elderly with special reference to the early detection of dementia. *Brit. J. Psychiat*, **149**, 698–709.

Shader, R. I., Harmatz, J. S. and Salzman, C. A. (1974). A new scale for clinical assessment in geriatric populations; Sandoz Clinical Assessment Geriatric (SCAG). *J. Am. Geriatric Soc.* **22**, 107–113.

Searle, R. T. (1984). A community based follow up of some suspected cases of early dementia in an interim report. *Bull. Br. Psychol. Soc.* **37**, A20–A21.

Shapiro, M. B. and Nelson, E. H. (1955). An investigation of the nature of cognitive impairment in co-operative psychiatric patients. *Br. J. Med. Psychol.* **4**, 205–280.

Slater, R. and Lipman, A. (1977). Staff assessment of confusion and the situation of confused residents in homes of old people. *Gerontologist* **17**, 523–530.

Spitzer, R. L.; Fleiss, J. L., Burdock, E. J. and Hardesty, A. S. (1964). The Mental Status Schedule: rationale, reliability and validity. *Compr. Psychiatry* **5**, 384–395.

Thompson, P. and Blessed G. (1987). Correlation between the 37 item mental test score and the abbreviated 10 item mental test score by psychogeriatric day patients. *Br. J. Psychiatry* **151**, 206–209.

Tinkleberg, J., Taylor, J., Peabody, C., Redington, D. and Gibson, E. (1984). Dual task performance measures in geriatric studies. *Psychopharmacol. Bull.* **20**, 441–444.

Tsai, L. and Tsuang, M. T. (1979). The Mini Mental State test and computerised tomography. *Am. J. Psychiatry* **136**, 436–438.

Wade, J. P. and Hachinski, V. C. (1987). Multi-infarct dementia. In *Dementia* (B. Pitt, ed.), Churchill Livingstone, Edinburgh.

Walton, D. and Black, D. A. (1957). The validity of a psychological test of brain damage. *Br. J. Med. Psychol.* **30**, 270–279.

Weiss, I. K., Nagel, C. L. and Aronson, M. K. (1986). Applicability of depression scales to the old person. *J. Am. Geriatric Soc.* **34**, 215–218.

Weissman, M. M., Myers, J. K., Tischler, G. L., Holzer, C. E., Leaf, P. J., Ovaschel. H. and Brody, J. A. (1985), Psychiatric Disorders (DSM-III) and cognitive impairment among the elderly in a US urban community. *Acta Psych. Scand.* **71**, 366–379.

Wilkinson, I. M. and Graham-White, J. (1980). Psychogeriatric dependence rating scales (PGDRS). A method of assessment for use by Nurses. *Br. J. Psychiatry* **137**, 558–565.

Wing, J. K., Cooper, J. E. and Sartorius, N. (1974). *The description and classification of psychiatric symptoms. An Instruction manual for the PSE and CATEGO System*, Cambridge University Press, London.

Yesavage, J. A., Adey, M. and Werner, P. D. (1981). Development of a geriatric behavioural self assessment scale. *J. Am. Geriatric Soc.* **29**, 285–288.

Yesavage, J. A., Brink, T. L., Rose, T. L., Lum, O., Huang, V., Adey, M. and Leirer, O. (1983). Development and evaluation of a geriatric depression screening scale; A preliminary report. *J. Psychiatr. Res.* **17**, 37–39.

Zung, W. W. K. and Green, R. L. (1973). Detection of affective disorders in the aged. In *Psychopharmacology and Ageing* (C. Eisdendopfer and W. E. Fann, eds), Plenum Press, New York, pp. 213–223.

Zung, W. W. K. (1975). *The Measurement of Depression* (O. H. Columbus, ed.), Merrill.

Index